Return to:

AMBLYOPIA
Basic and Clinical Aspects

AMBLYOPIA
Basic and Clinical Aspects

Kenneth J. Ciuffreda, O.D., Ph.D.
Dennis M. Levi, O.D., Ph.D.
Arkady Selenow, O.D.

Butterworth–Heinemann
Boston   London   Singapore   Sydney   Toronto   Wellington

Every effort has been made to ensure that the drug dosage schedules within this text are accurate and conform to standards accepted at time of publication. However, as treatment recommendations vary in the light of continuing research and clinical experience, the reader is advised to verify drug dosage schedules herein with information found on product information sheets. This is especially true in cases of new or infrequently used drugs.

 Recognizing the importance of preserving what has been written, it is the policy of Butterworth–Heinemann to have the books it publishes printed on acid-free paper, and we exert our best efforts to that end.

Library of Congress Cataloging-in-Publication Data
Ciuffreda, Kenneth J., 1947–
    Amblyopia: basic and clinical aspects/ Kenneth J. Ciuffreda,
Dennis M. Levi, Arkady Selenow.
      p.   cm.
    Includes index.
    ISBN 0-409-95171-4 (casebound)
    1. Amblyopia.   I. Levi, Dennis M.   II. Selenow, Arkady.
III. Title.
    [DNLM: 1. Amblyopia.   WW 276 C581a]
RE92.C58   1991
617.7′62—dc20
DNLM/DLC   90-2017
for Library of Congress   CIP

British Library Cataloguing in Publication Data
Ciuffreda, Kenneth J.
    Amblyopia.
    1. Man. Eyes. Strabismus
    I. Title II. Levi, Dennis M.   III. Selenow, Arkady
    617.762
    ISBN 0-409-95171-4

Butterworth–Heinemann
80 Montvale Avenue
Stoneham, MA 02180

10 9 8 7 6 5 4 3 2 1

Printed in the United States of America

To my beautiful daughters Gabrielle and Marcelline
for their love and affection.
To my mother, for all she sacrificed.

K.J.C.

This book is dedicated to my wife Diana
and children Megan, Christopher, and Joseph
for their support and love.

A.S.

This book is dedicated to Marilyn
for her help and support and to my daughter
Ronli who was conceived during its
preparation.

D.M.L.

Contents

Preface

Amblyopia was first described by Le Cat almost three centuries ago. While we have learned a great deal over the years, most particularly over the last half of this century, there is much we still do not understand about the mechanisms and pathophysiology of amblyopia or about the specific effects of clinical therapies.

In our present understanding, amblyopia, derived from the Greek (*amblyos*, "blunt"; *opia*, "vision"), is a developmental anomaly of spatial vision. It occurs early in life and is almost always associated with the presence of strabismus, anisometropia, or both. During the 20 years since Schapero's excellent book on the topic, there has been an explosion in our knowledge of both normal and abnormal vision development. Technological improvements in physiology, psychophysics, and eye-movement recording have all contributed to our vastly increased knowledge base. Thus we now have a better characterization of the functional capacities of the amblyopic visual system, as well as of some of the anatomic and physiologic consequences of amblyopia. We also have learned a great deal about the normal development of spatial vision. These gains in our basic knowledge have led to the advance, and sometimes the decline, of new treatment methods. However, as yet we do not have either a complete picture of the natural history of amblyopia or a comprehensive understanding of the pathophysiology, and in some respects, our treatment regimens are not too much advanced from those described by Conte De Buffon in 1742.

The size and scope of this book give some indication of the volume of recent work on the topic of amblyopia. Much of the interest in this area over the past 25 years or so stems from the pioneering work of Hubel and Wiesel, who first demonstrated the striking neural consequences of deprivation on the developing visual nervous system, as well as the vital role of its plasticity. Another factor contributing to the explosion of information is the development of new techniques for studying both normal and abnormal visual development in humans. It is interesting to note that some of this information has spilled over into the development of new ideas and methods for the clinical management of amblyopia.

Given the current, fluid state of our knowledge, it is not our intention to provide the "complete story." There is a considerable way to go before that will be told. Rather, our intent is to provide a status report, or a waystation for both basic scientists and clinicians who are interested in amblyopia. The first chapter reviews the history, classification, some of the prevailing theories, and the biostatistics of amblyopia. Chapter 2 provides a brief overview of normal development and its functional capacities and describes some of the consequences of abnormal visual input on the developing visual nervous system. Other chapters review the sensory (Chapter 3) and oculomotor (Chapters 5, 6, and 7) capacities of amblyopes and what is known of the effects of amblyopia on the geniculo-striate pathway (Chapter 4). The last third of the book is devoted to diagnosis (Chapter 8) and treatment (Chapters 9 and 10). It is our hope that this book will serve clinicians and scientists in developing a better understanding of the fascinating condition of amblyopia.

Kenneth J. Ciuffreda
Dennis M. Levi
Arkady Selenow

New York City and Houston
March 1990

Acknowledgments

We thank Mrs. Pat Sullivan for typing the manuscript many times over and for her assistance with various administrative aspects of the book, and Karen Jensen for her help with library research.

This work was supported in part by NIH Grants RO1-EY03541 (to K.J.C.) and RO1-EY01728 (to D.M.L.).

AMBLYOPIA
Basic and Clinical Aspects

Chapter 1

History, Definitions, Classifications, and Prevalence

Restoration of Visual Acuity. There have been devised many ingenious contrivances to force the use of the squinting eye, and thus bring up the acuity of the vision or prevent the loss of vision, in the squinting eye. As early as the seventh century, Paulus AEgineta devised a mask with central perforations which was to be worn as a goggle. Ambroise Pare, in 1509, had constructed of horn a pair of goggles with central perforations to be used by squinters [Figure 1.1].

(Wilkinson 1943)

HISTORY OF AMBLYOPIA

Le Cat (1713) is credited with providing the first accurate clinical description of human amblyopia. However, credit for first describing any treatment for amblyopia is given to George Louis Leclerc, Conte De Buffon (1707–1788) (Figure 1.2), who in 1742 suggested that the good eye be fully occluded to force use of the squinting amblyopic eye, both to improve its vision and to cure the strabismus. Buffon also discovered the usefulness of optically correcting the amblyopic eye, as well as the efficacy of penalization therapy by placing a convex lens in front of the good eye. As noted by MacKenzie (1833),

> Buffon recommended, therefore, that the patient should wear a pair of spectacles with a plane glass opposite to the bad eye, and a convex glass opposite to the good eye. In this way, the vision of the good eye would be rendered less distinct, and consequently it would be less in a state to act independently of the other. As the weak eye is often short-sighted, the same advantage might perhaps be derived from placing a plane glass before the good eye, and a concave glass before the distorted one.

Therefore, Buffon was the first to realize the two most important elements in amblyopia therapy: *occlusion and full optical correction*. Preceding Buffon,

1

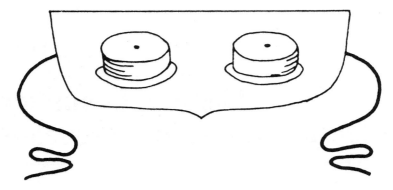

Figure 1.1   *Strabismus goggles with central perforations used for the treatment of strabismus by Ambroise Pare in 1509. (Reprinted, by permission of the publisher, from Revell MJ.* Strabismus: A History of Orthoptic Techniques. *London: Barrie and Jenkins, 1971.)*

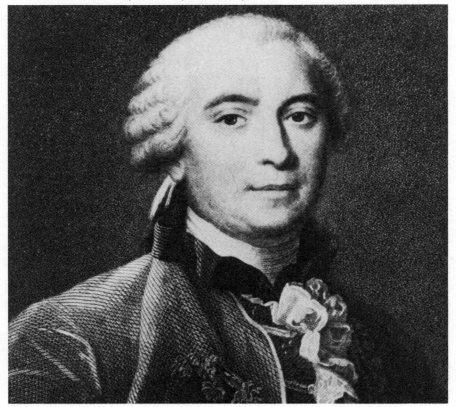

Figure 1.2   *George Louis Leclerc, Conte De Buffon (1707–1788). (Reprinted, by permission of the publisher, from Duke-Elder S.* Textbook of Ophthalmology, Vol. 6: Ocular Motility and Strabismus. *St. Louis: Mosby, 1973.)*

amblyopia was always mentioned in the same breath as strabismus. Buffon was astute enough to note the existence of amblyopia secondary to anisometropia. Buffon stated,

> But the most general cause, the most ordinary, of squint, and of which nobody that I know has made mention, is the inequality of strength of the eyes. A small degree of inequality will cause an object seen by the stronger eye to be as distinctly perceived as if it were seen by the stronger eye alone; and finally, a great deal of inequality will render the object seen by both eyes so confused that in order to see distinctly one will be obliged to turn the weak eye, and put it in a position where it cannot hinder.

MacKenzie (1833) also noted Erasmus Darwin's method, published in 1778, of treating an esotrope with use of a large artificial nose. By Darwin's advice,

> A gnomon of thin brass was made to stand over the patient's nose, with half a circle of the same metal to go round his temples. These were covered with black silk, and by means of a buckle behind his head, and a cross-piece over the crown of his head, this gnomon was worn without inconvenience, and projected before his nose about two inches and a half. By the intervention of this instrument, he soon found it less inconvenient to view oblique objects with the eye next to them, instead of the eye opposite to them. After this habit was weakened by a week's use of the gnomon, two bits of wood, about the size of a goose-quill, blackened all but a quarter of an inch at their summits, were frequently presented for him to look at, one being held on one side of the extremity of the gnomon, and the other on the other side of it.

Thus, in effect, the patient practiced bifixation before a mirror and achieved intermittent simultaneous alignment of both eyes.

Erasmus Darwin (1801), the physician grandfather of the eminent scientist Charles Darwin, suggested that a piece of gauze be stretched on a circle of whalebone to cover the "best eye in such a manner as to reduce the distinctness of vision of this eye to a similar degree of imperfection with the other," and he further stated that it "should be worn some hours every day, or the better eye should be totally darkened by a tin cup covered with black silk for some hours daily." This was the first suggestion of relative occlusion for the treatment of amblyopia. Similarly, Beer (1802) indicated that by binding up the sound eye every day for only a few hours, amblyopia therapy was successful.

MacKenzie (1833) stated that the treatment of amblyopia in squint should begin with "tying up the sound eye and thus obliging the patient to exercise only the eye which squints." Realizing the efficacy of part-time patching in conjunction with active amblyopia therapy over full-time patching alone, MacKenzie suggested,

The patient need not keep the sound eye covered during the whole day. At first, this may be done for ½ an hour or an hour at a time, and then for longer periods. During the blindfolding of the sound eye, the weak one is to be exercised both on distant and on near objects, but especially on the former. If the patient be a child, he must be encouraged to exercise the weak eye in playing at ball or shuttlecock, viewing extensive prospects in the country, reading books printed in a large type, looking at prints, etc.

MacKenzie also discovered the tremendous plasticity of the young visual system and the need for alternate occlusion in some cases,

This plan of curing strabismus is often attended by a diminished power both of motion and of vision in the sound eye; and that it has sometimes happened, that the squinting eye being cured by perseverance in this method, the sound eye has then become distorted. If both eyes squint from the first, they must be blind-folded alternately, each for several days at a time.

This is one of the earliest references to occlusion amblyopia.

Another example of "exercising" the amblyopic eye is a procedure used by MacKenzie (1833) that was recommended by Dr. Jurin:

Having placed the patient before us, we bid him close the undistorted eye, and look at us with the other. When we find the axis of this eye fixed directly upon us, we bid him endeavor to keep it in that situation, and open his other eye. Immediately, the distorted eye turns away from us towards his nose, and the axis of the other is pointed at us. But with patience and repeated trials, he will, by degrees, be able to keep the distorted eye fixed upon us, at least for some little time after the other is opened.

This is an early example of forcing alternation in a unilateral strabismic with amblyopia, which is extremely important for maintaining vision improvement in the amblyopic eye after the termination of therapy. In effect, this is the ultimate form of biocular occlusion.

The famous French ophthalmologist and father of orthoptics, Louis Emile Javal (1839–1907), used the *louchette*, or occluder, extensively to improve vision in the amblyopic eye, as well as to break down suppression by prolonged occlusion. Javal (1896) originally used a disk of hardened leather with a surrounding soft leather rim. Since this was uncomfortable in warm weather, he later used fine metal gauze lined with paper. By primarily occluding the good eye, Javal reported on a patient in 1866 whose visual acuity improved significantly while the strabismus was alleviated. According to Javal, "The principal point, on which I do not know how to insist enough, is the necessity of absolutely permanent use of the louchette." Wechert (1932) ensured total occlusion by stitching the eyelids together, a bit of a drastic measure but certainly peek-proof! In this same vein, Hiles and Galket (1974) reported on the use of elbow casts in young children to prevent them from bending their arms to remove their eye patch, another ridiculously drastic measure (Figure 1.3).

Most ophthalmologists were reluctant to accept the notion that amblyopia was reversible (Revell 1971). Acceptance was especially slow by those who thought of amblyopia as being a congenital defect (Frost 1887, Holthouse 1897). In describing his method of dealing with strabismus, Holthouse (1897) advised not attempting to correct the amblyopia with occlusion, and said, "There is certainly no general recognition of the benefit obtainable by such means." This group did not observe any significant results with occlusion. Unfortunately, "at the turn of the century, dogma often overruled practical experience" (Revell 1971). A. von Graefe (1877) argued that if occlusion were carried out faithfully, its value would be apparent even to the proponents of the congenital theory. As late as 1921, Poulard stated that he had never noticed any improvement (or worsening) of amblyopia following treatment. He considered orthoptic therapy to be an "unnecessary torture." Gifford (1935) felt that occlusion was capable of causing psychological trauma, leading to disorders such as stammering. Bangerter (1953) opposed occlusion for the same reason; however, he has modified his viewpoint (1962). Occlusion was abandoned and indeed rejected for many years when amblyopia was thought to be a congenital, hereditary anomaly. This view was defended as late as 1927 by Uhthoff. The extent of the controversy was obvious in Keiner's (1951) citation of Van der Hoeve. On this point Van der Hoeve wrote,

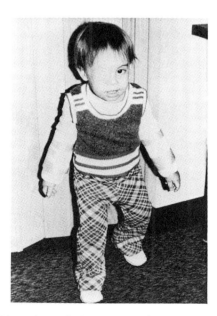

Figure 1.3 *Patient with ocular occlusion wearing plaster cast arm restraints held in place with filament tape. (Reprinted, by permission of the publisher, from Hiles DA, Galket RJ. Plaster cast arm restraints and amblyopia therapy. J. Pediatr. Ophthalmol. 11:151–2, 1974.)*

There exists a voluminous literature, the authors of which—although they include some of the most eminent members of our profession—have not always remained objective. Many adopt an attitude of unitarism: They assume the existence of primary squint and reject the possibility of primary amblyopia altogether, or they reject primary squint and show themselves protagonists of primary amblyopia.

With the birth of the concept of amblyopia as a *functional anomaly* developing as a *sensory adaptation to strabismus*, occlusion was resumed and has since remained the mainstay of amblyopia treatment for both optometrists and ophthalmologists.

Amblyopia: Central versus Peripheral

Javal (1896) is credited with first recognizing that the seat of the anomaly in amblyopia lies centrally and that its effect was not equally distributed across the retina. Of Javal's work, Parinaud (1899) said,

> He made a careful study of the conditions of the amblyopic eye. He found that the amblyopia is not equally distributed on the retina, the peripheral parts are nearly normal, while the center or yellow spot is the real focus of the affection; therefore, we might say that an amblyopic eye sees only with its periphery: its acuity of vision after correction, 1/60 to 3/60, is in accordance with this. Therefore, it is clear why the eye wanders around when the better eye is covered; it has lost its tendency to fixate because the function of the yellow spot is replaced by that whole periphery.

The development of our understanding of the pathophysiology of amblyopia began with a controversy at the turn of the nineteenth century between two theories regarding its etiology (Revell 1971):

1. Donders (1864; along with others such as Meyer 1930, Lagrange 1907, and Delard 1921) believed amblyopia to be secondary to habitual suppression. Therefore, the squint caused the amblyopia.
2. The opposing viewpoint was taken by Schweigger (1881; reviewed by Holthouse 1897, de Schweinitz 1906, and Poulard 1921), who considered the amblyopia to be a congenital defect that precedes and is therefore the cause of the squint. Priestley-Smith (1898) took a middle-of-the-road approach: "Of course it may be that these highly amblyopic eyes squint earlier than others just because they are amblyopic, but I think we ought not to leave out of consideration the possibility that the early onset of squint may arrest the visual development of the eye. The question is important in relation to educative treatment."

THEORY 1. **Squint** is primary → **Amblyopia** is secondary
THEORY 2. **Amblyopia** is primary → **Squint** is secondary
(congenital)

It remained for Worth (1901) to clear up the controversy. He compared the visual acuity of the squinting eye after occlusion therapy to the age of onset of the squint. In Worth's three tables (see Tables 1.1 through 1.3), he showed that congenital amblyopia was extremely rare and was never responsible for the extreme blindness found in untreated unilateral squinters. This is especially obvious if one compares Tables 1.1 and 1.3. In addition, Worth showed that strabismic amblyopia occurs rapidly in infants, but rarely if the onset of the strabismus was after the sixth year of life. Consequently, Worth's analysis has strongly influenced current thinking regarding amblyopia *prevention* before age 6 years. His work demonstrated that amblyopia was due to a true loss of vision, not to a failure of the function to develop. In addition, Worth's fraction became

Table 1.1 Cases That Worth First Saw When the Patient Had Squinted Constantly during Less than One-Eighth of His or Her Life

	Age of Onset of the Deviation			
Vision of the Deviating Eye	*Before 12 Months*	*1 to 3 Years*	*After 3 Years*	*Total*
6/6	23	62	80	165
6/9 and 6/12	2	6	9	17
6/18 and 6/24	1	3	5	9
6/36 and 6/60	0	1	1	2
Less than 6/60	0	0	0	0
Fixation lost irrecoverably	0	0	0	0

Table 1.2 Cases That Worth First Saw When the Patient Had Squinted Constantly More than One-Eighth and Less than One-Half of His or Her Life

	Age of Onset of the Deviation			
Vision of the Deviating Eye	*Before 12 Months*	*1 to 3 Years*	*After 3 Years*	*Total*
6/6	5	17	51	73
6/9 and 6/12	3	26	32	61
6/18 and 6/24	0	14	14	28
6/36 and 6/60	0	5	9	14
Less than 6/60	0	1	4	5
Fixation lost irrecoverably	0	2	5	7

Table 1.3   Cases That Worth First Saw When the Patient Had Squinted Constantly during More than One-Half of His or Her Life

Vision of the Deviating Eye	Age of Onset of the Deviation			
	Before 12 Months	*1 to 3 Years*	*After 3 Years*	*Total*
6/6	0	3	11	14
6/9 and 6/12	2	7	19	28
6/18 and 6/24	4	32	54	90
6/36 and 6/60	8	53	41	102
Less than 6/60	55	103	21	179
Fixation lost irrecoverably	56	110	25	191

a prognostic indicator for visual acuity improvement with treatment. As the fraction approached 1, prognosis improved.

$$\text{WORTH'S FRACTION} = \frac{\text{Age (months) when permanent squint was apparent}}{\text{Age (months) when therapy began}}$$

Thus Donder's (1864) viewpoint, i.e., that squint caused the amblyopia, not vice versa, became the state-of-the-art theory, and subsequently, occlusion became the treatment of choice. Maddox (1907) eloquently summarized approval of the first theory in his statement, "It is not for want of use that vision suffers but through seeing too much. The eye becomes a nuisance and the brain blinds it."

Arrest and Extinction

In 1939, Chavasse further elaborated on Worth's active central nervous system inhibition concept. Chavasse attributed the development of amblyopia and facultative suppression to the process of "adaptive inhibition in the face of dissociation." This is now known as the theory of "amblyopia of arrest" versus "amblyopia of extinction." Chavasse proposed the following:

1.   When corresponding retinal points are stimulated by dissimilar images, there is an inhibition of the macula of one eye that he called *facultative inhibition, suppression*, or *facultative amblyopia*. This inhibition of one eye occurs *only* when the other eye is in use. If one eye continues to be preferred over the other, the suppression becomes fixed, leading toward an *obligatory inhibition or true amblyopia*. Thus the inhibition remains even after its cause (i.e., the use of the other eye) is terminated. The earlier the age at which the inhibition first begins to take effect, the more profound is the amblyopia.

2.   Chavasse further divided amblyopia into two types: amblyopia of arrest and amblyopia of extinction. In *amblyopia of arrest*, there is a cessation of development of vision in the involved eye that must occur before the age of 6 years. Chavasse felt that 20/20 vision reflected a conditioned reflex that develops with normal visual stimulation and is firmly established by age 6 years. In addition to the arrest of development of visual acuity, there also could be an extinction of an unused or nonreinforced conditioned reflex. In other words, amblyopia of arrest was considered irreversible, whereas *amblyopia of extinction* could be improved, but only up to the best vision that was obtained *before* the onset of the anomalous visual experience (i.e., squint or anisometropia). Therefore, suppression occurring during the first 6 years of life arrested the full development of vision. This decrease in vision was yet further depressed by active suppression, so that amblyopia of extinction overlaid the amblyopia of arrest. Occlusion therapy, therefore, could only remove the effects due to the amblyopia of extinction. Unfortunately, this theory assumed that the development of 20/20 visual acuity occurred by 6 years of age. Chavasse's visual acuity levels were the lowest present in infants, as tested by the Worth ivory ball test (Chavasse 1939). The acuity values are approximations based on gross subjective methods of evaluation (Chavasse 1939; see Figure 1.4). Chavasse was aware of the underestimation of these values: "Before the age of three years, estimation of visual acuity can only be based on manual responses which cannot be accurate and in any case tend to give an underestimate." However, more recent objective methods have demonstrated 20/20 visual acuity to be obtainable by about 6 to 12 months of age with certain testing procedures (Dobson and Teller 1978) (Figure 1.5). Therefore, amblyopia of arrest can only exist when the anomalous visual experience occurs before age 6 months or so. Consequently, *the majority of amblyopia is of the extinction type and is therefore potentially reversible.*

Example:

1.   Onset of abnormal visual experience is at age 1 year.
2.   Best visual acuity at age 1 year:
     Chavasse: 20/120
     Dobson and Teller: 20/20
3.   Best visual acuity now (after age 6 years and without previous treatment): 20/200

Chavasse (1939)	*Dobson and Teller* (1978)
20/200 to 20/120 = deficit due to extinction and therefore fully reversible	20/200 to 20/20 = deficit due to extinction and therefore fully reversible
20/120 to 20/20 = deficit due to arrest and therefore nonreversible	

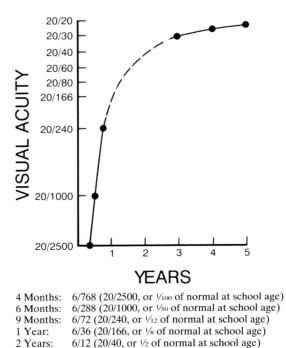

4 Months: 6/768 (20/2500, or 1/100 of normal at school age)
6 Months: 6/288 (20/1000, or 1/50 of normal at school age)
9 Months: 6/72 (20/240, or 1/12 of normal at school age)
1 Year: 6/36 (20/166, or 1/8 of normal at school age)
2 Years: 6/12 (20/40, or 1/2 of normal at school age)
3 Years: 6/9 (20/30, or 2/3 of normal at school age)
5 Years: 6/6 (20/20, or same as at school age)

Figure 1.4 *Chavasse's visual acuity levels.*

It also should be noted that in selected patients and with the proper therapy, one *can* achieve a visual acuity that is better than the best developed visual acuity predicted *before* onset of the anomaly (squint or anisometropia). For example, if a person is born without strabismus and with a normal visual system and then develops a constant unilateral strabismus at age 3 months when the developing visual acuity is expected to be 20/200, this unilateral strabismus causes an amblyopia to occur. If 1 year later this infant receives successful direct occlusion therapy, one can expect a final visual acuity of better than 20/200. Therefore, one can obtain a better acuity than was achieved *before* onset of the anomaly. This demonstrates that *even the amblyopia of arrest may be reversible.*

DEFINITIONS OF AMBLYOPIA

Amblyopia is the condition in which the observer saw nothing and the patient very little (Von Graefe 1888).

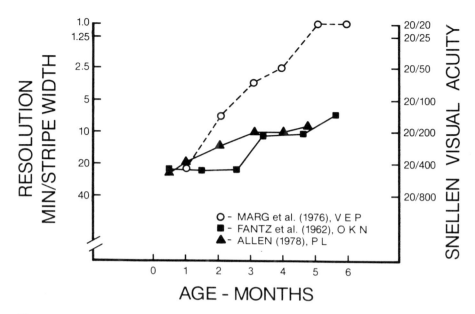

Figure 1.5 *Comparison of systematic acuity data obtained with OKN, PL, and VEP for infants between birth and 6 months of age. O—Marg et al. (1976), VEP;* ■ *Frantz et al. (1962), OKN;* ▲—*Allen (1978), PL. (Adapted from Dobson V, Teller DY. Visual acuity in human infants: A review and comparison of behavioral and electrophysiological studies. Vis. Res. 18:1469–1483, 1978.)*

Over the years, a number of definitions of amblyopia have been proposed. This has led to much confusion, however. Without a common definition, all data concerning such factors as etiology, prevalence, and treatment are difficult to compare. The following is a review of some of the more popular and commonly used definitions of amblyopia. We will then combine these to develop a working definition of amblyopia that will be used throughout the remainder of the book.

1. *Keiner* (1951): Impaired visual acuity in which no anatomic defect of the maculocerebral system can be detected.
2. *Burian* (1956a): A unilateral or bilateral decrease of vision for which no obvious cause can be detected by physical examination of the eye and which in appropriate cases is correctable by therapeutic measures.
3. *Fuchs* (1898): Disturbance of vision without apparent lesion, including only those patients with normal ophthalmoscopic findings and whose vision is uncorrectable by glasses.
4. *Schapero* (1971): Amblyopia may then be defined as low or reduced central vision not correctable by refractive means and not attributable to obvious

structural or pathologic anomalies of the eye. The level of vision that constitutes amblyopia may be set by one of two criteria:

    a.   A difference in level of vision in one eye versus the other; that is, an eye with 20/30 vision is considered to be amblyopic if vision in the other eye is 20/15. Generally, this difference is two lines of acuity or more.

    b.   Clinically significant departure from the expected 20/20 vision. Other commonly used visual acuity criteria are

        (1) *Feldman and Taylor* (1942): less than 20/50.

        (2) *Burian* (1953), *McCulloch* (1950), *Costenbader, Bair*, and *McPhail* (1948): 20/40 or less.

        (3) *Schapero* (1961): 20/30 or less.

        (4) *Bourquin* (1953): 20/25 or less.

        (5) *Bangerter* (1953): 20/25 or less than is indicated by the eye's state of health.

        (6) *Ramsay* (1950): less than 20/20.

5. *Duke-Elder* (1973): The term *amblyopia* ("blunt eye") is generally used in a restricted sense to denote reduced vision in an eye in the absence of any ophthalmoscopically detectable retinal anomaly or any disorder of the afferent visual pathways that might cause the defect. In its widest sense, the term may be used to include a defect of vision owing to the absence of adequate symmetrical stimuli to the two eyes so that the binocular reflexes cannot be developed.

6. *Ciuffreda* (1977): *Amblyopia* refers to a reduction (generally unilateral) of visual acuity that cannot be attributed to uncorrected refractive error, ocular or neurologic disease, or obvious structural abnormalities in the visual pathways.

7. *Flynn* and *Cassady* (1978): Visual acuity of 20/50 or less in the amblyopic eye in the presence of 20/20 acuity in the normal eye, or a difference of three lines of acuity between the amblyopic and the normal eye when the acuity of the normal eye is poorer than 20/20.

8. *Von Noorden* (1985): A decrease of visual acuity in one or both eyes which upon physical examination appear normal and which, if treated early in life, is completely or partially reversible.

The most commonly used definitions of amblyopia are those of Schapero and Burian. Although these definitions are adequate in the general sense, there are some inherent problems. A thorough definition of functional amblyopia should help the clinician make a differential diagnosis between functional and organic amblyopia. Schapero's definition operates by exclusion. Since we know that binocular vision anomalies can cause functional amblyopia, a definition should specify that a best corrected subnormal seeing eye (or eyes) is (are) amblyopic only if associated with one or more of the following:

1. Significant anisometropia
2. Constant unilateral esotropia or exotropia
3. Significant isometropia

4.   Image degradation

Therefore, functional amblyopia *must* be associated with one of the above anomalous conditions. If a patient has reduced visual acuity, *without* one or more of the above conditions, then he or she *does not* have functional amblyopia, even in the absence of any obvious pathological ocular abnormality.

By our present definitions, one can have reduced best corrected visual acuity without obvious pathology and without one of the causes of functional amblyopia and still be labeled a functional amblyope. Treatment in this case may be fruitless.

If one uses Schapero's second criterion of a clinically significant departure from the expected 20/20 by some of the criteria in 4b, a patient with abnormal visual acuity is *not* considered amblyopic. If the best corrected unilateral or bilateral acuity is slightly worse than 20/20, it is up to the clinician to determine the possible cause. The differential diagnosis includes functional amblyopia, provided that one or more amblyogenic factors is present. A working definition of amblyopia must allow the exclusion of functional amblyopia as a reason for the decreased visual acuity. Once this has been accomplished, organic causes of decreased visual acuity can be investigated. In addition, a working definition should allow for the possibility of functional amblyopia superimposed on some overt organic ocular disease (Kushner 1981).

The Burian definition is too general. It does not specify the extent of vision loss necessary to constitute amblyopia. Further, it assumes that all the amblyopia can be reversed with proper treatment if it is functional. The reversibility of amblyopia may not be appropriate in the definition, since this recovery of vision depends on the following:

1.   Stage of maturation of the visual system during onset of the vision anomaly
2.   Duration of deprivation
3.   Age when previous treatment was instituted and the appropriateness of the treatment

New Definition of Amblyopia

Amblyopia can be defined as a unilateral (or infrequently bilateral) condition in which the best corrected visual acuity is poorer than 20/20 in the absence of any obvious structural or pathologic anomalies but with one or more of the following conditions occurring before the age of 6 years:

1.   Amblyogenic anisometropia
2.   Constant unilateral esotropia or exotropia
3.   Amblyogenic bilateral isometropia
4.   Amblyogenic unilateral or bilateral astigmatism
5.   Image degradation

Whenever visual acuity is less than 20/20, it is clinically significant and therefore needs to be investigated further. If one of the five conditions associated with amblyopia is not present, then possible organic changes should be investigated.

There are four possible outcomes when evaluating a patient with vision loss:

- Organic change present without amblyogenic factors → therefore, none of the vision loss is of a functional nature.
- Organic changes present and amblyogenic causes also present → therefore, the functional amblyopia is superimposed on the organic amblyopia (see Chapter 10 on treatment for evaluating the percentage contribution of each).
- Amblyogenic factors present without any visible organic changes → therefore, it is a purely functional amblyopia (see Chapter 10).
- Neither obvious organic or amblyogenic factors apparent → therefore, one needs further testing for (postorbital) organic cause; this is *not* functional amblyopia.

A major problem with the present definitions of amblyopia is that they all revolve primarily around the decrease in visual acuity. It seems backwards to use the amount of vision loss as the primary criterion for whether or not a condition exists. Any other anomaly is defined not by the amount of vision loss, but rather by the cause and/or anatomic location of the anomaly. For example,

1. Myopia:
   a. Refractive
   b. Axial
2. Cataract:
   a. Posterior subcapsular
   b. Nuclear
3. Corneal opacity:
   a. Central versus peripheral
   b. Epithelial, stromal, etc.

We therefore propose the same type of reasoning for amblyopia:

Effect	*Possible Causes*
Decreased visual acuity	Strabismus (constant unilateral)
	Cataract
	Senile macular degeneration
	Anisometropia (significant amount)
	Optic atrophy

The advantage of this working definition is that (1) it is an excellent way of ruling out organic amblyopia, (2) it stresses the etiology of the amblyopia, and (3) any vision loss due to an amblyogenic factor is included.

CLASSIFICATION OF AMBLYOPIA

The classification of amblyopia has undergone a gradual shift in terminology over the years (see Table 1.4). One of the pioneers in this area was Fuchs (1898), who placed amblyopia under the heading of "disturbances of vision without any apparent lesion." He included only those patients whose vision was not corrected with spectacles and who had normal ophthalmoscopic findings. Fuchs used a broad classification of amblyopia, dividing it into two categories:

1. *Congenital.* This included those having a long-standing history of decreased vision, with other congenital anomalies likely to be present. It was typically unilateral, with the patient having a high probability of developing squint. Note that this definition does not mention the presence or absence of any obvious pathology.
2. *Ex anopsia (from disuse).* This included those whose reduced vision was due to physical obstacles such as corneal and lens opacities, as well as strabismic amblyopia due to suppression of the retinal image in the deviated eye.

Thus all amblyopia was considered either congenital or exanopic, implying an organic or functional etiology, respectively. Recall that in Fuchs' time, amblyopia was thought to be purely congenital and to be the cause of squint, not vice versa.

De Schweinitz (1906) agreed with Fuchs on the definition of amblyopia ex anopsia. However, he redefined congenital amblyopia to include those instances of defective vision with essentially an uncomplicated fundus picture. He noted that in some cases, however, "the papilla is discolored, and there is a scotoma." This seems to be a somewhat vague, middle-of-the-road position. According to Duke-Elder (1973), congenital (e.g., organic) amblyopia occurs from birth without any apparent retinal or central nervous system lesion, but he implied the

Table 1.4 History of Classification of Amblyopia

1. **Fuchs** (1898):		b. Aniseikonic
a. Congenital		c. Ametropic
b. Ex anopsia		d. Strabismic
2. **Von Noorden** (1967):	5.	**Amos** (1977):
a. Strabismic		a. Ex anopsia (stimulus
b. Anisometropic		deprivation)
c. Ametropic		b. Refractive
d. Ex anopsia (form deprivation)		(1) Anisometropic
3. **Schapero** (1971):		(2) Isometropic
a. Light deprivation		c. Strabismic
b. Isometropic		d. Aniseikonic
c. Amblyopia ex anopsia	6.	Our proposed classification (1990):
(1) Strabismic		a. Strabismic
(2) Anisometropic		b. Anisometropic
4. **Duke-Elder** (1973):		c. Isometropic
a. Anisometropic		d. Image degradation

presence of an undetectable lesion. He also used this term to include the patient in whom the initial visual improvement during therapy suddenly stopped, again suggesting an organic component.

Keiner (1951) felt that the term *amblyopia* was used much too loosely in the literature. His definition included only those cases of "impaired visual acuity in which no anatomic lesion of the maculocerebral system is detectable," thus separating out those patients with solely nonorganic losses of vision.

We agree with Keiner (1951) that the terminology in this area has been inconsistent and often misused. The following examples will help us understand where the confusion lies:

Amblyopia ex anopsia. The main problem in using this term is that it suggests disuse or lack of use as the cause, again pointing to amblyopia of arrest as the etiology. However, in the majority of the functional amblyopias, the onset occurs *after* full vision development (see Chapter 2), and therefore there must be an active inhibitory process that suppresses the already developed vision. As pointed out by Burian (1956a), amblyopia of disuse implies atrophy such as occurs in muscle fibers when they are not used for an extended amount of time. This is not the case in amblyopia.

Light-deprivation amblyopia. This term is often used when physical obstacles to normal retinal stimulation, such as congenital cataracts, ptosis, or corneal opacities, are present (Schapero 1971). As shown in animal studies (see Chapter 4), the main cause of amblyopia is degraded and/or dissimilar foveal images (von Noorden 1990, Bishop 1987). Consequently, it is the deprivation of a focused, high-contrast retinal image and not simply the deprivation of light per se that is responsible for the pathophysiology of this type of amblyopia.

Ametropic amblyopia. This term is often used with respect to amblyopia secondary to uncorrected refractive error (von Noorden 1967). However, this term does not specify the nature of the ametropia (i.e., isometropia versus anisometropia).

Refractive amblyopia. This term includes both anisometropia and isometropia since it is believed that both have a common mechanism (Amos 1977). However, the mechanisms are probably very different. One is secondary to an active competitive inhibition, while the other involves a more passive bilateral image (contrast) deprivation.

Bilateral ametropic amblyopia. This term is used when speaking of amblyopia secondary to bilateral isometropic uncorrected refractive error (von Noorden 1967). However, it also suggests a *bilateral* amblyopia, which is not always the case. Therefore, this classification does not cover the not so infrequent case of amblyopia occurring only in one eye despite the presence of equal refractive errors (that is, OD +5.00 sphere with 20/40 visual acuity and OS +5.00 sphere with 20/20 visual acuity). [*Note:* This type of case generally has a small-angle squint associated with it. We therefore prefer to use the term *isometropic amblyopia* because it can be used with either unilateral or bilateral amblyopia with equal bilateral refractive errors. In addition, it is conceivable that the patient may have been anisometropic at one time. A recent study of strabismic amblyopes suggests that over time the amblyopic eye either remained emmetropic or shifted toward hyperopia, while the fellow dominant eye became more myopic (Nastri et al. 1984).]

Aniseikonic amblyopia. Although Duke-Elder (1973) proposed aniseikonia as a separate type of amblyopia, it is doubtful whether one can find an aniseikonic amblyope in the absence of either significant anisometropia or constant unilateral esotropia. Therefore, this should be classified under either anisometropic or strabismic amblyopia. Phillips (1959) compared two groups of strabismics. The first had intermittent strabismus, and the second had constant strabismus. Phillips found no significant difference in the amount of aniseikonia in the two groups. Therefore, aniseikonia does not appear to be a significant cause of strabismus.

We will therefore use the following clinical classification of amblyopia which we believe circumvents past problems:

- Strabismic
- Anisometropic
- Isoametropic
- Image degradation

Strabismic Amblyopia

Strabismic amblyopia is associated with an early-onset (before age 7 years or so), constant, unilateral deviation at distance *and* at near. The cause of the strabismic amblyopia is presumably an active cortical inhibition of impulses originating in the fovea of the deviated eye. When a constant unilateral deviation of the visual axis occurs to produce a strabismus, the visual system has two important problems to deal with: *diplopia* and *confusion* (see Figure 1.6).

Diplopia

This occurs when the object of regard falls on the fovea in the dominant eye and on a nonfoveal point in the deviating eye. Since these retinal points are not corresponding, the object will be perceived in two different visual directions, resulting in diplopia, or "double images." One would then develop suppression to avoid one of the diplopic images ("distasteful diplopia").

Confusion

This inconsistency occurs when the fovea of the squinting eye is stimulated by some target other than the object of fixation (+) (Figure 1.6). Since both foveas are primary corresponding points, objects O and + are seen as being superimposed, thereby creating confusion and retinal rivalry. One would then develop

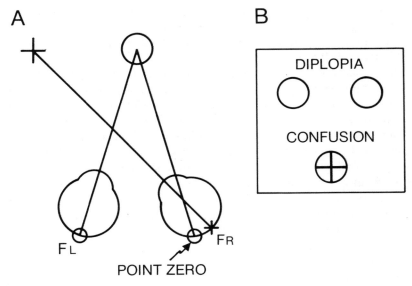

Figure 1.6   *(a) Schematic diagram of a right esotropia (FL = fovea of left [dominant] eye; FR = fovea of right [esotropic] eye; Point Zero = point in deviated eye that the object of fixation falls on; + = object falling on the fovea of the deviated eye.) (b) Patient's view of diplopia and confusion.*

suppression to prevent simultaneous perception of the two different objects in a common visual direction. *Suppression*, wherein all or part of the ocular image of one eye is prevented from contributing to the binocular percept, is the visual system's primary mechanism of eliminating the diplopia and/or confusion. Since strabismic amblyopia occurs as a result of constant suppression, Figure 1.6 shows how suppression secondary to diplopia and confusion occurs.

1.   The object of fixation (O) is imaged on the fovea of the dominant left eye.
2.   Since the patient has a right esotropia, the object (O) impinges on the nasal retina of the deviating eye and is therefore seen to the right, resulting in uncrossed (homonymous) diplopia.
3.   To eliminate the diplopia, the retinal image in the deviated eye must be suppressed. This is the "zero measure" point (Jampolsky 1955).
4.   Since the dominant left eye has the circle imaged on its fovea while the deviated right eye has the cross imaged on its fovea, the cross and circle are seen superimposed and perceived in identical visual directions, thus creating confusion. To eliminate or avoid this confusion, suppression of the fovea of the deviated eye must occur. Foveal suppression is deeper than suppression at point zero (Jampolsky 1955). According to Jampolsky, the suppression zone (at least theoretically) extends from a sharp vertical border through the fovea to an oval border at point zero, resembling a stretched

capital letter D. The area of suppression is greater horizontally than vertically (Figure 1.7). Since there are two areas and etiologies for the suppression (fovea *and* point zero), we do not know with certainty whether diplopia or confusion is the primary amblyogenic factor. While patients complain of diplopia and not confusion, the critical factor in triggering suppression is probably confusion. One reason why diplopia may not be the main amblyogenic factor is that the diplopic image (except in microstrabismus) is far off from the fovea. However, with confusion, there are decorrelated images *on the foveas*, which leads us to assume indirectly that confusion is a greater amblyogenic factor. With the coexistence of both conditions (i.e., confusion and diplopia), the amblyopia is typically deeper than when only one of the anomalous sensory conditions is present. For example, Brock (1952) examined 200 anisometropic amblyopes, 100 with and 100 without strabismus. The amblyopes with both strabismus and anisometropia had deeper amblyopia (Table 1.5).

When mention is made of strabismic amblyopia, it is esotropia and not exotropia that is typically assumed to be the case (Table 1.6). It is important to note that by itself (i.e., without the coexisting amblyogenic anisometropia), primary esotropia and *not* exotropia typically is associated with amblyopia. This is true because under most conditions, exotropia presents as an intermittent

Table 1.5 Degree of Amblyopia Found in 100 Nonsquinters as Compared to That Found in 100 Strabismic Individuals

Degree of Amblyopia	Nonsquinters	Squinters
20/40 to 20/50	33	5
20/60 to 20/100	35	19
6/40 to 6/100	23	44
6/120 and up	9	32

Source: Brock (1952).

Table 1.6 Incidence of Amblyopia: Percent Esotropia versus Exotropia in Different Populations of Amblyopes with Strabismus

	Percent ET[*]	Percent XT[*]	Miscellaneous
Glover and Brewer (1944)	68.9	31.1	
Theodore et al. (1944)	80.5	19.4	
Downing (1945)	72.5	27.8	
Frandsen (1960)	95.8	4.2	
Helveston (1965)	83.3	16.7	
Flynn and Cassady (1978)	79.7	16.1	4.2

[*]ET = esotropia; XT = exotropia.

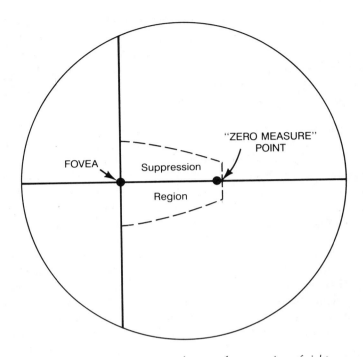

Figure 1.7 *Funduscopic view of areas of suppression of right eye.*

and/or alternating deviation rather than a constant unilateral deviation, which seems to be a prerequisite for the development of significant amblyopia. Therefore, the following sequence of events probably occurs (before age 7 years): constant unilateral esotropia with subsequent unilateral amblyopia in the absence of previous anisometropia. In contrast, the following sequence is extremely rare: constant unilateral exotropia with subsequent unilateral amblyopia in the absence of previous anisometropia. The chance of a constant unilateral exotropia occurring is greater when it is secondary to a preexisting unilateral decrease in vision, such as anisometropic or organic amblyopia, as shown below:

Anisometropic or → Constant unilateral exotropia → Unilateral functional
organic amblyopia   (onset before age 7)   amblyopia superimposed
(without squint)   on anisometropic or
                                                       organic amblyopia

Therefore, if a patient presents with an exotropia and reduced unilateral visual acuity in the absence of anisometropia or a history of retinal image degradation, the clinician should suspect organic amblyopia. Remember, there may be a functional amblyopia superimposed over the organic amblyopia, with the cause of the functional amblyopia being the secondary exotropia.

Types of Primary Strabismus and Presence or Absence of Amblyopia

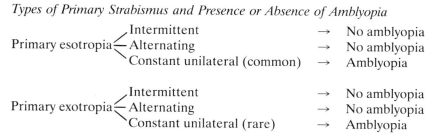

Primary esotropia
- Intermittent → No amblyopia
- Alternating → No amblyopia
- Constant unilateral (common) → Amblyopia

Primary exotropia
- Intermittent → No amblyopia
- Alternating → No amblyopia
- Constant unilateral (rare) → Amblyopia

Anisometropic Amblyopia

Anisometropia is frequently considered to be the most common cause of amblyopia, occurring twice as frequently as strabismic amblyopia (Glover and Brewer 1944, Theodore et al. 1944, Agatson 1944, Sugar 1944, Downing 1945, Helveston 1965, Schapero 1971). In this condition, there is either a difference in retinal image clarity (and contrast) if the anisometropia is uncorrected or a difference in retinal image size (i.e., aniseikonia) if the refractive anisometropia is corrected (Jampolsky et al. 1955). As in strabismic amblyopia, there is a dissimilarity of retinal images. However, the difference is one of clarity, size, and contrast (instead of form), and therefore, the suppression mechanism in the two cases may be very different. Although the causes of strabismic and anisometropic amblyopia are different, there is a common factor leading to the amblyopia:

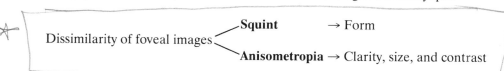

Dissimilarity of foveal images
- **Squint** → Form
- **Anisometropia** → Clarity, size, and contrast

As previously mentioned, the dissimilarity of images (defocus-related) is the etiology of anisometropic amblyopia. Although it has been traditionally assumed that suppression leads to amblyopia, recent research shows that deep amblyopes may have less suppression than alternating strabismics with good visual acuity, thus suggesting a negative correlation between the depth of amblyopia and the degree of suppression (Holopigian et al. 1988).

Anisometropic amblyopia has been found to occur twice as frequently as strabismic amblyopia (Table 1.7). Unfortunately, fixation status was not tested in any of these studies. Therefore, microtropes with anisometropia would be classified as anisometropic amblyopes. In a more recent retrospective study, Flynn and Cassady (1978) analyzed 544 amblyopes referred to their clinic (Table 1.7). Of these, 48% were strabismic, 32% were strabismic and anisometropic, and 20% were purely anisometropic. The importance of fixation testing is made

Table 1.7   Incidence of Amblyopia: Strabismic versus Nonstrabismic

Author	Percent Strabismic	Percent Nonstrabismic
Glover and Brewer (1944)	25	75
Theodore et al. (1944)	34	66
Agatston (1944)	30	70
Sugar (1944)	36	62
Downing (1945)	55	45
Helveston (1965)	48	52
Flynn and Cassady (1978)	80	20

Note: This table compares a more recent study (Flynn and Cassady 1978) in which fixation status was assessed with older studies in which some microtropes were probably grouped under nonstrabismic amblyopia.

Source: Adapted in part from Shapero (1971).

obvious by the fact that 20% of their strabismics had microtropia. The advantage of this study was that microtropia was tested and categorized under strabismus. Unfortunately, anisometropia was defined as a 1-diopter or greater difference between eyes. However, significant "amblyogenic" anisometropia is different for myopic versus hyperopic anisometropia. This distinction should be addressed to obtain a true strabismic versus nonstrabismic frequency value. For example,

> OD   plano   20/20
> OS   − 2.00 sph. 20/100 with left esotropia

Although this hypothetical patient has both anisometropia and strabismus, he or she should be categorized under strabismic amblyopia, since the myopic anisometropia is probably not a significant amblyogenic factor. There exists a controversy as to how one categorizes a patient having both significant anisometropia *and* unilateral constant strabismus. We feel that with such coexistence, the initial amblyopia is probably caused by the anisometropia, which then leads to the strabismus and a further deepening of the amblyopia. In partial support of this notion is a study by Pistocchi and Lamberti (1962), who looked at the relationship between amblyopia, degree of anisometropia, and strabismus. They found that in those patients with greater than 5 diopters of anisometropia, over two-thirds had amblyopia, a quarter of whom also had strabismus. However, in those patients with less than 2 diopters of anisometropia, less than 20% had amblyopia and only 1% had a strabismus. Unfortunately, myopic and hyperopic anisometropes were *not* differentiated. In contrast to this notion, there is some evidence that emmetropization *depends* on normal visual experience. In one study of 61 children with amblyopia, it was found that the refractive error developed at a different rate in the amblyopic eyes than in the dominant eyes, with the dominant eyes becoming more myopic while the amblyopic eyes stayed the same or became more hyperopic (Nastri et al. 1984). If this were true, then, theoretically, the sequence of events in a case of coexistence could be unilateral esotropia causing amblyopia followed by the development of anisometropia leading to further amblyopia.

There is some suggestion in the literature that incidence and depth of amblyopia may be dependent on the degree and type of anisometropic refractive error. Jampolsky et al. (1955) and Phillips (1959) noted that the incidence of amblyopia was lower in myopic than in hyperopic anisometropia. These authors confirmed Copps' (1944) earlier observation that amblyopia accompanying anisometropia is greater in hyperopic than myopic eyes. Feldman (1949) showed that the degree of anisometropia and amblyopia is *not* correlated with posttherapy visual acuity. Helveston (1966) concluded from his data that there was no relationship between the amount of anisometropia and the depth of the amblyopia. However, he did not differentiate between myopic and hyperopic anisometropes in his analysis. Several studies confirm that myopic anisometropia occurs more frequently in the general population than does hyperopic anisometropia. However, amblyopia is more prevalent in patients with hyperopic than myopic anisometropia. The confusion stems from the use of an inadequate definition of anisometropic amblyopia, which is applied to those cases of amblyopia in which there is a difference between corresponding major meridians of the two eyes of at least 1 diopter (Schapero 1971).

While a 1-diopter interocular difference in refractive error may be an adequate criterion for anisometropia, it is not for specification of anisometropic amblyopia, since the amount of anisometropia required to cause amblyopia is different for myopic versus hyperopic anisometropes. The hyperopic anisometrope will accommodate just enough to form a clear retinal image in the less hyperopic eye at all distances. Since the accommodative response is controlled by the less hyperopic eye, the fellow eye *never* receives a clear image and thus suffers from what can be regarded as a mild monocular form of contrast deprivation. In particular, the high spatial frequency component of the stimulus will be degraded. On the other hand, the myopic anisometrope often uses either eye to fixate: the less myopic eye for distance and the more myopic eye for near. Thus the patient with a refractive error of OD plano and OS +3.00 diopters is likely to be amblyopic, whereas the patient with OD plano and OS −3.00 diopters should not be amblyopic, since the myopic eye theoretically receives a clear image from objects 33 cm and closer. Tanlamai and Goss (1979) found the incidence of amblyopia to be 100% among hyperopic anisometropes (least hyperopic meridian) of 3.5 diopters and greater and among myopic anisometropes of 6.5 diopters and greater. An incidence of 50% was found for hyperopic anisometropes of 2.0 diopters and myopic anisometropes of 5.0 diopters (Table 1.8).

Some studies have shown a lack of relationship between the amount of anisometropia and the amount of amblyopia (Horwich 1964, Helveston 1966). Unfortunately, Helveston did not divide his sample into myopic and hyperopic anisometropes. Jampolsky (1955), however, did divide his 200 patients by refractive error type and found a strong correlation in the hyperopic anisometropic group.

Table 1.8 Comparison of Differences in Criteria for Anisometropia versus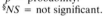
Anisometropic Amblyopia

	Myopic Criteria	*Hyperopic Criteria*
Anisometropia	> 1-diopter difference	> 1-diopter difference
Anisometropic Amblyopia	> 6.5-diopter difference (100% incidence)	> 3.5-diopter difference (100% incidence)
Anisometropic Amblyopia	≥ 5-diopter difference (50% incidence)	≥ 2-diopter difference (50% incidence)

Table 1.9 Summary of Other Authors' Data Regarding Initial Vision versus Degree of Anisometropia

Author	Analysis by Author	Patients	n*	rd†	p‡
Ingram et al. (1985)	Statistics	Children	50	—	<0.01
Dolezalova (1974)	Table	Children	184	0.42	0.001
Robinson (1961)	None	Children	41	0.38	<0.02
Sullivan (1976)	None	Children	21	0.31	NS§
Jampolsky (1955)	Statistics	?Adults	200	—	<0.001 to <0.01
Sugar (1944)	None	Adults	108	0.28	<0.01
Helveston (1966)	Graph	Adults	37	0.21	NS

*n = number of patients.
†rd = rank-difference coefficient.
‡p = probability.
§NS = not significant.

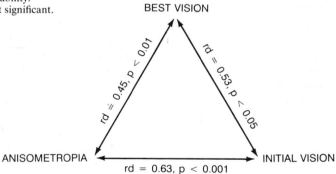

Source: Kivlin and Flynn (1981).

The greater the hyperopic anisometropia, the greater was the degree of amblyopia. Kivlin and Flynn (1981), who also divided their anisometropic amblyopes into myopic and hyperopic groups, found a significant correlation between the degree of anisometropia and the amount of amblyopia (Table 1.9). Still, it is not unusual to see a patient with a small amount of anisometropia, absence of strabismus, and deep amblyopia. This suggests that *dissimilarity* of foveal images and not *deprivation* of form per se (from inadequate stimulation) is the main amblyogenic factor. Further proof of this is the relatively mild amblyopia associated with isometropic amblyopia, where the two eyes are equally deprived of form. It will be argued (see Chapter 3) that abnormal binocular interaction produced by the difference in image clarity between the two eyes is the key amblyogenic factor in anisometropic amblyopia.

The area and depth of suppression in anisometropic amblyopia are significantly different from those in strabismic amblyopia. Contrary to the deep and more well-defined suppression of strabismic amblyopia, the suppression in anisometropic amblyopia is milder and more variable in area (Jampolsky 1955, Pratt-Johnson et al. 1968).

An exhaustive number of papers have attempted to show the relationship of amblyopia to esotropia versus exotropia, strabismus versus anisometropia, hyperopic versus myopic anisometropia, and various other coexisting visual conditions [see Schapero (1971) for an excellent review]. The following is a summary of why these relationships are difficult to establish.

1. Many of the early studies of suppression do not distinguish the effect of suppression from the amblyopia per se.

2. When analyzing data on the incidence of amblyopia with esotropia versus exotropia, those with significant anisometropia are often *not* excluded from the data. However, when significant anisometropia and squint coexist, the sequence of events may be anisometropia → anisometropic amblyopia → esotropia or exotropia. Therefore, when comparing esotropia versus exotropia as amblyogenic factors, one cannot use patients with significant anisometropia, since the anisometropia itself may be the initial amblyogenic factor.

3. There is a 3:1 ratio of esotropes versus exotropes with amblyopia (Schapero 1971). This has been regarded as a manifestation of the higher frequency of esotropia versus exotropia in general. However, to determine if this ratio is indeed accurate, one must use nonanisometropic, constant, unilateral esotropes and exotropes. Since constant *primary* unilateral exotropia probably does not exist, one would then conclude that exotropia is *not* a primary amblyogenic factor.

4. It has been found that amblyopia occurs almost twice as frequently when strabismus is present. However, most studies do not report visuoscopy results, and even if they do, they fail to include anisometropes with eccentric fixation (i.e., microtropes) in the strabismic category.

5. When comparing the prevalence of myopic versus hyperopic anisometropic amblyopia or the relationship between degree of anisometropia and depth of amblyopia, anisometropia is defined as being present when there is a 1 diopter or greater interocular refractive difference. Instead, a criterion of anisometropia sufficient to cause amblyopia should be used (see Table 1.8). This is different for myopic versus hyperopic anisometropic amblyopia. Such a notion explains why studies show that clinically significant myopic anisometropia occurs more frequently in the general population than does hyperopic anisometropia, although the prevalence of amblyopia is greater in hyperopic than in myopic anisometropes.

Isometropic Amblyopia

Isometropic amblyopia occurs secondary to a significant bilateral refractive error which, even when properly corrected, does not immediately result in normal vision. Visual acuity usually improves once the corrective lenses have been worn for a period of time (a few months). Typical for this type of amblyopia is a relatively mild vision loss that is amenable to vision therapy, since abnormal binocular interaction is not a factor. This once again supports the importance of abnormal binocular competition as an amblyogenic factor. With isometropic amblyopia, the retinal images (with and without corrective lenses in place) are generally equal in clarity and size. In addition, strabismus secondary to the amblyopia is much less likely to occur because of the bilateral nature of the amblyopia. Actually, *esotropia* is more likely to occur in lower amounts of bilateral hyperopia. Since the visual system can compensate for the excessive accommodative demand but the fusion system cannot handle the excessive vergence demand, strabismus will result if the AC:A (accommodative convergence to accommodation) ratio is high. A typical example is a young patient with moderate bilateral hyperopia and unilateral amblyopia secondary to an accommodative esotropia.

If visual acuity is not normalized once the proper corrective lenses are constantly worn for an extended period of time, then vision therapy is indicated, with an emphasis on accommodative and ocular-motor procedures (see Chapter 10). It is interesting to note that in these cases, stimulation by contours in the normal environment is *not* sufficient for subsequent development of normal visual acuity. This provides justification for active versus passive (i.e., patching only) therapy.

The isometropia can be either hyperopic, myopic, or astigmatic in nature. As in anisometropic amblyopia, the uncorrected isometropic (myopic) refractive error has to be greater than a hyperopic one because of the myope's ability to have a clear image when viewing at near.

Clinically, isometropic amblyopes typically exhibit visual acuities in the range of 20/30 to 20/70 in each eye when first corrected. Myopes and astigmats show their best acuities through full correction, whereas hyperopes show better acuities when slightly undercorrected. When dealing with hyperopes, a careful binocular evaluation is imperative, since a large exophoric or tropic deviation may become manifest as the full correction is gradually accepted, with the amount of deviation being dependent on the AC:A ratio. The lower the refractive error, the greater is the chance of the patient achieving 20/20 visual acuity shortly after the proper corrective lenses have been worn (Abraham 1964, Ingram, 1986).

Schapero (1971) considers any visual reduction that remains after full correction has been provided to be "organic or congenital amblyopia." However, visual acuities of 20/20 or better are frequently achieved even in adulthood with vision therapy (Birnbaum et al. 1977, Selenow and Ciuffreda 1986, Ciuffreda 1986). Even if vision does not normalize, it seems to be incorrect to consider all nonreversible acuity deficits to be organic. Perhaps more intense and/or prolonged therapy would produce full (or greater) reversibility of acuity; also, perhaps beyond a certain age, complete reversibility is no longer possible, but this does not mean that the amblyopia was or is of an organic nature. It should be mentioned that isometropic amblyopia is generally detected and treated earlier than anisometropic amblyopia (Griffin 1982). This is due to the patient's inability to see clearly out of *either* eye. Fortunately, the prevalence of isometropic amblyopia is decreasing in countries where early vision care is emphasized (Griffin 1982).

The cause of isometropic amblyopia is the occurrence of bilateral uncorrected refractive error during all or part of the first 7 or so years of life. The resultant bilaterally blurred retinal images deprive the visual system of the necessary stimulation (i.e., contours, contrast, spatial frequencies, etc.) found in focused retinal images. The suppression characteristics of isometropic amblyopes differ significantly from those of anisometropic and strabismic amblyopes. Pratt-Johnson (1967) investigated the suppression characteristics of five isometropic amblyopes. Three subjects had no suppression scotoma in either eye, one had a suppression scotoma in either eye, and the remaining subject showed a suppression scotoma only in the amblyopic eye. An undetected strabismus is a possible explanation for the latter subjects.

It has been shown that grating visual acuity in adult astigmatic subjects is meridionally dependent, with acuity losses occurring for gratings oriented along the habitually blurred meridian (Mitchell et al. 1973). This so-called meridional amblyopia is observed clinically in patients who show a mild reduction in visual acuity even when the full astigmatic correction is in place. Although the meridional amblyopia is presumably due to the presence of a habitually blurred meridian early in life, there is evidence that meridional amblyopia does not develop during the first year of life (Gwiazda et al. 1985), despite the high incidence of significant astigmatism during the first year of life (Mohindra et al. 1978). This is in contrast to the development of strabismic amblyopia that has been found to occur during this same time period (Jacobson et al. 1981), again suggesting that these different visual anomalies may have dissimilar "critical period" timetables.

Owing to inconsistencies in criteria, it is difficult to determine precisely the prevalence of isometropic amblyopia. However, it appears to be about 0.03% (wartime Army drafted population) (Theodore et al. 1944, Agatson 1944). In a population of 5129 nonsquinting amblyopes, only 1.1% had amblyopia due to uncorrected isometropia (Theodore et al. 1944). Fortunately, the effects of bilateral loss of clear form vision are not as damaging as asymmetrical visual inputs (von Noorden 1967). Consequently, the depth of isometropic amblyopia, and its resistance to therapy, is less. It should be mentioned that high degrees of myopia are frequently associated with retinal thinning and macular pigment abnormalities. Consequently, when dealing with a high bilateral (or unilateral) myopic amblyope, one may be uncertain about the percentage of vision loss that may be organic versus functional in nature.

Image Degradation

Image degradation refers to amblyopia secondary to the occurrence of a physical obstruction along the line of sight that prevents the formation of a well-focused, high-contrast image on the retina. This obstruction can occur in either one or both eyes and must take place before the seventh year of life for amblyopia to develop, with the degree of amblyopia being dependent on the time of onset and the extent of the degradation. Some of the conditions that can lead to this type of amblyopia are cataracts, corneal opacities, congenital ptosis, and early total occlusion (Leibfelder 1963, von Noorden and Maumenee 1968). Clinically, congenital cataracts are the most common cause of image-degradation amblyopia. The prognosis for improvement of vision is less favorable in those with complete congenital cataracts than in those with partial congenital cataracts, even when the media are postoperatively clear (Ryan et al. 1965). The same is true for unilateral versus bilateral cataracts (Brent et al. 1986).

Traditionally, the management of congenital cataracts had been conservative. Even with significant reductions in surgical complications, the improvement in vision had been disappointing. Recently, with a less conservative approach, the outcomes have been much more favorable. This includes early surgery (before 8 weeks of age), short intervals between operations on the fellow eye (48 hours or less), total bilateral occlusion between operations, and early correction of aphakia (within 1 week of surgery) with extended-wear contact lenses (Gelbart et al. 1982). As might be expected, the amblyopia is much more severe with unilateral versus bilateral deprivation. Parks (1982) followed the vision changes of 99 aphakic eyes. He found the prognosis to be dependent on the cataract type (lamellar was best and axial was worst) and age at treatment (before age 4 months was best). In a group of 51 aphakic infants who were fit with contact lenses (Taylor et al. 1979), it was found that much of the visual defect in cases of congenital cataract was due to functional amblyopia and therefore *could be prevented and treated*. These researchers stressed the importance of *early* treatment and optical correction, since the effect of deprivation begins at about 4 months of age, increases rapidly up to 8 months, and then declines gradually over the first decade of life. Crawford (1972) studied the effect of unilateral and bilateral incomplete congenital cataracts. He found that visual acuity was related to the density of the cataract, not the size or type. In terms of visual acuity, the prognosis was the same (poor) for a unilateral incomplete versus a bilateral incomplete congenital cataract. One must remember that congenital cataracts are often associated with organic ocular diseases such as microphthalmia, coloboma, and optic atrophy. In these cases, there is no hope for vision improvement. Nonetheless, one must rule out the possibility of functional amblyopia if superimposed on the organic amblyopia. Von Noorden and Maumenee (1968) believe that such image-deprivation amblyopia is caused by lack of normal retinal stimulation and not by inhibition secondary to interference with normal binocular vision. Unilateral aphakia is an example of the most marked degree of anisometropia and aniseikonia. The depth of amblyopia here depends on the following:

1. Age at which the cataract began
2. Length of time the cataract was present
3. Age at which the cataract was removed
4. Time between aphakia and optical correction
5. Presence of squint either before or after the cataract was removed

The concept of occlusion amblyopia in human infants is now well established. It is well known that even short periods (less than 1 week) of direct occlusion in a young amblyope can result in dramatic changes in monocular acuities and a tradeoff between the acuities of the two eyes (Thomas et al. 1979, Awaya et al. 1979, Levi 1976). Fortunately, visual acuity in these cases generally can be rapidly recovered. The topic of occlusion amblyopia will be further discussed in Chapter 2.

Awaya et al. (1979) have divided 100 cases of stimulus-degradation amblyopia into three cause-related categories: (1) short-term complete, (2) long-term complete, and (3) long-term incomplete. The incidence of poor recovery was highest when the degradation occurred between the sixth and ninth months of age. Recovery of visual acuity was good when degradation occurred after the eighteenth month of age.

PREVALENCE OF AMBLYOPIA

The reported prevalence of amblyopia varies tremendously. The purpose of this section is (1) to present the numerous variables that can contribute to discrepancies in these prevalence values, (2) to determine the most accurate or representative prevalence value for each major population group, and (3) to formulate suggestions for further amblyopia screenings and studies of its prevalence in different populations. Most studies report *prevalence* (the number of cases of a disease in *existence* at a certain time in a designated area) rather than *incidence* (the number of *new* cases of a disease occurring during a certain period in a designated area). It is difficult to obtain reliable age-specific incidence data, since it is hard to pinpoint the precise age of onset of the amblyopia. In addition, since amblyopia can only develop during the first 7 years or so of life, incidence values are confined to this relatively short time frame. Therefore, unless otherwise noted, we will be discussing the *prevalence* of amblyopia.

The populations used for these studies fall into three main categories (Table 1.10) (with prevalence ranges):

1. Preschool and school-age children (1% to 4.8%)
2. Ophthalmic patients seeking eye care (1.7% to 5.6%)
3. Military personnel (1% to 4.0%)

The following variables all can contribute to discrepancies in prevalence values.

Differences in Criteria

There are no standard criteria for establishing a diagnosis of amblyopia. The following are some of the criteria used:

Table 1.10   Prevalence of Amblyopia by Population

Preschool and school-aged children:

1. **McNeil** (1955):
   a. Prevalence: 2.7%
   b. Criteria: 20/30 or less
   c. Sample: Children 9 to 15 years of age examined in an ophthalmic clinic in an English borough as compared with the total estimated population of children in this borough in this age bracket (n = 6965). Majority of children referred to clinic due to periodic vision testing in the borough's schools (unspecified referral criteria). Diagnosed 189 children as having amblyopia of 20/30 or worse.
   d. Comments: McNeil noted that his estimates may be low because attendance at the ophthalmic clinic was not mandatory. However, estimates may be high, since one does not know how many children who attended the clinic came from outside the borough's schools.
2. **Frandsen** (1960):
   a. Prevalence: 2.6%
   b. Criteria: 20/30 or less *and* presence of squint
   c. Sample: 10,537 normal Danish school children aged 7 years and over
   d. Comments: Children with amblyopia but no squint were omitted.
3. **DaCunha and Jenkins** (1961):
   a. Prevalence: 1.7%
   b. Criteria: Two or more lines difference in visual acuity between the two eyes
   c. Sample: 301 normal 3-year-olds examined at a maternity and child welfare center in England
   d. Comments: (1) Testing done: (A) Sjogren hand test (31% failed to respond), (B) cover test, and (C) retinoscopy. (2) 20/60 visual acuity in each eye was considered normal for 3-year-olds. (3) A total of five children failed, three on the visual acuity test and two due to poor fixation on the cover test.
4. **Russell et al.** (1961):
   a. Prevalence: 1.3%
   b. Criteria: Two or more lines of difference between the two eyes, or 20/50 or worse in either or both eyes for 3-year-olds, 20/40 or worse for 4-year-olds. Doctor's criteria unknown.
   c. Sample: 1572 children between 3 and 6 years of age examined by lay volunteers using illiterate E's
   d. Comments: Failures of screening sent for eye examination, 50% of whom actually received professional attention. Ten of these diagnosed as having amblyopia, criteria unknown. Extrapolation for 50% attendance is 1.3%.
5. **Cholst et al.** (1962):
   a. Prevalence: 4.7%
   b. Criteria: Not stated
   c. Sample: 2986 children, 90% 7 years of age or older, at two health centers of the Bureau for Handicapped Children in New York City
6. **Vereecken et al.** (1966):
   a. Prevalence: 3.5%
7. **Flom and Neumaier** (1966):
   a. Prevalence: 1.09%
   b. Criteria: 30/40 or less and more than one line difference between the two eyes.
   c. Sample: 2762 children screened in two California school districts (1561 kindergarteners and 1201 children in grades 1 through 6) using projected single E target. Screening administered by optometrists.

Table 1.10   (*Continued*)

Preschool and school-aged children:

7. (*continued*)
   d. Comments: Owing to crowding phenomenon, single E's would tend to underestimate number of amblyopes. When taking into account that 0.2% are missed by screening with single letters and 0.6% with previous successful therapy, the prevalence value becomes 1.89%.
8. **Franceschetti et al.** (1966):
   a. Prevalence: 11.8%
   b. Criteria: 20/30 or worse
   c. Sample: 314 preschool children in 13 kindergartens in Geneva
   d. Comments: Refractive error not checked; therefore, the unusually high prevalence value includes uncorrected unilateral and bilateral refractive errors.
9. **Woo** (1968):
   a. Prevalence: 3.85%
   b. Criteria: 20/40 or less (one or more letters missed on 20/30 line considered 20/40); 3.20% were 20/40 or less (less than half of the 20/30 line correct considered as 20/40).
   c. Sample: 5354 children ages 5 to 17 years in northern and eastern Ontario, Canada, using an illiterate E and Snellen chart; all subjects examined by Woo.
10. **Vaughan et al.** (1960):
    a. Prevalence: 0.6%
    b. Criteria: Two or more lines of difference between the two eyes
    c. Sample: Reviewed health records of 25,000 children in San Jose, California, public school grades kindergarten through 12. If criteria were met (nurse screening), the child was sent to orthoptic technician ($n = 489$), who made diagnosis of amblyopia in 132. An additional 71 were sent to Vaughan and Cook (ophthalmologists), who diagnosed 24 as having amblyopia. Therefore, $132 + 24/25,000 = 0.6\%$.
    d. Comments: Does not include children already under care for amblyopia. Therefore, the 0.6% prevalence is of newly discovered amblyopia.
11. **Gilman** (1964):
    a. Prevalence: 0.2%
    b. Criteria: 20/40 or less
    c. Sample: 6553 kindergarteners and first graders in Marin County, California
    d. Comments: Purpose of study was to determine number of amblyopes missed by school nurse screening. Final examination and criteria by eye specialists.
12. **Rantanen and Tommila** (1971):
    a. Prevalence: 1.8%
    b. Criteria: 20/33
    c. Sample: 2100 7-year-old pupils in the first grade in Finland. Research carried out by bachelor of medicine research group under the direction of Dr. Rantanen from the Eye Hospital.
13. **Newmann et al.** (1971):
    a. Prevalence: .55%
    b. Criteria: Constant unilateral squint
    c. Sample: 6400 children aged 1 to 2½ years attending child welfare clinics in Israel
    d. Comments: Low prevalence due to missing mild and nonsquinting amblyopes.

(continued)

Table 1.10   (*Continued*)

Preschool and school-aged children:

14. **Nawratzki and Oliver** (1972):
     a. Prevalence: Group A, 0.5%; group B, additional 0.4% for total of 0.9%; group C, 2.2%
     b. Criteria: Unilateral squint, or difference in behavior with one eye occluded, or difference in visual acuity of at least two lines (when possible)
     c. Sample: Group A, 1½ to 3 years old (*n* = 1910); group B, 1176 children of group A examined 1 year later; group C, 4½- to 5½-year-olds (*n* = 1161)
     d. Comments: (1) Poor cooperation in youngest group; only 11.4% and 1.3% on picture chart and matching picture tests, respectively; and, (2) low prevalence value in group A due to detecting only severe amblyopes. All amblyopes in group C had squint; therefore, purely anisometropic amblyopes were missed. By using behavior under occlusion as a criterion, milder amblyopes may be missed and young normal children who do not like to be occluded would be classified as amblyopes.
15. **Friedman et al.** (1978):
     a. Prevalence: Group 1, 0.5%; group 2, 0.2%
     b. Criteria: Group 1, constant unilateral squint; group 2, greater than 5 diopters of bilateral hypermetropia, 3.5 diopters of bilateral astigmatism, or 2.0 diopters or more of anisometropia
     c. Sample: Group 1, 38,000 children aged 1 to 2½ years attending child welfare clinic in Israel; group 2, 15,084 children aged 1 to 2½ years attending same clinic, but without squint or pathology.
     d. Comments: Both groups screened by orthoptist, with failures referred to eye clinic for further examination. Second group screened with rapid spot retinoscopy.
16. **Haase and Muhlig** (1979):
     a. Prevalence: 4.1%
     b. Criteria: 20/40 or worse
     c. Sample: 830 children medically examined at the time of beginning school in Hamburg, Germany
     d. Comment: Strict criteria that include bilateral amblyopia

Ophthalmic patients seeking eye care:

1. **de Roeth** (1945):
    a. Prevalence: 4.5%
    b. Criteria: Less than 20/40
    c. Sample: 1000 consecutive new patients in private practice in Spokane, Washington; most over 40 years of age
    d. Comment: Only 5% of patients in study had *no* ocular defect.
2. **Irvine** (1948):
    a. Prevalence: 4.0%
    b. Criteria: Not stated
    c. Sample: 5000 Air Corps personnel for whom spectacles were prescribed
    d. Comment: These are considered ophthalmic patients, since they had vision complaints alleviated by ophthalmic prescription.

Table 1.10   (*Continued*)

Ophthalmic patients seeking eye care:

3. **Cole** (1959):
   a. Prevalence: 5.3%
   b. Criteria: 20/50 or less for one eye with the other eye at least two Snellen lines better
   c. Sample: 10,000 consecutive patients examined in his private practice in Nottingham, England
   d. Comments: Examination free, but most had some form of ocular complaint. Additional young children suspected of having amblyopia were referred to him as a result of his informing his colleagues of the implications of amblyopia.
4. **Flom and Neumaier** (1966):
   a. Prevalence: 1.7%
   b. Criteria: 20/40 or less and more than one line difference between the two eyes
   c. Sample: 7017 clinic patients at the University of California School of Optometry, Berkeley, ages 10 to 50 years
   d. Comments: (1) Low prevalence may be due to large number of visually normal persons, especially students, who come to the university clinic. (2) Examinations performed by optometry students.
5. **Abraham** (1966):
   a. Prevalence: 5.64%
   b. Criteria: Less than 20/25 in one or both eyes
   c. Sample: 7225 patients examined in private practice
   d. Comment: Strict criteria and inclusion of bilateral amblyopia contribute toward high prevalence value.

Military personnel:

1. **Glover and Brewer** (1944):
   a. Prevalence: 2.3%
   b. Criteria: 20/70 or less with corrective lenses
   c. Sample: 21,466 draftees in Pennsylvania between the ages of 17 and 44 years
   d. Comment: Mentioned that amblyopia did not appear to be associated with either family income or nationality.
2. **Theodore et al.** (1944):
   a. Prevalence: 4.04%
   b. Criteria: 20/50 or less with best possible correction
   c. Sample: 190,912 inductees previously screened and accepted for service
   d. Comments: (1) Authors stressed that data did not represent a "cross section of the eyes of American men between the ages of 18 and 36." (2) Most of the "not obvious" amblyopes were checked for malingering. "Not obvious" was defined as not having squint or high refractive error.
3. **Agatston** (1944):
   a. Prevalence: 1.8%
   b. Criteria: 20/40 or less

(continued)

Table 1.10   (*Continued*)

Military personnel:

3. *(continued)*
    c. Sample: 2400 consecutive draftees personally examined and screened for malingering
    d. Comment: Estimated that 0.5% to 3.0% of inductees *were* malingering. This was accounted for in the prevalence value.
4. **Downing** (1945):
    a. Prevalence: 3.2%
    b. Criteria: 20/50 or less with optimum correction
    c. Sample: 60,000 *selectees* in Minnesota personally examined by Downing
    d. Comment: Reports testing for suspected malingerers
5. **Irvine** (1948):
    a. Prevalence: 1.0%
    b. Criteria: Not stated
    c. Sample: 10,000 Air Force officers and enlisted men at discharge
6. **Irvine** (1948):
    a. Prevalence: 4.0%
    b. Criteria: Not stated
    c. Sample: 5000 Air Force personnel examined for glasses
    d. Comment: Discrepancy in prevalence values of two populations (see No. 5) can be attributed to inherent bias toward amblyopia in second population.
7. **Helveston** (1965):
    a. Prevalence: 1.0%
    b. Criteria: 20/50 or less
    c. Sample: 9000 men, *primarily enlistees* but some selectees, between ages of 17 and 25 years, in Minnesota, in same induction center as Downing; all amblyopes personally examined by Halveston
    d. Comments: Were examined for duty in all branches of the armed forces except the Coast Guard during peacetime.
8. **Evens and Kuypers** (1967):
    a. Prevalence: 1.8%

1. Reduced visual acuity in one eye. This in itself usually varies from 20/25 to 20/70.
2. Difference in visual acuity of two or more lines between the eyes.
3. Presence of strabismus.
4. Noticeable difference in the person's behavior when one eye is occluded. Primarily used with toddlers and other nonverbal individuals.

An example of the effect of one's criterion on the prevalence of amblyopia is obvious in the Flom and Neumaier (1966) study (see Table 1.11). Prevalence values ranged from 1.2% to 3.5% and 0.7% to 1.4% in the clinic and pediatric populations, respectively, depending on the acuity value used and inclusion of the criterion of a greater than one-line visual acuity differential.

Table 1.11 Amblyopia Prevalence Based on Criteria

	With *Greater Than One Line Acuity Difference Between Eyes*	Without *the Differential Acuity Criterion*
General clinic population:		
20/30 or worse	2.3%	3.5%
20/40 or worse	1.7%	2.0%
20/50 or worse	1.2%	1.2%
Preschool and school-aged population:		
20/40 or worse	1.0%	1.4%
20/50 or worse	0.7%	0.9%

Source: Adapted from Flom and Neumaier (1966).

Various Populations

Many of the populations studied have inherent problems. These include the following:

1. *Ophthalmic patients seeking eye care.* The prevalence values in most clinic populations are of necessity inflated due to self-selection. In other words, those with vision problems seek eye care more often than those without apparent visually related complaints. Consequently, a greater percentage of vision anomalies (including amblyopia) can be expected to be found in a typical ophthalmic patient base. An example is the study by de Roeth (1945), who found the prevalence of amblyopia to be 4.5% in 1000 consecutive new private patients. Of the 1000, only 5% had *no* ocular problems. This is further evident in Irvine's study (1948). The prevalence of amblyopia was 1% for all Air Force officers and enlisted men routinely examined at discharge and 4% for Air Force personnel specifically examined for possible need of optical correction and thus probably having some complaint regarding vision. A main advantage of the ophthalmic patient population-based studies is that fully corrected visual acuities are taken.
2. *Military personnel.* Most prevalence values for military personnel are flawed for one or more of the following reasons (Flom and Kerr 1965):
   a. *Malingering.* Agatston (1944) attempted to determine the degree of malingering in World War II inductees. He estimated that 0.5% to 3.0% were malingering. Only Agatston (1944) and Helveston (1965) carefully controlled for malingering in their studies, which tends to be greater in draftees versus enlistees (for obvious reasons). Helveston (1965) minimized most of the factors responsible for inflated prevalence figures in military populations. This included more careful examination techniques and a specific effort to detect malingerers. His sample consisted of 9000 men, primarily enlistees, but some selectees who were examined

during peacetime in all branches of the armed forces except the Coast Guard. Helveston used the same criteria as Downing (1945) and even worked at the same examining station, but he reputedly carefully controlled for malingering by personally examining anyone with 20/40 or worse vision. Helveston found a prevalence of 1.0% compared with Downing's 3.2%. Helveston's value is probably the more accurate one. Another possible reason for Helveston's lower value is that a greater number of his population represented previously successful amblyopia therapy.

b.   The screening process was very rapid during World War II, thus allowing for a greater number of errors.

c.   Unsuccessful attempts to enlist in one or more of the special branches of the military (such as the Navy, Marine Corps, or Coast Guard) because of failure to meet their higher vision standards usually resulted in waiting to be drafted into the Army (Flom and Kerr 1965). Therefore, these Army *selectees* probably represented a biased sample of men with vision problems, including amblyopia.

3.   *Preschool and school-aged children.* With the emphasis on early detection, studies conducted over the past 20 years have concentrated on school and preschool populations. These mass screening programs allow a more accurate estimate of the prevalence of amblyopia; however, inaccuracies in rates still do occur because of the following:

a.   The examination techniques are relatively crude and usually conducted by volunteers. This is especially true when dealing with preschoolers, where an accurate subjective visual acuity assessment is difficult to obtain. Often, single letter E's are used, which are known to overestimate acuity in amblyopia (Flom et al. 1963). Some studies use the presence of squint as a criterion for the presence of amblyopia. However, one can have amblyopia without squint as well as squint without amblyopia.

b.   Magnitude of refractive error is typically not assessed.

c.   Children previously amblyopic owing to successful vision therapy are *not* included in the amblyopia prevalence values. Since the success of therapy varies between populations, these prevalence values may actually reflect to some extent the success of previous amblyopia detection and therapy. Flom and Neumaier (1966) took most of these factors into consideration. Their population consisted of 2762 children screened in two California school districts (1561 kindergarteners and 1201 children in grades 1 through 6). Administered by optometrists, the screening consisted of an assessment of monocular visual acuity (single projected E's), refractive error (retinoscopy), binocular coordination at distance and at near (cover test), and ocular health (ophthalmoscopy and external examination). They found the prevalence of amblyopia to be 1.0%. By using single rather than multiple acuity targets, they estimated their prevalence values to be low by 0.2%. In addition, they estimated that 0.6% of the children received previous visual therapy that may have prevented or eliminated an amblyopia. Taking these factors into consideration increases the

estimated prevalence to 1.8%. This is probably the most accurate prevalence value for a preschool and school-aged population in the literature.

Other factors specific to the preceding three populations are

1. *Motivation and attention.* These are probably better in adults than children and in military enlistees than in draftees.
2. *Fully corrected visual acuity.* This is more likely to be true in ophthalmic patient samples but not in children's screenings.

Type of Visual Acuity Test

Amblyopes perform significantly better on some visual acuity charts than others (Flom 1967). Some examples are whole-chart, single-line, single-letter, multiple E's, and Allen cards (listed in order of hardest to easiest). In addition, there is no standardization or consensus as to the percent correct level of visual acuity that is considered passing in most clinic situations. This is particularly important in amblyopic eyes, where a few letters correct on *each* of several lines may be found (Flom 1966), making the true level of visual acuity difficult to assess.

Omission of Successfully Treated or Prevented Amblyopia

The extent of those patients having received previous successful orthoptic or vision therapy is not included in the prevalence values.

Incomplete Examination

There are few studies with a complete vision examination included to rule out uncorrected refractive error and ocular disease as a cause of decreased vision. Taking all these factors into consideration, the most accurate estimates of the prevalence of amblyopia for the three populations are

1. Military personnel, 1.6%
2. Preschool and school-aged children, 1.8%
3. Ophthalmic patients, 2.3%

SUGGESTIONS FOR FUTURE STUDIES

To obtain more accurate values for the prevalence of amblyopia, the following is required:

1. A large school-aged population
2. Standardization and verification of screening techniques for amblyopia and not refractive error, since our present screenings are designed for detecting refractive error
3. Use of a full vision examination, including history, objective and subjective refractive error, binocular status, and assessment for presence of ocular disease

REFERENCES

Abraham SV. (1964) Bilateral ametropia amblyopia. *J. Pediatr. Ophthalmol.* 1:57–61.

Abraham SV. (1966) *Nonparalytic Strabismus, Amblyopia and Heterophoria*. Encino, CA: Pan American.

Agatston H. (1944) Ocular malingering. *Arch. Ophthalmol.* 31:223–31.

Amos J. (1977) Refractive amblyopia: Its classification, etiology, and epidemiology. *J. Am. Optom. Assoc.* 48:409–97.

Awaya S, Sugawara M, Niyake S. (1979) Observations in patients with occlusion amblyopia: Results of treatment. *Trans. Ophthalmol. Soc. U.K.* 99:447–54.

Bangerter A. (1953) Uber Pleoptk. *Mener Klini. Wochen-Schrift.* 65:966.

Bangerter A. (1962) Notre Dendir Ehvers Les Ehfants Amblyopes. Bulletin des Societes d'ophthalmologie de France. 62:332–40.

Beer V. (1979) Pflege gesunder und geschwachter augen. Frankfurt, 1802, p. 41; cited by MacKenzie W. *A Practical Treatise on the Diseases of the Eye*. Boston: Krieger.

Birnbaum MH, Koslowe K, Sanet R. (1977) Success in amblyopic therapy as a function of age. *Am. J. Optom. Physiol. Opt.* 54:269–75.

Bishop P. (1987) Binocular Vision. In *Adler's Physiology of the Eye*. St. Louis: Mosby.

Bourquin AL. (1953) Incidence des maladies sur les yeux amblyopes. *Ophthalmologie* 125:405–9.

Brent HP, Lewis TL, Maurer D. (1986) Effect of binocular deprivation from cataracts on development of Snellen acuity. *Invest. Ophthalmol. Vis. Sci.* (Suppl.) 27:51.

Brock FW. (1952) Visual training. *Optometry Weekly.* 43:1641–45, 1683–87.

Buffon GL. (1943) Dissertation sur la cause der strabisme, Memories d' Acadamie des sciences pour 1743, Amsterdam, 1748; cited by Wilkinson O. *Strabismus: Its Etiology and Treatment*. Boston: Meador.

Burian HM. (1953) Adaptive mechanisms. *Trans. Am. Acad. Ophthalmol. Otolaryngol.* 57:131–44.

Burian HM. (1956a) Thoughts on the nature of amblyopia ex anopsia. *Am. Orthop. J.* 6:5–12.

Burian HM. (1956b) Treatment of amblyopia ex anopsia with eccentric fixation. *J. Iowa State Med. Soc.* 449–55.

Chavasse B. (1934) Thermoplasty of the extraocular muscle and posterior partial myotomy. *Trans. Ophthalmol. Soc. U.K.* 54:506–24.

Chavasse B. (1939) *Worth's Squint*, 7th Ed. Philadelphia: Blakiston.

Cholst MR, Cohen IJ, Losty MA. (1962) Evaluation on amblyopia problems in the child. *N.Y. State J. Med.* 62:3927–30.

Ciuffreda KJ. (1977) Eye Movements in Amblyopia and Strabismus. Ph.D. dissertation, School of Optometry, University of California, Berkeley.

Ciuffreda KJ. (1986) Visual System Plasticity in Human Amblyopia. In Hilfer SR, Sheffield JB (Eds), *Development of Order in the Visual System*, pp. 211–44. New York: Springer-Verlag.

Cole RBW. (1959) The problem of unilateral amblyopia. *Br. Med. J.* 1:202–6.

Copps LA. (1944) Vision in anisometropia. *Am. J. Ophthalmol.* 27:641–44.

Costenbader FD, Bair D, McPhail A. (1948) Vision in strabismus: A preliminary report. *Arch. Ophthalmol.* 40:438–53.

Crawford JS. (1972) Prevention of amblyopia caused by incomplete congenital cataract. *Isr. J. Med. Sci.* 8:1488–91.

DaCunha, Jenkins EM. (1961) Amblyopia in three-year-olds. *Med. Officer* 106:146–48.

Darwin E. In Zoomonia, 1801; cited by Wilkinson O. (1943) *Strabismus: Its Etiology and Treatment.* Boston: Meador.

Delard. (1921) *Arch. Ophthalmol.* 38:597–600. Cited in Revell, 1971.

de Roeth A. (1945) Statistical analysis of 1000 consecutive new eye patients. *Am. J. Ophthalmol.* 28:1329–34.

De Schweinitz GE. (1906) *Diseases of the Eye.* Philadelphia: Saunders.

Dobson Y, Teller DY. (1978) Visual acuity in human infants: A review and comparison of behavioral and electrophysiological studies. *Vis. Res.* 18:1469–83.

Dolezalova V. (1974) Beziehung der anisometropie zum Grad der Amblyopie. *Klin. Mbl. Augenheilk*, 169:382–385.

Donders F. (1864) *Accommodation and Refraction of the Eye.* London: The New Syndenham Society.

Downing AH. (1945) Ocular defects in sixty thousand selectees. *Arch. Ophthalmol.* 33:137–43.

Duke-Elder S. (1973) *Textbook of Ophthalmology*, Vol. 6: *Ocular Motility and Strabismus.* St. Louis: Mosby.

Evens L, Kuypers C. (1967) Frequence de l'amblyopia en Bolgique. *Bull. Soc. Belge Ophthalmol.* 147:445.

Fantz RL, Grady JM, Udelf MS. (1962) Malfunction of pattern vision in infants during first six months. *J. Comp. Physiol. Psychol.* 55:907–17.

Feldman JB. (1949) Further studies in amblyopia. *Am. J. Ophthalmol.* 32:1394–98.

Feldman JB, Taylor AF. (1942) Obstacle to squint training—amblyopia. *Arch. Ophthalmol.* 27:851–868.

Flom MC. (1966) New concepts in visual acuity. Optometric Weekly. 57:63–68.

Flom MC, Kahneman D. (1963) Visual resolution and contour interaction. *J. Optical Soc. Amer.* 53:1026–1032.

Flom MC, Kerr KE. (1965) Amblyopia: a hidden threat? *J. Amer. Optom. Assoc.* 36:906–912.

Flom MC, Neumaier RW. (1966) Prevalence of amblyopia. *Public Health Rep.* 81:329–41.

Flynn JT, Cassady JC. (1978) Current trends in amblyopia therapy. *Ophthalmology* 85:428–50.

Franceschetti A, Hudson-Shaw S. (1966) The Social Importance of Amblyopia: The Possibilities of Early Detection. In *International Strabismus Symposium* (edited by A. Arruga), pp. 1–7. Basel: S. Karger.

Frandsen AD. (1960) Occurrence of Squint. Ph.D. Dissertation. University of Copenhagen.

Friedman Z, Neumann E, Hyams SW, Peleg B. (1978) Ophthalmic screening of 38,000 children aged 1 to 2½ years in child welfare clinics. *J. Pediatr. Ophthalmol. Strabismus.* 17:261–67.

Frost A. *Br. Med. J.*, Sept. 24, 1887, p. 663; cited by Revell MJ. (1971) *Strabismus: A History of Orthoptic Techniques*. London: Barrie and Jenkins.

Fuchs E. (1898) *Textbook of Ophthalmology*. New York: Appleton (translated from the second German edition by A. Duane). (As interpreted by Henderson J.) (1962) *Symposium of New Orleans Academy of Ophthalmology*. St. Louis: Mosby.

Gelbert SS, Hoyt CS, Jastrebski G, Marg E. (1982) Long-term visual results in bilateral congenital cataracts. *Am. J. Ophthalmol.* 93:615–621.

Gifford SR. (1935) Some notes on the treatment of strabismus. *Paris J. Ophthalmol.* 19:148.

Gilman E. (1964) The importance of preschool vision testing for amblyopia. *Chron. Dis. Quart.* 4:970–76.

Glover LP, Brewer WR. (1944) An ophthalmologic review of more than twenty thousand men at the Altoona Induction Center. *Am. J. Ophthalmol.* 27:346–48.

Graefe A. (1888) Hanbuok Ges. Augenhk. 6:141; cited by Revell MJ. (1971) *Strabismus: A History of Orthoptic Techniques*. London: Barrie and Jenkins.

Griffin JR. (1982) *Binocular Anomalies: Procedures for Vision Therapy*. Chicago: Professional Press.

Gwiazda J, Mohindra I, Brill S, Held R. (1985) Infant astigmatism and meridional amblyopia. *Vis. Res.* 25:1269–76.

Haase W, Muhlig HP. (1979) Schielhaufigkeit bei Hamburger Schulanfangerr (The incidence of squinting in school beginners in Hamburg). *Klin. Mbe. Augenheilk.* 174:232–35.

Helveston EM. (1965) The incidence of amblyopia ex anopsia in young adult males in Minnesota in 1962–63. *Am. J. Ophthalmol.* 60:75–77.

Helveston EM. (1966) The relationship between the degree of anisometropia and the depth of amblyopia. *Am. J. Ophthalmol.* 62:757–59.

Hiles DA, Galket RJ. (1974) Plaster cast arm restraint and amblyopia therapy. *J. Pediatric Ophthalmol.* 11:151–152.

Holopigian K, Blake R, Greenwald MJ. (1988) Clinical suppression and amblyopia. *Invest. Ophthalmol. Vis. Sci.* 29:444–451.

Holthouse E. (1897) Convergent strabismus and its treatment, p. 173. Cited in Revell, 1971. London.

Horwich H. (1964) Anisometropic amblyopia. *Am. Orthop. J.* 14:99–104.

Ingram RM, Walker C, Wilson JM, Arnold PE, Dally S. (1986) Prediction of amblyopia and squint by means of refraction at age 1 year. *Br. J. Ophthalmol.* 70:12–15.

Ingram RM, Walker C, Wilson JM, Arnold PE, Lucas J, Dally S. (1985) A first attempt to prevent amblyopia and squint by spectacle correction of abnormal refractions from age 1 year. *Br. J. Ophthalmol.* 69:851–53.

Irvine SR. (1948) Amblyopia ex anopsia: Observations on retinal inhibition, scotoma, projection light difference discrimination and visual acuity. *Trans. Am. Ophthalmol. Soc.* 46:527–75.

Jacobson S, Mohindra I, Held R. (1981) Age of onset of amblyopia in infants with esotropia. *Doc. Ophthalmol.* 30:210–16.

Jampolsky AB. (1955) Characteristics of suppression in strabismus. *Arch. Ophthalmol.* 54:683–96.

Jampolsky AB, Flom BC, Weymouth FW, Moses LE. (1955) Unequal corrected visual acuity as related to anisometropia. *Arch. Ophthalmol.* 54:893–905.

Javal E. (1896) *Manuel der Strabisme*, p. 64. Paris: Masson.

Keiner GBJ. (1951) *New Viewpoints on the Origin of Squint*. The Hague: Martinus Nijhoff.

Kivlin JD, Flynn JT. (1981) Therapy of anisometropic amblyopia. *J. Pediatr. Ophthalmol.* 18:47–56.

Kushner BJ. (1981) Functional amblyopia associated with organic ocular disease. *Am. J. Ophthalmol.* 91:39–45.

Lagrange F. (1907) *Arch. Ophthalmol.* 27:209, cited in Revell, 1971.

Le Cat: Cited by Camper P. (1713) *De Oculorum Fabrica et Morbis,* Amsterdam: Opuscula Selecta.

Leibfelder PJ. (1963) Amblyopia associated with congenital cataract. *Am. J. Ophthalmol.* 55:527–29.

Levi DM. (1976) Occlusion amblyopia. *Am. J. Optom. Physiol. Opt.* 53:16–19.

MacKenzie W. (1833) *A Practical Treatise on the Diseases of the Eyes.* Boston: Cartes Hendee.

Maddox E. (1907) *Tests and Studies of Ocular Muscles.* Philadelphia: Keystone.

Marg E, Freeman DN, Peltzman P, Goldstein P. (1976) Visual acuity development in human infants: Evoked potential measurements. *Invest. Ophthalmol.* 15:150–3.

McCulloch C. (1950) Discussion of Ramsey. *Arch. Ophthalmol.* 43:188.

McNeil NL. (1955) Patterns of visual defects in children. *Br. J. Ophthalmol.* 39:688–701.

Meyer E. Cited by Schieck F, Bruckner A. (1930) *Kurzes hanbuck der ophthalmologie,* Vol. 3, p. 527. Berlin: Springer.

Mitchell DE, Freeman RD, Millodot M, Haegstrom G. (1973) Meridional amblyopia: Evidence for modification of the human visual system by early visual experience. *Vis. Res.* 13:535–57.

Mohindra I, Held R, Gwiazda J, Brill S. (1978) Astigmatism in infants. *Science* 202:329–31.

Nastri G, Caccia Perugini G, Savastano S, Polzella A, Sbordone G. (1984) The evolution of refraction in the fixing and amblyopic eye. *Doc. Ophthalmol.* 56:265–74.

Nawratski I, Oliver M. (1972) Screening for amblyopia in children under 3 years of age. *Sight Sav. Rev.* 42:14–19.

Neuwmann E, Eibschitz N, Hyams SW, Friedman Z. (1971) Ophthalmic screening in child welfare clinics in Israel with particular reference to strabismus and amblyopia. *J. Pediatr. Ophthalmol.* 8:257–60.

Parinaud H. (1899) *Le Strabisme et son Traitement;* cited by Wilkinson O. (1943) *Strabismus: Its etiology and treatment.* Boston: Meador.

Parks MM. (1982) Visual results in aphakic children. *Am. J. Ophthalmol.* 94:441–9.

Phillips CI. (1959) Strabismus, anisometropia and amblyopia. *Br. J. Ophthalmol.* 43:449–60.

Pistocchi P, Lamberti O. (1962) Further statistical investigation on the relationship of refraction, ocular motility, and amblyopia. *Arch. Ophthalmol.* 1:253–58.

Poulard A. (1921) Amblyopie par strabisme. *Ann. Ocul.* 158:95–100.

Pratt-Johnson JA, Lunn CT, Pop AE, Wee HS. (1968) The significance and characteristics of ametropic amblyopia. *Trans. Pacific Coast Otol. Ophthalmol. Soc.* 49:231–42.

Pratt-Johnson JA, Wee HS, Ellis S. (1967) Suppression associated with esotropia. *Can. J. Ophthalmol.* 2:284–91.

Priestly-Smith E. (1898) *Trans. Ophthalmol. Soc. U.K.* 8:17. Cited in Revell, 1971.

Ramsay RM. (1950) Amblyopia ex anopsia. *Arch. Ophthalmol.* 43:188–89.

Ratanen A, Tommila Y. (1971) Prevalence of strabismus in Finland. *Acta Ophthalmol.* 47:506–7.

Revell MJ. (1971) *Strabismus: A History of Orthoptic Techniques.* London: Barrie and Jenkins.

Robinson J. (1961) Simple anisometropia and amblyopia. *Br. Orthoptic J.* 18:13–26.

Russell EL, Kada JM, Hufhines DM. (1961) Orange County vision screening project, Part 2. Ophthalmological evaluation. *Sight Sav. Rev.* 31:215–19.

Ryan JS, Blanton FM, von Noorden GK. (1965) Surgery of congenital cataracts. *Am. J. Ophthalmol.* 60:583–87.

Schapero M. (1961) Amblyopia ex anopsia. *Am. J. Optom.* 38:509–30.

Schapero M. (1971) *Amblyopia*. Philadelphia: Chilton.

Schweigger KE. (1881) *Klinische Untersuchungen uber das Schielin*. Berlin. Cited in Revell, 1971.

Selenow A, Ciuffreda KJ. (1986) Visual function recovery during orthoptic therapy in an adult esotropic amblyope. *J. Am. Optom. Assoc.* 57:132–40.

Sugar HS. (1944) Suppression amblyopia. *Am. J. Ophthalmol.* 27:469–76.

Sullivan M. (1976) Results in the treatment of anisometropic amblyopia. *Amer. Orthoptic J.* 26:37–42.

Tanlamai T, Goss DA. (1979) Prevalence of monocular amblyopia among anisometropes. *Am. J. Optom. Physiol. Opt.* 56:704–715.

Taylor D, Vaegen, Morris JA, Rodgers JE, Warland J. (1979) Amblyopia in bilateral infantile and juvenile cataract. *Trans. Ophthalmol. Soc. U.K.* 99:1170–175.

Theodore FH, Johnson RM, Miles NE, Bonser WH. (1944) Causes of impaired vision in recently inducted soldiers. *Arch. Ophthalmol.* 31:399–402.

Thomas J, Mohindra I, Held R. (1979) Strabismic amblyopia in infants. *Am. J. Optom. Physiol. Opt.* 56:197–201.

Uhthoff. (1927) *Klin. Monatsbl. Augenhk.* 78:453. Cited in Keiner, 1951.

Vaughan D, Cook R, Bock R. (1960) *Eye Tests for Preschool and School Age Children*. Stockton, Calif.: California Medical Eye Council.

Vereecken E, Feron A, Evens L. (1966) Importance de la detection precoce du strabisme ede L' amblyopie. *Bull. Soc. Belge. Ophthalmol.* 143:729–742.

von Noorden GK. (1967) Classification of amblyopia. *Am. J. Ophthalmol.* 63:238–44.

von Noorden GK. (1985) Proctor lecture: Amblyopia: A multidisciplinary approach. *Invest. Ophthalmol. Vis. Sci.* 26:1704–16.

von Noorden GK. (1990) Binocular Vision and Ocular Motility, 4th edition. St. Louis: C.V. Mosby.

von Noorden GK, Maumenee AE. (1968) Clinical observations on stimulus deprivation amblyopia (amblyopia ex anopsia). *Am. J. Ophthalmol.* 65:220–24.

Wechert H. (1932) *Zbl. Augenhk*, pp. 227–39; cited by Revell MJ. (1971) *Strabismus: A History of Orthoptic Techniques*. London: Barrie and Jenkins.

Wilkinson A. (1943) *Strabismus: Its Etiology and Treatment*. Boston: Meador.

Woo G. (1968) Incidence of Amblyopia in Grade School Children in Relation to Age and Sex. Paper read before the annual meeting of the American Academy of Optometry, Los Angeles.

Worth C. (1901) *Squint: Its Causes, Pathology and Treatment*. London: J. Bale, Sons, and Danielsson, Ltd.

Chapter 2

Amblyopia as a Developmental Disorder

Amblyopia may be considered to be a developmental disorder of spatial vision that is associated with the presence of strabismus, anisometropia, or form deprivation *early in life*. If the same disorders (i.e., strabismus, anisometropia, or form deprivation) occur late in life, amblyopia does not develop. The powerful notion of amblyopia as a developmental disorder was first articulated by Worth (1903), who formulated the theory that the reduced vision of the amblyopic eye represented arrested sensory development (see Chapter 1). Specifically, Worth suggested that the presence of a "sensory obstacle" (e.g., unilateral strabismus) arrested the development of visual acuity ("amblyopia of arrest"), so that the patient's acuity remained at the level achieved at the time of onset of strabismus. In this view, the depth of amblyopia is a direct function of the age of onset of the "sensory obstacle." Worth further suggested that if amblyopia of arrest were allowed to persist, that "amblyopia of extinction" could occur as a result of binocular inhibition. In Worth's view, only this "extra" loss of sensory function (i.e., the amblyopia of extinction) could be recovered by treatment. Although this latter notion appears to be untenable in the light of present knowledge (see Chapter 10), the ideas of Worth (1903) have had a powerful influence on both clinicians and basic scientists. Thus, as we shall see, many of our currently held concepts, such as plasticity, sensitive periods, and abnormal binocular interaction, were already known almost a century ago. In this chapter we examine the notion of amblyopia as a developmental disorder. We first briefly review what is known regarding normal visual development and then examine the effects of abnormal sensory experience as it pertains to amblyopia.

NORMAL VISUAL DEVELOPMENT

A complete review of normal visual development is well beyond the scope of this chapter. The interested reader should consult the following recent sources for a detailed treatment: normal development, Maurer and Maurer (1988); and normal and abnormal visual development, Movshon and Van Sluyters (1981), Banks and Salapatek (1983), Boothe et al. (1985), Mitchell and Timney (1984), and Teller and Movshon (1986). In this chapter we focus primarily on the development of the primate visual system and, in particular, that of humans.

Figure 2.1, from Teller and Movshon (1986), illustrates vividly the historical view of the development of visual structure and function, with visual acuity beginning at birth (at 0) and gradually rising to adult levels (by 5 to 8 years) as various anatomic functions (depicted below) mature. The present view no longer holds the world of the newborn to be the "blooming, buzzing confusion" envisioned by William James a century ago (James, 1890). Figure 2.2 provides a more modern picture of the development of visual acuity. Figure 2.2 summarizes the development of acuity based on the recent "sweep" visual evoked potential

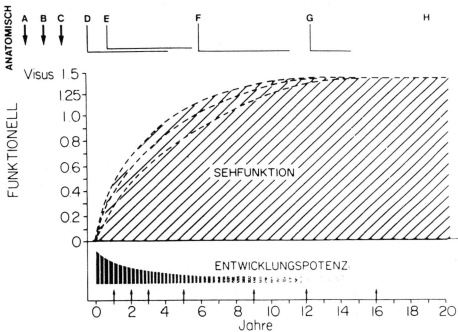

Figure 2.1   *A fanciful depiction of the development of visual function, its correlation with anatomic landmarks, and the remaining "developmental potential" at each age. (Redrawn from Bangerter 1959, by Teller and Movshon 1986.)*

study of Norcia and Tyler (1985). While it may be argued that cortical evoked potential data do not provide a direct estimate of an infant's perception, the presence of a reliable evoked response indicates that the visual pathway has resolved the stimulus pattern, at least up to the primary visual cortex. As is evident from these data, visual acuity is about 4.5 cycles per degree (MAR = 6.7 minutes, or 20/133) at age 1 month and reaches 20 cycles per degree (MAR = 1.5 minutes, or 20/30) by the end of the first year. While the 20 cycles per degree acuity attained at 1 year approaches the acuity of adults (24 cycles per degree) tested under the same conditions, it remains almost a factor of 3 below the limit of adult acuity obtained psychophysically with stationary high-contrast gratings or optotypes. Indeed, there are components, notably the C2 component of the visual evoked potential (VEP) that do not fully mature until much later (Regan and Spekreijse 1986, De Vries-Khoe and Spekreijse 1982), and VEP latencies to high spatial frequency stimuli are longer than those of adults until 5 years of age (Moskowitz and Sokol 1983), perhaps related to the myelination of the cortex. Nonetheless, the data of Figure 2.2 demonstrate a far higher level of pattern resolution in infants than suggested by Figure 2.1 (or than suggested by studies using forced-choice preferential looking techniques) and suggest that the visual system may be susceptible to the influence of degraded or defocused images earlier than previously thought. (See also Figure 1.5.) In the next section we briefly consider the optics of the eye and the anatomic structures and physiologic functions that may limit spatial vision during development.

Optics

Primates are born with clear optical media. While no quantitative data on the optical image quality of the eyes of human infants are presently available, optical line-spread functions obtained from infant monkeys suggest that optical image quality is very good at birth and reaches adult levels by about 9 weeks after birth (Williams and Boothe 1981). The optical changes that occur are small compared with the dramatic alterations in visual acuity and contrast sensitivity that occur during this period, so it seems unlikely that the optics limit normal development of spatial vision. Both infant monkeys and humans tend to be hyperopic at birth. Full-term human infants are, on average, about +2 diopters (Banks 1980). This hyperopia increases until about 6 months of age and then decreases, while accommodation appears to be more or less "on target" by 3 to 4 months of age (Haynes et al. 1965, Banks 1980). This is shown in Figure 2.3 from Banks (1980). Young infants also frequently demonstrate significant amounts of astigmatism (Mohindra et al. 1978, Atkinson et al. 1980, Howland and Sayles 1984), which is highly correlated with the curvature of the infant's cornea (Howland 1982). The astigmatism lessens between 1.5 and about 4 years (Gwiazda et al. 1984, Dobson et al. 1984, Howland and Sayles 1984).

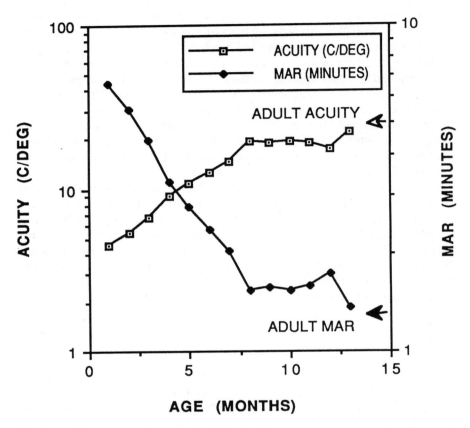

Figure 2.2 *The development of acuity based on the recent "sweep" visual evoked potential study of Norcia and Tyler. Plotted here are acuity in cycles per degree (left axis), or minimum angle of resolution in minutes (right axis) as a function of age. (From Norcia and Tyler 1985.)*

Anatomy and Physiology

The Retina

The primary postnatal changes in the retina concern differentiation of the macular region (Boothe et al. 1985). After birth, foveal receptor density and cone outer-segment length both increase as foveal cones become thinner and more elongated. There is a dramatic migration of ganglion cells and inner nuclear layers from the foveal region as the foveal pit develops during the first 4

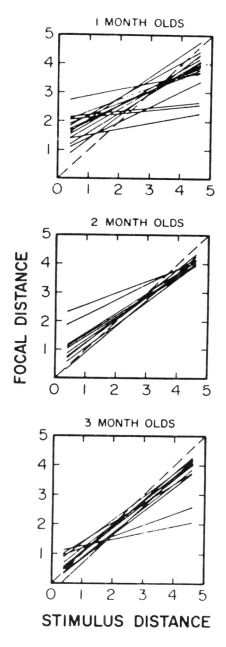

Figure 2.3   *The accommodative stimulus-response relationship for infants aged 1, 2, and 3 months. Note that by age 3 months, most of the infants accommodate quite accurately. (From Banks 1980.)*

months of life, and it is not until about 4 years of age that the fovea is fully adult-like (Youdelis and Hendricksen 1986). Figure 2.4 from Youdelis and Hendricksen (1986) demonstrates the sequence of foveal development from birth to 72 years of age. During this period, cone density increases in the central region as a result of both migration of receptors and decreases in their dimensions. Both these factors result in finer cone sampling (by decreasing the distance between neighboring cones). It is likely that alterations in cone spacing and the light-gathering properties of the cones during early development contribute a great deal toward the improvements in acuity and contrast sensitivity during the first months of life. The massive migration of retinal cells and the alterations in the size of retina and eyeball (along with changes in interpupillary distance) may necessitate the plasticity of cortical connections early in life.

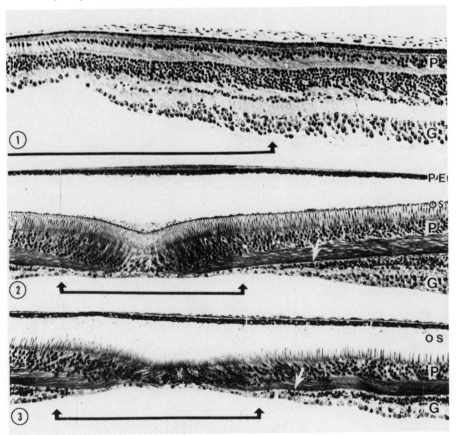

Figure 2.4 *Low-power light micrographs of the developmental stages of the postnatal human fovea at birth (above), 45 months (center), and 72 years (below). Sections are from the center of the foveola. The black lines mark the width of the rod-free foveola (at birth it is so wide that only half can be seen in this figure). (From Youdelis and Hendricksen 1986.)*

The Lateral Geniculate Nucleus

The lateral geniculate nucleus (LGN) is a laminated structure, with the left and right eye afferents already segregated into separate laminae at birth (Hitchcock and Hickey 1980). The parvo and magnocellular layers of the LGN develop at different rates. In humans, for example, the parvocellular layers reach adult levels near the end of the first year, while neurons in the magnocellular layers continue to grow until at least 2 years of age (Hickey 1977). The LGN has a preponderance of spines and filopodia on the dendrites of immature neurons. The number of spines increases after birth, to a maximum around 4 months postnatal, and declines to adult levels by about 9 months in humans (Garey and De Courten 1983). In the next section we shall argue that a number of significant developmental events occur around age 4 months in the human visual system and that they may be closely related to the alterations in numbers of spines in the LGN and cortex.

The circles in Figure 2.5, from Blakemore and Vital-Durand (1979), show how the spatial resolution of neurons (X cells) from the foveal representation of the LGN of monkeys improves with age. Monkey development is thought to more or less parallel that of humans, but at a rate approximately 4 times faster. Thus 30 "monkey days" are roughly equivalent to 120 "human days" (Boothe et al. 1985). Interestingly, Blakemore and Vital-Durand found that in the peripheral retina (beyond about 10 degrees), spatial resolution in the LGN of newborn monkeys was similar to that of adults. Development of resolution of the LGN and of cortical neurons closely parallels the development of behaviorally determined acuity in the monkey (Blakemore and Vital-Durand 1979). The stars in Figure 2.5 show the resolution of neurons in the LGN receiving input from an eye that was deprived of normal visual input from birth. These results will be discussed in the following section.

Striate Cortex

As in the LGN, there is an overabundance of spines in the immature striate cortex, and these spines first increase and then are pruned back to adult levels. Huttenlocher et al. (1982, 1987) estimated that the number of synapses in the human visual cortex at birth is similar to that of adults, but that it essentially doubles by 8 months, before declining to adult levels. Thus it appears that early in development, neurons connect with all possible neighbors, perhaps as an aid or assurance to making the "right" connections. Figure 2.6, from Leuba and Garey (1987), also shows the steep decline in neuronal density in area 17 of humans over the first 4 months postnatally.

In the cortex of newborn macaque monkeys, many of the properties of the receptive fields seem to be established. For example, cells can be classified as simple, complex, or hypercomplex, and they demonstrate orientation tuning and

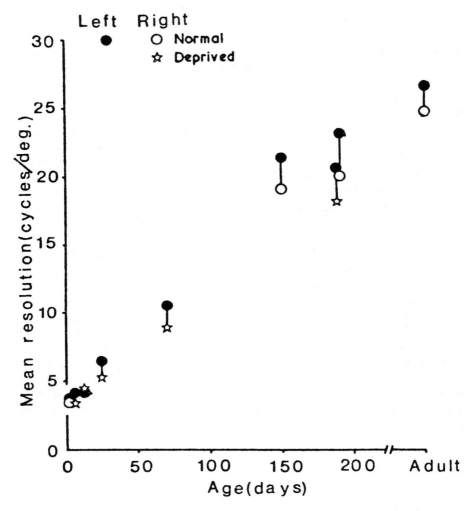

Figure 2.5   *Mean spatial resolution of foveal LGN cells with age in normal and monocularly deprived monkeys. The stars depict recordings from the LGN ipsilateral to the deprived eye. Filled circles plot resolution of cells driven by the left eye. Open circles plot comparable data from the right eye. Data from the two eyes of a single animal are connected by vertical lines. Monocular deprivation from birth until the day of recording does not affect the development of spatial resolution in the LGN. (From Blakemore and Vital-Durand 1979.)*

binocular input, as is the case with adults (Wiesel 1982). Whether these properties of striate cortical neurons are quantitatively similar to those of adults remains to be determined, and it seems likely that the properties of the smallest foveal receptive fields (those with the highest spatial resolution), as well as their

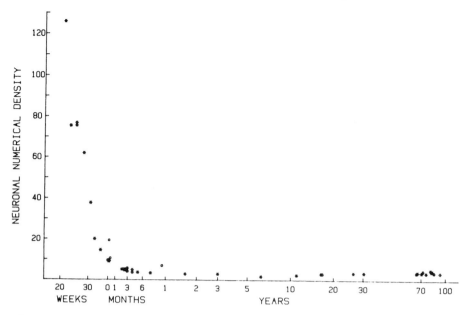

Figure 2.6 *Neuronal numerical density (× 10⁴) in area 17 of humans between 21 weeks of gestation and 93 years of age. Age is given in gestational weeks, postnatal months, and years on a logarithmic scale. (From Leuba and Garey 1987.)*

spatial resolution, develop over the first few months of life (Blakemore and Vital-Durand 1979).

One of the most striking features of the mature primate striate cortex is its organization into ocular dominance columns (see Figure 4.7), where input from the two eyes is segregated into discrete bands. In the monkey striate cortex until about 3 weeks prior to birth, when segregation into ocular dominance columns begins, there is complete overlap of terminals from left and right eye laminae of the LGN. At birth, ocular dominance columns are present (Rakic 1976, LeVay et al. 1980), and segregation is complete by about 6 weeks of age. If the 1:4 rule, which seems to hold for the development of visual function in monkeys as compared with humans, also holds for anatomic development, then we might anticipate that human ocular dominance columns are completely formed by about 6 months. This point and its possible behavioral consequences will be discussed further.

While little is known about the development of functional cortical circuitry, several evoked potential studies suggest that in human visual cortex certain types of cortical inhibitory interactions do not appear until 6 months of age. For example, Morrone and Burr (1986) showed that there was no orientation-dependent masking in the VEP until 6 months of age (see also the section on evoked potentials in Chapter 4). Many sensory functions, including orientation and spatial frequency tuning, and binocular interactions are critically dependent on inhibitory interactions in the cortex.

DEVELOPMENT OF VISUAL FUNCTION

> *"Things start out badly, then they get better; then, after a long time, they get worse again."—Movshon's last law.*
>
> (Teller and Movshon 1986)

The purpose of this section is *not* to provide a detailed summary of the burgeoning literature on infant visual development, but rather to provide a broad overview of particular aspects of development that may be relevant to an understanding of the development of amblyopia. Since amblyopia appears to affect certain aspects of visual function selectively, it is of particular interest to ask whether certain functions develop before others and then to try to relate these to the structural and physiologic changes described earlier.

The "Light Sense": Functional Properties of Rods and Cones

The rod system appears to be functional in early infancy (Powers et al. 1981, Werner 1982; also see Teller and Bornstein 1986). However, while rods and rhodopsin are functional early, postreceptoral mechanisms may mature later, since dark-adapted spatial summation areas of infants are considerably enlarged compared with those of adults (Hamer and Schneck 1984).

Most of the investigations of cone-mediated vision have focused on the development of mechanisms of color vision. It is now reasonably well established that by 2 to 3 months postnatally, infants must have three functioning cone types. The question of when each of the three cone types functions normally is less clear. Infants less than 1 month of age fail to make chromatic discriminations; however, what remains unclear is whether these failures reflect immature cones or postreceptoral mechanisms (Teller and Bornstein 1986, Teller and Movshon 1986) or simply lack of attention and/or motivation.

Temporal resolution for uniform fields is highly developed in young infants. For example, the critical fusion frequency (CFF) at 1 month is about 40 Hz and is approximately adult-like by 3 months (Regal 1981).

Spatial Vision: Acuity, Contrast, Sensitivity, and Hyperacuity

Much effort over the past decade or so has focused on the development of spatial vision in human infants, and this seems of particular relevance to the development of amblyopia. Figure 2.2 showed that VEP acuity approached the adult level of 24 cycles per degree by the end of the first year of life, considerably earlier than behavioral (forced-choice preferential looking, FPL) techniques suggest. The discrepant estimates of these techniques have not been resolved (Dobson and Teller 1978, Teller and Movshon 1986), but the VEP data shown in Figure 2.2 may be considered to provide a lower bound on the spatial resolution of the afferent visual pathway up to striate cortex. Interestingly, Wilson's (1988) analysis of acuity and cone spacing in the infant retina suggests that VEP acuity at age 1 month is consistent with limitations imposed by cone sampling, whereas FPL acuity is considerably lower. Moreover, it seems likely that development of the highest spatial frequency mechanisms (those responsible for acuities approaching 60 cycles per degree in adults) continue to develop well beyond the first year of life (Regan and Spekreijse 1986). Figure 2.7 from Wilson (1988) shows forced-choice preferential looking acuity data from several laboratories. This figure also shows a line labeled "theory." This line is based on the notions (1) that the alterations in cone spacing during development lead to a change in "spatial scale" and (2) that growth of foveal cone outer segments causes an increase in mechanism sensitivity. These ideas will be discussed in

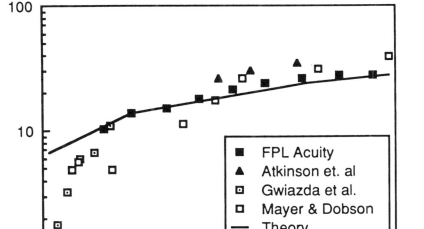

Figure 2.7 *Comparison of theoretical foveal acuity (solid line) with FPL acuity. Theory and data agree well from 10 months on, suggesting that foveal immaturity is the primary factor limiting FPL acuity during this period. For the youngest infants, however, theoretical thresholds are far above the FPL data, suggesting that immaturity at a level beyond the striate cortex produces additional limits on FPL acuity. (From Wilson 1988.)*

greater detail later. For now, it is worth noting that Wilson's theory provides a reasonable fit to the data beyond about 10 months of age. However, the FPL acuity of the neonate is so low that it is likely that it reflects constraints beyond those imposed by retinostriate immaturity. This may reflect immaturity of higher visual areas or simply failure of neonates to attend to the high spatial frequency targets.

While studies of the development of contrast sensitivity in infants are sparse, the emerging picture suggests that contrast sensitivity increases and the peak of the contrast sensitivity function (CSF) shifts toward higher spatial frequencies with age. In addition, the low spatial frequency fall-off characteristic of adult CSFs is absent at 1 month (Banks and Salapatek 1983), suggesting the possibility of postnatal development of lateral inhibition. Moreover, several studies have suggested that the CSF data of 1-month-olds is consistent with either a single channel or an absence of bandpass tuning (Banks and Stephens 1982, Wilson 1988), while that of older infants (perhaps as early as 1.5 months) is consistent with a multiple-bandpass spatial frequency channel model (Banks and Stephens 1982, Fiorentini et al. 1983). Much of the developmental change in visual resolution and contrast sensitivity can be understood on the basis of developmental changes in the retina and cortex. For example, Wilson (1988) has suggested that the growth of foveal cone outer segments causes an increase in mechanism sensitivity, while migration of foveal cones produces a change in spatial scale and a progressive shift of mechanism tuning toward higher spatial frequencies. This is illustrated in Figure 2.8 from Wilson (1988). Development of cortical inhibition is thought to contribute significantly to the development of bandpass spatial frequency and orientation tuning. From the perspective of amblyopia, it is relevant to note that sensitivities to different spatial frequencies develop at different rates, with low frequencies reaching adult levels of sensitivity sooner than high spatial frequencies. Thus the CSF progressively shifts upward (higher sensitivity) and to the right (higher spatial frequencies) with age (Boothe et al. 1985). The poor spatial and good temporal resolution of 1-month-olds suggests that mechanisms tuned to lower spatial frequencies and higher temporal frequencies mature earliest. Since sensitivity to high spatial frequencies develops last, it may not be surprising that amblyopia, which develops early in life, primarily influences the sensitivity of high spatial frequency mechanisms and that sensitivity to large objects (low spatial frequency) and high temporal frequencies is reasonably intact. It would be interesting to determine if the degree of loss at low spatial frequencies present in some amblyopes is closely related to the age of onset of the amblyopia. Figure 2.9 (on page 56) from Norcia et al. (1988) provides a clear illustration of the development of contrast sensitivity for different spatial frequencies. Note that sensitivity to the lowest spatial frequency (0.25 cycles per degree) is asymptotic by about 9 weeks, while sensitivity to higher spatial frequencies continues to grow beyond 33 weeks (the oldest age tested).

Two laboratories have attempted to map the development of Vernier acuity, and two contrasting pictures have emerged. Shimojo et al. (1984, 1987) suggest that Vernier acuity is initially worse than grating acuity and then shows a dramatic improvement (relative to grating acuity) between about 2 and 8 months. At 8 months, Vernier acuity was about twice as good as grating acuity.

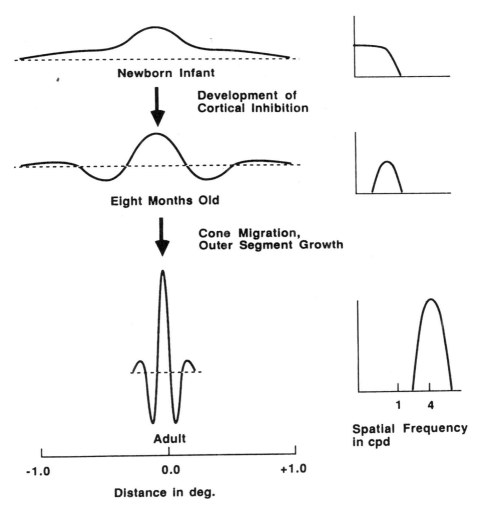

Newborn Infant

Development of
Cortical Inhibition

Eight Months Old

Cone Migration,
Outer Segment Growth

Adult

1   4

Spatial Frequency
in cpd

-1.0   0.0   +1.0

Distance in deg.

Figure 2.8 *Schematic representation of the proposed development of infant mechanism receptive fields. Spatial profiles of the receptive fields are shown on the left, and their Fourier transforms are on the right. The first stage is the development of spatial inhibition that transforms low-pass into bandpass tuning. This is followed by a prolonged stage of cone migration and outer segment growth that shifts the spatial tuning curve toward higher frequencies and increases the sensitivity (below, right). (From Wilson 1988.)*

Shimojo and Held (1987) interpreted their results on the basis of undersampling in young infants and the rapid development of cortical organization; however, there are alternative explanations. For example, poor Vernier acuity of the youngest infants may reflect the effects of crowding, since the stimulus was a repetitive grating. In contradistinction, Manny and Klein (1984) suggested that Vernier acuity and grating acuity developed in parallel between birth and 6

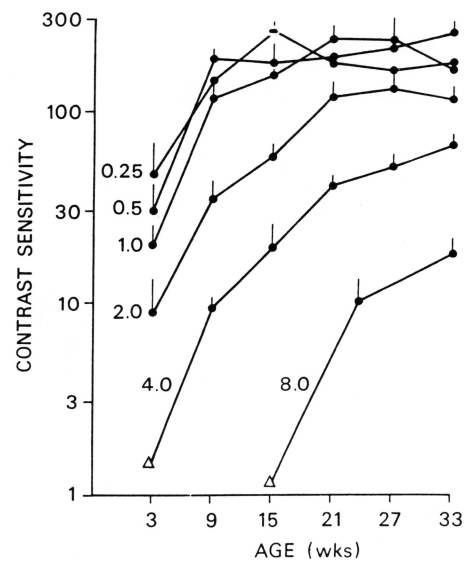

Figure 2.9 *Development of contrast sensitivity as measured by sweep VEP. This figure provides a clear illustration of the development of contrast sensitivity for different spatial frequencies. Note that sensitivity to the lowest spatial frequency (0.25 cycles per degree) is asymptotic by about 9 weeks, while sensitivity to higher spatial frequencies continues to grow beyond 33 weeks (the oldest age tested). (From Norcia et al. 1988.)*

months, with Vernier acuity being about twice as good as grating acuity at all ages. The discrepancies in the results are likely due to the very different stimuli utilized by the two laboratories (Manny and Klein 1985), one with motion and one with no motion. Nonetheless, we still know almost nothing about the development of adult levels of hyperacuity—which is 6 to 10 times better than grating acuity. It seems likely that this very high level of spatial processing develops well beyond the age range studied to date and may coincide with the late development of finely sampled foveal high spatial frequency mechanisms in the cortex. The critical point is that Vernier acuity and grating acuity must have a different developmental time course from birth until they reach adult levels of performance. As noted in Chapter 3, strabismic and anisometropic amblyopes show different relative losses of grating and Vernier acuity, and this raises the intriguing question of whether strabismus and anisometropia exert their effects on the developing visual nervous system at different times during development.

Binocular Vision: Binocular Correlation, Stereopsis, and Rivalry

A substantial number of different studies point to the emergence of binocular processing between 3 and 6 months of life consistent with the segregation of inputs from the two eyes to form the ocular dominance columns of the striate cortex. For example, before 3 months of age, infants (1) fail to respond to binocular correlation (Braddick et al. 1980), (2) fail to demonstrate stereopsis (Fox et al. 1980, Held 1986, Petrig et al. 1983), (3) fail to show aversion to rivalrous stimuli (Birch et al. 1983), and (4) demonstrate asymmetric optokinetic nystagmus (OKN) (Atkinson 1979). Both stereopsis and binocular rivalry probably encompass an important role for cortical inhibition, and it seems important to determine how development of these functions relates to the development of cortical inhibition.

Summary

Visual function develops postnatally; however, the studies reviewed here suggest that different functions may emerge at different times and develop at different rates. Thus, for example, flicker sensitivity appears to be adult-like by 3 months of age, while acuity and contrast sensitivity for high spatial frequencies develop slowly and do not reach adult levels until several years of age. The preceding brief description of the visual capacities of infants provides at least a qualitative sense that many aspects of the abnormal visual functions of amblyopes (see Chapter 3) can be understood on the basis of arrested or abnormal development. Structures and functions that develop earliest are most robust to the effects of abnormal visual input, while those which develop more slowly seem most susceptible. Thus the amblyopic visual system resembles in many respects the immature visual system. Both show normal or near-normal receptoral functions (light sense), relatively normal function at low spatial and high temporal frequencies, reduced acuity and contrast sensitivity particularly at high spatial frequencies, and reduced hyperacuity. In addition, many amblyopes, like infants, show absent or reduced binocular interactions. While there seems to be reasonable qualitative agreement, not everything fits so neatly. For example, while several studies suggest a more rapid anatomic development of the parvocellular (discussed earlier) than of the magnocellular layers of the LGN, it is the former that appear to be most susceptible to the effects of abnormal visual input in both monkeys (Movshon et al. 1987) and humans (von Noorden et al. 1983). Given the finer resolution and grain of the parvocellular system in the central field, this does not seem too surprising.

THE INFLUENCE OF AMBLYOGENIC FACTORS ON POSTNATAL DEVELOPMENT

One of the most influential ideas suggested by Worth (1903) was that "sensory obstacles" could disrupt and arrest normal visual development and lead to amblyopia. These sensory obstacles, retinal image degradation (due to cataract, lid closure, or high uncorrected refractive error) and binocular misregistration (due to strabismus), are now considered to be *amblyogenic factors*—that is, factors that are sufficient but not necessary to produce amblyopia (von Noorden 1977). In this section we will discuss further the necessary and sufficient conditions for developing amblyopia. The ideas of Worth received their major experimental validation from the landmark studies of Wiesel and Hubel (1963) and Wiesel (1982). Their work provided several clear pointers regarding the role of visual experience in the development of visual function:

1. Disruption of binocular input completely disrupts the pattern of cortical excitatory binocular interaction.
2. Monocular deprivation has a dramatic effect on the anatomy, physiology, and function of the striate cortex.
3. Binocular deprivation has less effect than monocular deprivation.
4. The physiologic consequences of deprivation are more or less confined to the striate cortex.
5. The effects of abnormal visual experience occur only during a "sensitive" period early in life.
6. The physiologic consequences of deprivation can be reversed during a "critical" period early in life.

While each of these points has received a good deal of critical attention and refinement over the past 25 years, the key findings remain largely intact and represent "basic principles of central nervous system development" (Teller and

Movshon 1986). Several of these points are discussed in Chapter 3. Here we shall pay particular attention to what is known about the development of amblyopia in humans, the notion of a "sensitive" period or periods, and the issue of plasticity.

DEVELOPMENT OF AMBLYOPIA

The presence of amblyopia is always associated with an early history of a "sensory obstacle": binocular misregistration (strabismus) or image degradation (high refractive error, anisometropia, cataract, ptosis, or lid closure consequent to treatment). These amblyogenic factors were discussed in detail in Chapter 1. In Chapter 3, the issues of deprivation, binocular competition, and suppression will be discussed. Suffice it to state here that the severity of the amblyopia appears to be associated with the degree of imbalance between the two eyes (e.g., dense unilateral cataract results in severe loss), as well as the age at which the amblyogenic factor occurred. Precisely how these factors interact is as yet unknown. In humans with naturally occurring amblyopia, the age of onset of the amblyogenic condition(s) is difficult to ascertain, and the effects of intervention combine to make it difficult to obtain a clear picture of the natural history of amblyopia development. Thus much of our current understanding of the development of amblyopia accrues from animal studies (see Boothe et al. 1985 for a review) and from retrospective studies of clinical records (e.g., von Noorden 1980). Recent technological improvements in infant testing (such as forced-choice preferential looking and rapid VEP methods) are also beginning to provide more direct data on the development of naturally occurring amblyopia in humans (Mohindra et al. 1979, Maurer et al. 1983, Jacobson et al. 1981, Birch et al. 1983) and monkeys (Kiorpes et al. 1984, 1989). All of these studies provide strong evidence for a sensitive period for the development of amblyopia. We shall examine the notion of sensitive periods in more detail.

Clinicians are well aware that amblyopia does not develop after age 6 to 8 years of age (Worth 1903, von Noorden 1980). Since the most severe amblyopias are generally associated with monocular pattern degradation, both laboratory and clinical studies have focused on the period of susceptibility for developing amblyopia due to pattern degradation. This is somewhat unfortunate, since this is the least common form of amblyopia in humans. The data suggest that in human infants, even 1 week of monocular patching (following entropian surgery) can result in severe amblyopia at the peak of the period of susceptibility (Awaya et al. 1980, von Noorden 1981). For older children, brief periods of deprivation are less likely to result in visual loss; however, prolonged deprivation may. For example, von Noorden (1981) reported that several months of monocular occlusion at 5 years of age can result in uncorrectable loss of acuity. This seems to be close to the upper limit of the period when visual acuity is susceptible to the effects of deprivation. However, recent studies suggest that there may be multiple sensitive periods. There is now clear evidence from anatomic and physiologic studies that the sensitive period in layer IVc (the input layer) of the cortex of monkeys is considerably shorter than that of other layers (LeVay et al. 1980). The behavioral studies of lid-sutured monkeys by Harwerth et al. (1987) provide strong evidence for different sensitive periods for different visual functions. For example, they found that early lid suture (age 3 to 6 months) had a marked influence on scotopic and photopic spectral sensitivity and essentially abolished pattern and binocular vision. A later onset of deprivation (up to about 25 months) had no influence on spectral sensitivity but resulted in reduced contrast sensitivity at high spatial frequencies and reduced binocular summation. Lid suture beyond 25 months had no effect on contrast sensitivity but still disrupted binocular functioning. These results are summarized in Figure 2.10. There are several points worth noting: first, to extrapolate these results to monocular pattern deprivation in humans, the 1:4 rule should be applied (i.e., 1 "monkey year" is equivalent to about 4 "human years"). Second, the effects of deprivation seem to be the "mirror image" of the developmental sequence. Thus, as noted earlier, different visual functions (and presumably their underlying anatomic and physiologic structures) develop at different rates. Those which develop earliest seem most robust to the influences of pattern deprivation, while those which develop last are most at risk and remain susceptible for the longest time.

Vaegan and Taylor (1980) attempted to define the upper limit of the period of susceptibility in humans with unilateral traumatic cataracts, with the age of onset known precisely. Figure 2.11 shows the visual acuity of each subject immediately following cataract surgery and careful optical correction. Note that deprivation in the first 3 years of life left only rudimentary vision. Patients with later onset of the cataract suffered less visual loss, and patients deprived after 10 years of age suffered no loss. One of the most interesting aspects of Vaegan and Taylor's study is that many of the patients showed substantial improvements in vision after proper optical correction and orthoptic treatment.

While the upper limit for susceptibility of excitatory binocular interactions is not yet certain, it appears to be later than that for acuity or contrast sensitivity in monkeys and may extend to at least 7 or 8 years (and possibly more) in humans. Psychophysical studies of interocular transfer in humans with a history of strabismus (Banks et al. 1975, Hohmann and Creutzfeldt 1975) provide an indirect estimate of the period of susceptibility of binocular connections. The results of both studies suggest that binocular connections are highly vulnerable during the first 18 months of life and remain susceptible to the effects of strabismus until at least age 7 years. While the period of susceptibility to strabismus or anisometropia in primates has received less attention, clinical wisdom suggests that it extends over a similar period.

The Natural History of Amblyopia Development

The stars in Figure 2.5 show the resolution of neurons (X cells) in the LGN of monkeys receiving input from an eye that was deprived of normal visual input from birth. Comparison of these results with those from normal monkeys (filled circles) suggests little effect of monocular occlusion on the development of spatial resolution in the LGN. While the effects of deprivation on the retina and

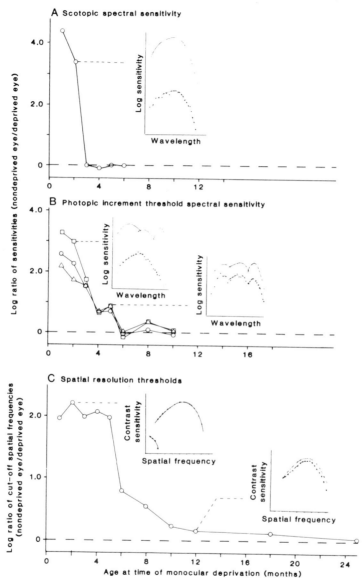

Figure 2.10   *Interocular sensitivity ratios are plotted as a function of age of the monkey at the time that monocular form deprivation was initiated. Each panel shows a different psychophysical task. (A) Dark-adapted spectral sensitivity. The test stimulus had a wavelength of 500 nm. The inset shows the complete scotopic spectral sensitivity curve for the animal deprived at age 2 months. (B) Photopic increment threshold spectral sensitivity obtained with a 3000-Td background. Data are shown for stimulus wavelengths of 440, 520, and 600 nm. The insets are the entire functions for animals deprived at 2 and 5 months of age. (C) Cutoff spatial frequency. The insets represent the CSF for animals deprived at 2 and 12 months. (From Harwerth et al. 1987.)*

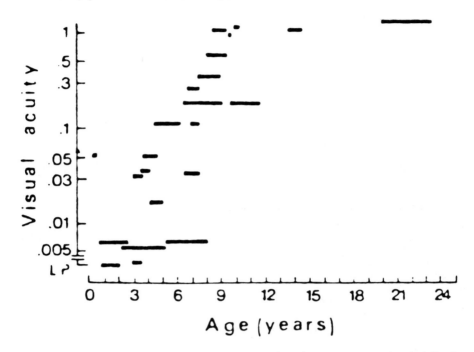

Figure 2.11 *Visual acuity of 23 humans with unilateral cataracts immediately following restoration of normal visual input on removal of the crystalline lens. Each subject is represented by a horizontal bar, whose length spans the period of monocular deprivation and whose position with respect to the ordinate defines first visual acuity score measured with careful optical correction following surgical removal of the lens. Ordinate shows decimal acuity score, where 1.0 represents 20/20 and 0.1 represents 20/200. LP indicates light perception only. (Adapted from Vaegan and Taylor 1980, by Mitchell and Timney 1984.)*

LGN remain controversial (Mitchell and Timney 1984, Boothe et al. 1985), this picture is consistent with the notion that the primary effects of abnormal visual experience early in life are cortical.

Several lines of evidence suggest that the period of susceptibility to deprivation in primates does not begin at birth, and this has raised interesting debates regarding when treatment should begin. For example, in monocularly deprived kittens, Hubel and Wiesel (1970) reported that the period of susceptibility began abruptly at about 4 weeks of age. In humans, neither congenital cataract nor congenital esotropia produce a loss of acuity prior to 2 months of age (Taylor et al. 1979, Maurer et al. 1983, Mohindra et al. 1979). This can be clearly seen in Figure 2.12. Thus it appears that the onset of amblyopia may not begin before the normal development of binocular interaction in striate cortex (Held 1984). Moreover, there is frequently a period of uninterrupted continued parallel acuity development in the two eyes following the onset of experimental strabismus. This also can be seen in the development of resolution in monkeys with experimental strabismus (Kiorpes et al. 1989), providing some support for the notion that the development of amblyopia involves binocular competition and suppression (von Noorden 1977).

One interesting and important question that remains unanswered is why some strabismics develop amblyopia while others do not (strabismic amblyopia is reported to occur in between 35 and 50% of children with strabismus). Several factors appear to be important in determining the development of strabismic amblyopia. These include the type of strabismus (more frequent in constant esotropia), the presence of high refractive error or a refractive imbalance, and age of onset (amblyopia is more likely to develop in early-onset strabismus than in the later-onset type). The difficulty is to determine the relative weighing of each of these factors and the possibility of other factors that have not yet been determined. Kiorpes et al. (1989) found that in monkeys with experimental strabismus, those with the earliest onset were most likely to develop amblyopia. Another factor that has received little attention but which seems important is the degree to which the amblyogenic factor results in neural deprivation. Consider, for example, anisometropia. If one eye has a high uncorrected hyperopic refractive error, the retinal image will be blurred, thus reducing high spatial

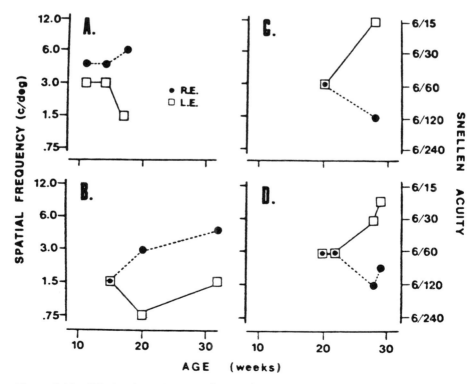

Figure 2.12   *FPL visual acuities (in cycles per degree) of four esotropic infants with onset of strabismus shortly after birth. (From Jacobson et al. 1981.)*

frequencies in the retinal image. This blur will not influence neural processing until it exceeds the "neural" blurring of the image by the developing visual nervous system. It is only at this stage that monocular defocus is likely to result in a binocular neural imbalance. Although little is known about the development of anisometropia, it seems at least plausible that anisometropic amblyopia may have its onset considerably later than amblyopia associated with, for example, congenital cataracts or strabismus. The mildest form of amblyopia, known as *meridional amblyopia* (see Chapter 1), is associated with high degrees of astigmatism early in life. Data from human infants suggest that it does not develop in the first year of life and perhaps not until age 3 (Mohindra et al. 1979, Teller et al. 1978).

INTERVENTION

A critical question for the practitioner is, "Is there a critical period for the effect of intervention or treatment of amblyopia?" Much of the evidence regarding the efficacy of treatment, the effects of age on prognosis, and the many factors that interact with amblyopia to influence the outcome of intervention or treatment is covered in detail in Chapter 10. It is clear from a review of this chapter that the end of the period of susceptibility for amblyopia *does not* mark the end of the period during which treatment may result in improved visual function. Rather, for many cases of functional amblyopia, some degree of residual plasticity remains present well into adulthood (Ciuffreda 1986).

REFERENCES

Atkinson J. (1979) Development of optokinetic nystagmus in the human infant and monkey infant. In RD Freeman (Ed.), *Developmental Neurobiology of Vision*, pp. 277–87. New York: Plenum Press.

Atkinson J, Braddick O, French J. (1980) Infant astigmatism: its disappearance with age. *Vision Res.* 20:891–93.

Awaya S, Sugawara M, Miyake S, Isomura Y. (1980) Form vision deprivation amblyopia and the results of its treatment—with special reference to the critical period. *Jpn. J. Ophthalmol.* 24:241–250.

Banks MS. (1980) The development of visual accommodation during early infancy. *Child Dev.* 51:646–66.

Banks MS, Aslin RN, Letson RD. (1975) Sensitive period for the development of human binocular vision. *Science* 190:675–7.

Banks MS, Salapatek P. (1983) Infant Visual Perception. In Haith M, Campos J (Eds.), *Biology and Infancy Handbook of Child Psychology*. New York: Wiley.

Banks MS, Stephens BR. (1982) The contrast sensitivity of human infants to gratings differing in duty cycle. *Vision Res.* 22:739–44.

Birch EE, Shimojo S, Held R. (1983) The development of aversion to rivalrous stimuli in human infants. *Invest. Ophthalmol. Vis. Sci.* 24(Suppl.):92.

Blakemore C, Vital-Durand F. (1979) Development of the neural basis of visual acuity in monkeys: Speculations on the origin of deprivation amblyopia. *Trans. Ophthalmol. Soc. U.K.* 99:363–8.

Boothe RG, Dobson V, Teller DY. (1985) Postnatal development of vision in human and nonhuman primates. *Ann. Rev. Neurosci.* 8:495–545.

Braddick O, Atkinson J, Julesz B, Kropfl W, Bodis-Wolner I, Raab E. (1980) Cortical binocularity in infants. *Nature* 288:363–5.

Ciuffreda KJ. (1986) Visual System Plasticity in Human Amblyopia. In SR Hilfer, JB Sheffield (Eds.), *Cell and Developmental Biology of the Eye: Development of Order in the Visual System*, pp. 211–44. New York: Springer-Verlag.

De Vries-Khoe L, Spekreijse H. (1982) Maturation of luminance and pattern EPs in man. *Doc. Ophthalmol.* 31:461–75.

Dobson V, Fulton AB, Sebris SL. (1984) Cycloplegic refractions of infants and young children: The axis of astigmatism. *Invest. Ophthalmol. Vis. Sci.* 25:83–7.

Dobson V, Teller DY. (1978) Visual acuity in human infants: A review and comparison of behavioral and electrophysiological studies. *Vision Res.* 18:1469–83.

Fiorentini A, Pirchio M, Spinelli D. (1983) Electrophysiological evidence for spatial frequency selective mechanisms in adults and infants. *Vision Res.* 22:739–44.

Fox R, Aslin RN, Shea SL, Dumais ST. (1980) Stereopsis in human infants. *Science* 207:323–4.

Garey LJ, de Courten C. (1983) Structural development of the lateral geniculate nucleus and visual cortex in monkey and man. *Behav. Brain Res.* 10:3–13.

Gwiazda J, Scheiman M, Mohindra I, Held R. (1984) Astigmatism in children: Changes in axis and amount from birth to six years. *Invest. Ophthalmol. Vis. Sci.* 25:88–92.

Hamer RD, Schneck ME. (1984) Spatial summation in dark-adapted human infants. *Vision Res.* 24:77–85.

Harwerth RS, Smith EL III, Duncan GC, Crawford MLJ, von Noorden GK. (1987) Multiple sensitive periods in the development of the primate visual system. *Science* 232:235–8.

Haynes H, White BL, Held R. (1965) Visual accommodation in human infants. *Science* 148:528–30.

Held R. (1984) Binocular Vision: Behavioral and Neuronal Development. In Mehler J, Fox R (Eds.), *Neonate Cognition: Beyond the Blooming, Buzzing Confusion.* Hillsdale, N.J.: Erlbaum Press.

Hickey TL. (1977) Postnatal development of the human lateral geniculate nucleus: Relationship to a critical period for the visual system. *Science* 198:836–8.

Hitchcock PF, Hickey TL. (1980) Prenatal development of the human lateral geniculate nucleus. *J. Comp. Neurol.* 194:395–411.

Hohmann A, Creutzfeldt OD. (1975) Squint and the development of binocularity in humans. *Nature* 254:613–14.

Howland HC. (1982) Infant eyes: Optics and accommodation. *Curr. Eye Res.* 2:217–24.

Howland HC, Sayles N. (1984) Photorefractive measurements of astigmatism in infants and young children. *Invest. Ophthalmol. Vis. Sci.* 25:93–102.

Hubel DH, Wiesel TN. (1970) The period of susceptibility to the physiological effects of unilateral eye closure in kittens. *J. Physiol.* (London) 206:419–36.

Huttenlocher PR, de Courten C. (1987) The development of synapses in striate cortex of man. *Hum. Neurobiol.* 6:1–9.

Huttenlocher PR, de Courten C, Garey LJ, van der Loos H. (1982) Synaptogenesis in human visual cortex: Evidence for synapse elimination during normal development. *Neurosci. Lett.* 33:247–52.

Jacobson SG, Mohindra I, Held R. (1981) Age of onset of amblyopia in infants with esotropia. *Doc. Ophthalmol.* 30:210–16.

James W. (1890) *The Principles of Psychology.* New York: Holt.

Kiorpes L, Boothe RG, Carlson MR. (1984) Acuity development in surgically strabismic monkeys. *Invest. Ophthalmol. Vis. Sci.* 25(Suppl.):216.

Kiorpes L, Carlson MR, Alfi D, Boothe RG. (1989) Development of visual acuity in experimentally strabismic monkeys. *Clin. Vis. Sci.* 4:95–106.

Leuba G, Garey LJ. (1987) Evolution of neuronal numerical density in the developing and aging human visual cortex. *Hum. Neurobiol.* 6:10–18.

LeVay S, Wiesel TN, Hubel DH. (1980) The development of ocular dominance columns in normal and visually deprived monkeys. *J. Comp. Neurol.* 191:1–51.

Manny RE, Klein SA. (1984) The development of vernier acuity in infants. *Curr. Eye Res.* 3:453–62.

Manny RE, Klein SA. (1985) A three-alternative tracking paradigm to measure vernier acuity of older infants. *Vision Res.* 25:1245–52.

Maurer D, Lewis TL, Tytla ME. (1983) Contrast sensitivity in cases of unilateral congenital cataract. *Invest. Ophthalmol. Vis. Sci.* 24(Suppl.):21.

Maurer D, Maurer C. (1988) *The World of the Newborn.* New York: Basic Books.

Mayer DL, Dobson DC. (1982) Visual acuity development in infants and young children as assessed by preferential looking. *Vision Res.* 22:1141–1151.

Mitchell DE, Timney B. (1984) Postnatal Development of Function in the Mamallian Visual System. In Darian-Smith I (Ed.), *American Physiological Society Handbook of Physiology*, Section 1: *The Nervous System*, Vol. 3: *Sensory Processes*, Part 1. Bethesda, MD: American Physiological Association.

Mohindra I, Held R, Gwiazda J, Brill S. (1978) Astigmatism in human infants. *Science* 202:329–31.

Mohindra I, Jacobson SG, Thomas J, Held R. (1979) Development of amblyopia in infants. *Trans. Ophthalmol. Soc. U.K.* 99:344–6.

Morrone C, Burr DC. (1986) Evidence for the existence and development of visual inhibition in humans. *Nature* 321:235–7.

Moskowitz A, Sokol S. (1983) Developmental changes in the human visual system as reflected by the latency of the pattern reversal VEP. *Electroencephalogr. Clin. Neurophysiol.* 56:1–15.

Movshon JA, Eggers HM, Gizzi MS, Hendrickson AE, Kiorpes L, Boothe RG. (1987) Effects of early unilateral blur on the macaque's visual system. III. Physiological observations. *J. Neurosci.* 7:1340-51.

Movshon JA, Van Sluyters RC. (1981) Visual neural development. *Ann. Rev. Psychol.* 32:477–522.

Norcia AM, Tyler CW. (1985) Spatial frequency sweep VEP: Visual acuity during the first year of life. *Vision Res.* 25:1399–1408.

Norcia AM, Tyler CW, Hamer RD. (1988) High visual contrast sensitivity in the young human infant. *Invest. Opthalmol. Vis. Sci.* 29:44–49.

Petrig B, Julesz B, Kropfl W, Baumgartner G, Anliker M. (1983) Development of stereopsis and cortical binocularity in human infants: Electrophysiological evidence. *Science* 213:1402–5.

Powers MK, Schneck M, Teller DY. (1981) Spectral sensitivity of human infants at absolute visual threshold. *Vision Res.* 21:1005-16.

Rakic P. (1976) Prenatal genesis of connections subserving ocular dominance in the rhesus monkey. *Nature* 261:467-71.

Regal DM. (1981) Development of critical flicker frequency in human infants. *Vision Res.* 21:549-556.

Regan D, Spekreijse H. (1986) Evoked potentials in vision research 1961-1986. *Vision Res.* 26:1461-80.

Shimojo S, Birch EE, Gwiazda J, Held R. (1984) Development of vernier acuity in infants. *Vision Res.* 24:721-4.

Shimojo S, Held R. (1987) Vernier acuity is less than grating acuity in 2- and 3-month-olds. *Vision Res.* 27:77-86.

Taylor DM, Vaegan, Morris JA, Rogers JE, Warland J. (1979) Amblyopia in bilateral infantile and juvenile cataract. *Trans. Ophthalmol. Soc. U.K.* 99:170-5.

Teller DY, Bornstein MH. (1986) Infant Color Vision and Color Perception. In P Salapatek and LB Cohen (Eds.), *Handbook of Infant Perception.* New York: Academic Press.

Teller DY, Allen JL, Regal DM, Mayer DL. (1978) Astigmatism and acuity in two primate infants. *Invest. Ophthalmol. Vis. Sci.* 17:344-49.

Teller DY, Movshon JA. (1986) Visual development. *Vision Res.* 26:1483-1506.

Vaegan, Taylor D. (1980) Critical periods for deprivation amblyopia in children. *Trans. Ophthalmol. Soc. U.K.* 99:432-39.

von Noorden GK. (1977) Mechanisms of amblyopia. *Adv. Ophthalmol.* 34:92-115.

von Noorden GK. (1980) *Burian and von Noorden's Binocular Vision and Ocular Motility: Theory and Management of Strabismus.* St. Louis: Mosby.

von Noorden GK. (1981) New clinical aspects of stimulus deprivation amblyopia. *Am. J. Ophthalmol.* 92:416-21.

von Noorden GK, Crawford MLJ, Levacy RA. (1983) The lateral geniculate nucleus in human anisometropic amblyopia. *Invest. Ophthalmol. Vis. Sci.* 24:788-9.

Werner JS. (1982) Development of scotopic sensitivity and the absorption spectrum of the human ocular media. *J. Opt. Soc. Am.* 72:247-58.

Wiesel TN. (1982) Postnatal development of the visual cortex and the influence of environment. *Nature* 299:583-91.

Wiesel TN, Hubel DH. (1963) Single-cell responses in striate cortex of kittens deprived of vision in one eye. *J. Neurophysiol.* 26:1003-17.

Williams R, Boothe R. (1981) Development of optical quality in the infant monkey (*Macaca nemestrina*) eye. *Invest. Ophthalmol. Vis. Sci.* 21:728-36.

Wilson HR. (1988) Development of spatiotemporal mechanisms in the human infant. *Vision Res.* 28:611-628.

Worth CA. (1903) *Squint: Its Causes, Pathology and Treatment.* Philadelphia: Blakiston.

Youdelis C, Hendricksen A. (1986) A qualitative and quantitative analysis of the human fovea during development. *Vision Res.* 26:847-55.

Chapter 3

Sensory Processing in Strabismic and Anisometropic Amblyopia

If we believed that we must try to find out what is not known, we should be better and braver and less idle than if we believed that what we do not know is impossible to find out and that we need not even try.

Socrates, "The Meno"

In clinical practice, the defining characteristic of amblyopia is reduced visual acuity in an otherwise healthy and properly corrected eye; however, in psychophysical studies, amblyopes demonstrate many, various, and often curious visual losses. The thrust of this chapter will be an attempt to define, describe, and explain the performance properties of the amblyopic visual system. To accomplish this, the overview presented here will be necessarily overly simplified.

An attempt will be made throughout this chapter to compare and, where possible, contrast the performance of strabismic and anisometropic amblyopes (other categories of amblyopes, e.g., stimulus deprivation, were considered in Chapter 1). This is easier said than done, since many studies have not paid attention to distinctions that may exist between amblyopias associated with different presumptive etiologies. Moreover, even studies that have attempted to make distinctions are confronted with two potential sources of ambiguity: (1) difficulty in clinical diagnosis (e.g., failure to discover microstrabismus in a patient with anisometropia); and (2) perhaps more critical, the difficulty in ascertaining an accurate and complete history of the amblyopia and its associated conditions. Despite these difficulties, there is now strong evidence that strabismic and anisometropic amblyopia represent two distinct syndromes with considerable overlap in their performance along several dimensions. Finally, we will consider the optical, oculomotor, and neural factors that may limit visual performance in normal vision and, in Chapter 4, the developmental alterations that may occur in the amblyopic visual system.

1. BASIC PROCESSES: LIGHT AND COLOR

1A. The "Light Sense"

The earliest psychophysical studies of amblyopia were concerned with the integrity of basic processes in the amblyopic visual system. Specifically, early workers were interested in learning about the status of rod and cone mechanisms in the amblyopic eye. More than a century ago, Bjerrum (1884) noted that there was essentially no difference in the "light sense" between the amblyopic and nonamblyopic eye. In their classic study, Wald and Burian (1944) measured dark adaptation and spectral sensitivity curves in a group of amblyopes. Their results showed essentially identical dark adaptation curves in the two eyes (Figure 3.1) and normal scotopic and photopic spectral sensitivity—both centrally and peripherally. These findings have been widely accepted, and while several investigators have noted slightly elevated cone thresholds in amblyopic eyes (e.g., Oppel and Kranke 1958), these losses were found in only some observers and were small in magnitude. The conclusion drawn by Wald and Burian, and now widely accepted, was that the basic retinal sensory mechanisms (rods, cones, and photopigments) are intact and normal in the amblyopic visual system. Wald and Burian argued further that amblyopia represents a dissociation between the "light sense" and the "form sense."

Other aspects of the light sense also appear to be normal or nearly normal in amblyopic eyes. For example, glare recovery is essentially normal in amblyopic eyes (Maraini and Cordella 1961). In addition, suprathreshold brightness perception as determined from interocular matching experiments is normal or nearly normal in amblyopic eyes (Levi and Harwerth 1974). It should be noted that some amblyopes report small differences in perceived brightness between

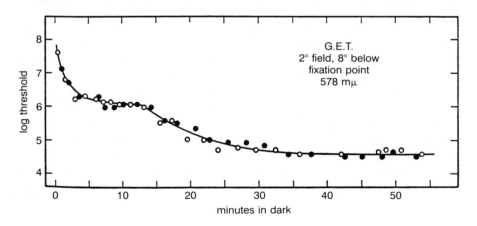

Figure 3.1 *Dark adaptation curves of the preferred* (open circles) *and amblyopic* (filled circles) *eye of a strabismic amblyope. Note the similarity between the two eyes. (From Wald and Burian 1944.)*

Normal D.A.C. in amblyopic eyes

the two eyes. In some cases, the amblyopic eye's image is slightly dimmed, as if the target were viewed through a filter. This "sunglass" effect may be more common in anisometropic amblyopes; however, it does not appear to be a general phenomenon, and these differences in perceived brightness between the two eyes are small when compared with the visual acuity differences. Moreover, some amblyopes actually show the opposite effect, that is, higher perceived brightness with the amblyopic eye. Interestingly, some amblyopes also show paradoxical suprathreshold contrast perception, with the amblyopic eye judging suprathreshold stimuli to be of higher contrast than the preferred eye (see section on suprathreshold contrast perception).

1B. Luminance Increment Thresholds

Both strabismic and anisometropic amblyopes show elevated luminance increment thresholds for small targets (Miller 1955, Grosvenor 1957) and increased spatial summation (Flynn 1967). The increment threshold task requires the observer to detect a target (e.g., a bar, slit, or spot) that is superimposed on a homogeneous background. Thus the task is actually one of contrast discrimination. While Miller, Grosvenor, and Flynn all interpreted their results in terms of altered retinal receptive field characteristics (i.e., increased receptive field size or reduced lateral inhibition), this explanation does not seem tenable in light of more recent studies. A more plausible alternative explanation will be discussed in the section on spatial frequency channels. This explanation does not depend on alterations in either the size or the shape of retinal receptive fields, but rather is based on the spatial frequency–specific loss of contrast sensitivity of the amblyopic eye.

1C. Stiles-Crawford Effect

Enoch (1957, 1967) was the first to suggest that the amblyopia could be a consequence of a specific retinal receptor abnormality (i.e., "receptor amblyopia"). Enoch's suggestion came from his studies of the Stiles-Crawford effect no. 1 in amblyopic eyes. His results showed that amblyopes may have slightly distorted Stiles-Crawford functions. Enoch hypothesized that tilting or malorientation of the retinal receptors could lead to both the abnormal Stiles-Crawford functions and the reduced central visual acuity characteristic of amblyopes. This conclusion has been questioned on a number of grounds. First, a marked malorientation of the receptors would produce only a minor reduction in acuity (Campbell and Gregory 1960). Second, undetected eccentric fixation in an amblyopic eye could mimic malorientation of the retinal receptors (Marshall and Flom 1970). More recently, Bedell (1980), working in Enoch's laboratory, has reconsidered the question of photoreceptor misalignment in amblyopic eyes. His results clearly demonstrated that the reduced vision of amblyopes cannot be attributed to disturbances in the physical or optical properties, nor in the malorientation of the retinal receptors. Bedell noted that all the amblyopic eye peaks were clustered within a subregion of the pupil, as occurs in normal eyes.

1D. Color Vision

Figure 3.2, from Harwerth and Levi (1978), illustrates the photopic luminosity curves for each eye of two amblyopes—one with anisometropia and the other with both strabismus and anisometropia. These data, obtained using flicker photometry, corroborate the earlier report of Wald and Burian (1944) that photopic (as well as scotopic) spectral sensitivity are essentially normal in the amblyopic eye. While the cone color mechanisms have not been studied in detail psychophysically in the amblyopic visual system, it is likely that they are normal. Thus Oppel (1960) and Francois and Verriest (1967) have found that the color vision of amblyopes is normal except for a few very severe cases of strabismic amblyopia (visual acuity worse than 20/200). These deficits are similar to those found in normal peripheral vision, as are many other aspects of visual performance in strabismic amblyopes.

1E. Increment Threshold Spectral Sensitivity

Amblyopes do, however, demonstrate anomalies in their increment threshold spectral sensitivity functions (Harwerth and Levi 1977). Increment threshold spectral sensitivity is measured by superimposing the test spot on a bright uniform white background, so the observer's task is to distinguish the test spot from the background. Figure 3.3 shows the increment threshold spectral sensitivity functions of the same two amblyopes as shown in Figure 3.2. These increment threshold curves are obtained by superimposing a small monochromatic test spot on a bright background. In normal (and nonamblyopic eyes of amblyopes), the increment threshold spectral sensitivity curve characteristically has three peaks. The peak in the blue region of the spectrum is thought to reflect the sensitivity of the blue cone mechanisms. However, the red and green peaks are too narrow to represent cone mechanisms and thus are thought to reflect opponent processing (Sperling and Harwerth 1971). Specifically, the dip between the red and green peaks is thought to reflect a subtractive neural interaction between red and blue cone mechanisms. While the photopic luminosity function is determined by the sensitivity of the *luminance* channels, the increment threshold spectral sensitivity function reflects processing by the *chromatic* channels. While the luminance channels respond to large stimuli that are rapidly changing in time (i.e., flickering), the chromatic channels respond more strongly to smaller stimuli that change slowly. The increment threshold results suggest that

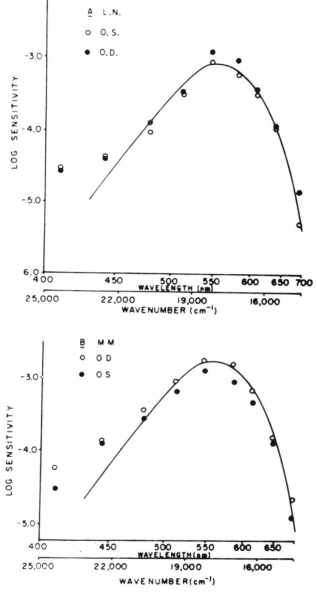

Figure 3.2 *Photopic luminosity curves for each eye of two amblyopes—one with an-isometropia (above) and the other with both strabismus and anisometropia (below). Open circles are the data of the preferred eyes, filled circles are those of the amblyopic eyes. These data were obtained using flicker photometry, and the solid lines are the CIE photopic-luminosity curve for the standard observer. (From Harwerth and Levi 1978.)*

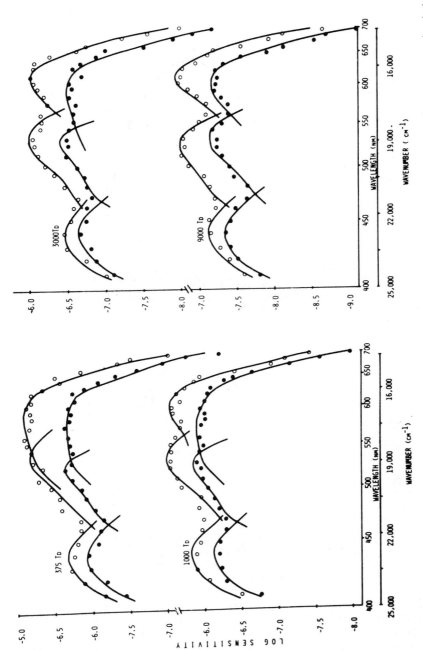

Figure 3.3   *Increment threshold spectral sensitivity functions of the same two amblyopes as shown in Figure 3.2. These increment threshold curves are obtained by superimposing a small monochromatic test spot on a white background (at the four levels indicated in the figure). Open and filled circles represent the data of the preferred and amblyopic eyes respectively. (From Harwerth and Levi 1977.)*

the chromatic channels are affected in the amblyopic visual system. For the amblyopic eyes, the increment thresholds were elevated for all wavelengths. Additionally, the dip between the red and green peaks (around 530 nm) was less pronounced in the amblyopic eye. Harwerth and Levi interpreted these results as showing an overall reduction in incremental sensitivity similar to that found for white light by Miller (1955) and Grosvenor (1957), that is, reduced contrast sensitivity. Moreover, they interpreted the reduced dip at 530 nm as evidence for abnormal neural interactions between red and green cone mechanisms.

However, it is important to point out that this finding does not necessarily imply a retinal anomaly. Even if chromatic processing occurs in the retina in normal vision, normal retinal signals could be degraded by the cortex in amblyopic vision. Recent studies suggest an alternative explanation for the increment threshold data of amblyopes. Rather than an alteration in the retinal receptive field properties, it is likely that when presented with a broadband spatial stimulus, the amblyopic visual system uses the most sensitive cortical receptive field. Because of the altered contrast sensitivity function (to be discussed later), this receptive field is larger than that used by the preferred eye for the same stimulus (see section on multiple spatial frequency channels) and thus presents a different profile. Therefore it is not necessary to postulate alterations in retinal (or cortical) receptive field shape or size to account for the extant increment threshold data. Recent experiments using sinusoidal gratings (Bradley et al. 1986) show that the contrast sensitivity of the amblyopic eye is similarly reduced for chromatic and achromatic sine wave gratings, suggesting that the reduction in increment threshold spectral sensitivity in the amblyopic eye can be understood in terms of its reduced spatial contrast sensitivity.

1F. Clinical Tests of Color Vision

In clinical practice, testing the color vision of each eye of amblyopes is routinely used to distinguish amblyopes from patients with retinal anomalies. Use of the Farnsworth-Maunsell 100-hue test or the D-15, which are sensitive to blue-yellow defects, is recommended to distinguish between amblyopia and acquired maculopathies. For a detailed discussion of clinical testing of color vision, see Pokorny et al. (1979).

Summary

The results of the psychophysical studies (reviewed earlier) and of electrophysiologic experiments (reviewed later) suggest, first, that the basic retinal receptor processes (rods and cones) of the amblyopic eye are essentially normal. In fact, there is little hard evidence for any primary retinal abnormality in the amblyopic eye. Second, Wald and Burian concluded in 1944 that amblyopia is an anomaly of the "form sense" rather than the "light sense." However, as was pointed out by Hecht and Mintz (1939), this distinction is specious. Rather, as will be seen later in this chapter, it may be more appropriate to describe the threshold abnormalities of strabismic and anisometropic amblyopes in terms of reduced contrast sensitivity for high spatial frequencies (i.e., fine detail). In the next section, this conclusion will be sharpened. Thus we will argue that amblyopia may be regarded as a developmental anomaly involving primarily those cortical mechanisms involved in form and shape perception.

2.   SPATIAL VISION IN AMBLYOPIA

2A. Visual Acuity

Since reduced visual acuity is the defining feature of amblyopia, it seems reasonable to begin with a brief discussion of factors that may limit normal visual acuity (for a more detailed theoretical treatment of visual acuity see Westheimer 1981a; see also Chapter 8 for a detailed clinical treatment) and then a description of visual acuity in amblyopic vision.

Visual acuity refers to a limit of spatial discrimination and is therefore specified by varying the spatial dimensions of the stimulus. In clinical practice, the size of Snellen letters is varied and the limit is expressed in terms of a Snellen fraction (e.g., 6/6 or 20/20) or the corresponding minimum angle of resolution (MAR) in minutes of arc. However, there are several accepted criteria for visual acuity (Westheimer 1981a):

1. Detection of a feature (i.e., minimum visible acuity)
2. Resolution of two features (e.g., minimum resolvable)
3. Identification of features in a target (or their orientation, i.e., minimum recognizable visual acuity)
4. Relative localization of features (i.e., the spatial minimum discriminable)

Minimum Visible Acuity

Minimum visual acuity refers to the smallest test object that can just be detected. Since the optics of the eye spread the image of a point or thin line over about a minute (i.e., the half width of the line-spread function), detection of a small, bright object on a dark background is based primarily on quantal absorption and may thus be considered a luminance threshold rather than a spatial discrimination. In amblyopic eyes, the absolute detection threshold is essentially normal (see section on the "light sense").

Detection of a thin line on a uniform background can be measured by varying the width of the line. Hecht and Mintz (1939) found that under ideal conditions, a dark line with a width of just 0.5 second of arc could be detected. Of course, on the retina, this thin line has a width of at least 1 minute, and increasing its width (up to about 1 minute) is equivalent to increasing its contrast. Thus the minimum visible acuity for a thin line on a uniform background represents a measure of local contrast sensitivity, and in their definitive study, Hecht and Mintz demonstrated that the minimum visible threshold could be fully accounted for on this basis. As will be discussed later, many studies have shown abnormal contrast sensitivity for grating patterns in the amblyopic eye (see section on contrast sensitivity). Recently, Klein and Levi (1986) have suggested that a local measure of contrast sensitivity based on detecting thin lines may be highly sensitive to the amblyopic deficit and to other visual abnormalities.

Minimum Resolvable Acuity

Minimum resolvable acuity refers to the smallest angular separation between neighboring targets (e.g., lines, dots, or the stripes of a grating) that can be resolved (i.e., appear separate). Under optimal conditions, this separation is on the order of 1 minute of arc (i.e., the distance between adjacent peaks or troughs of a sine-wave grating with a spatial frequency of 60 cycles per degree). This value is just what might be expected given the eyes' optics and the spacing of foveal cones (approximately 0.5 minute). In amblyopia, the minimum resolvable acuity is reduced; however, as will be seen in the section on contrast sensitivity, the minimum resolvable acuity of strabismic amblyopes often underestimates their functional losses. In particular, the grating resolution of strabismic amblyopes may be much less affected than their Snellen (minimum recognizable) acuity or their relative localization acuity. In the section on periphery as a model for amblyopia, it will be seen that the normal periphery also shows a decoupling of resolution and localization acuities.

Minimum Recognizable Acuity

Minimum recognizable acuity refers to the capacity to identify a form or its orientation. This type of acuity is generally associated with Snellen letters, Landolt C's, or illiterate E's and represents the standard clinical method. Normal Snellen acuity values of 20/10 to 20/20 (0.5 to 1 minute) refer to the size of the "critical detail" (e.g., the threshold size of the gap in a Landolt C or the threshold separation between the limbs of an E). These values are quite similar to those obtained in simple resolution tasks in normal foveal vision, and therefore, minimum recognizable acuity is often modeled as a resolution task. However, minimum recognizable acuity differs in several ways from simple resolution. First, it is very highly localized (a 20/20 letter subtends 5 minutes of arc at the posterior nodal point of the eye). Second, it is subject to localized interactions from nearby stimuli ("crowding"). Third, in normal peripheral vision, in patients with maculopathy, and in strabismic amblyopes, it is degraded to a greater extent than resolution (Loshin and White 1984). Thus, while the factors that limit resolution acuity and Snellen acuity may be the same in normal foveal vision (e.g., the optics of the eyes, the size and spacing of foveal cones, the density of the retinal ganglion cells, and the pooling of neural signals at various levels of the visual pathway), these two forms of acuity are differentially sensitive to physiologic or pathologic degradation.

With respect to amblyopia, the distribution of Snellen acuities provides some interesting insights into the differential effects of anisometropia and strabismus. Figure 3.4 shows in histogram form the distribution of Snellen acuities of 68 amblyopes taken from several laboratories. For the anisometropic amblyopes, the most frequent acuities fall between 2 and 4 minutes (20/40 and 20/80), with hardly any occurrence of acuity poorer than 8 minutes. Strabismic amblyopia is also most frequently associated with acuities between 20/40 and 20/80; however, strabismic amblyopes also show a preponderance of poorer Snellen acuities. Interestingly, amblyopes with both conditions also show poor acuities. For example, while 80% of strabismic amblyopes show acuities of better than 10 minutes, only 60% of those with both have acuities better than 10 minutes, suggesting that the effects of strabismus and anisometropia on Snellen acuity may be additive. Chapter 1 and various sections of this chapter will provide a detailed description of the minimum recognizable acuity deficits of amblyopic eyes.

2B. Spatial Contrast Sensitivity

Sine-Wave Gratings as Visual Stimuli

Amblyopia is generally defined by a decrease in visual acuity; however, visual acuity represents only one limit of visual capacity (i.e., the smallest high-contrast stimuli which can be detected). Most objects in everyday vision are larger than this limit, but they may have lower contrast. In fact, the ability to perceive spatial detail is determined to a great extent by one's ability to discern contrast (i.e., differences in brightness of adjacent areas). It is interesting to note that neurons in the primary visual cortex are quite indifferent to variations in luminance (e.g., Shapley 1986). Changes in adaptation level are handled by retinal gain-control mechanisms (e.g., Green 1986).

A remarkable facet of the normal visual system is that we are more sensitive to contrast for certain object sizes than for others (Campbell and Green 1965). This is in many ways analogous to the stimulus specificity of hearing. In auditory testing, the simplest sound signal is a pure sine wave that is varied in frequency (the number of cycles per second) and amplitude. The normal ear is sensitive to a range of frequencies from about 15 to 15,000 cycles per second; however, it is about 100 times more sensitive to sound at 2000 cycles per second than at either extreme. In vision, the simplest unidimensional light distribution is a grating pattern whose brightness varies sinusoidally (Figure 3.5). The contrast of the grating is specified as the modulation of its brightness about an average level,

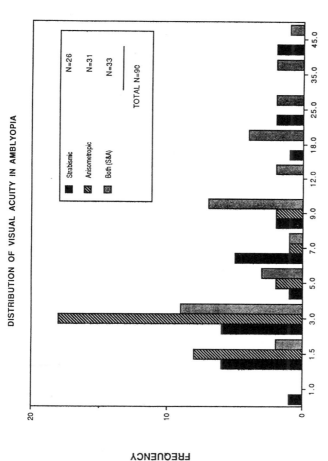

Figure 3.4 *The distribution of Snellen acuity in 90 amblyopes. For the anisometropic amblyopes, the most frequent acuities fall between 1.5 and 3 minutes (20/30 and 20/60), with hardly any occurrence of acuity poorer than 9 minutes. Strabismic amblyopia is also most frequently associated with acuities between 20/30 and 20/60; however, strabismic amblyopes also show a preponderance of poorer Snellen acuities. Interestingly, amblyopes with both conditions show even poorer acuities. (The data are from several studies in the authors' laboratories and studies by Hess and coworkers and Bedell and Flom.)*

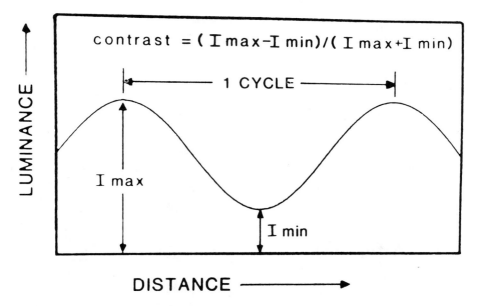

Figure 3.5   *In vision, the simplest unidimensional light distribution is a grating pattern whose brightness varies sinusoidally. The figure shows the luminance profile of the grating. The contrast of the grating is specified as the modulation of its brightness about an average level, and the grating size is specified as the number of whole light/dark cycles per degree of visual angle at the eye of the observer.*

and the grating size is specified as the number of whole light/dark cycles per degree of visual angle at the eye of the observer. This is termed the *spatial frequency* (in cycles per degree). Thus, in a grating of 30 cycles per degree, each light/dark cycle subtends 2 minutes of arc and the individual bars subtend 1 minute (i.e., 20/20 or 6/6), while the individual bars of a 3 cycles per degree grating subtend 10 minutes (equivalent to 20/200 or 6/60). By measuring contrast thresholds as a function of object size (spatial frequencies) over a wide range of sizes, it is possible to plot a *contrast sensitivity function (CSF)*.

Campbell and Green's seminal paper (1965) described the optical and neural contributions to the human foveal CSF, and over the past 20 years, sine-wave gratings have become perhaps the most widely used stimuli in visual science. There are a number of reasons for the popularity of the sine-wave grating. First, contrast sensitivity can be assessed at a fixed adaptation level. Second, the retinal stimulus waveform is known. It is also a sine wave. The optics of the eyes can, of course, degrade the contrast of the image, but they do not alter the waveform. Third, rather than relying on a single number (the acuity) to describe an individual's spatial vision, a curve (the CSF) provides a more complete description (some of the drawbacks of the sine-wave gratings will be discussed later).

$30c/0 = 20/20$

$3 c/0 = 20/200$

Abnormal contrast functions have long been implicated in the amblyopic eye. The studies of Miller (1955), Grosvenor (1957), Flynn (1967) all suggested that amblyopes have difficulty in detecting contrast variations in small stimuli. Lawwill and Burian (1966) actually measured the contrast required by each eye of amblyopes to read letters of various sizes. They found that at photopic luminance levels, amblyopic eyes needed considerably higher contrast to detect the letters than did the fellow eyes.

2C. The Contrast Sensitivity Function (CSF) in Amblyopia

The use of sine-wave gratings to measure contrast sensitivity in amblyopic eyes has a particular advantage. By using an extended stimulus, it is possible to ensure that the target is imaged on the fovea, even in amblyopes with eccentric fixation. Using this approach, it is now well established that strabismic and anisometropic amblyopia result in marked losses of threshold contrast sensitivity (Gstalder and Green 1971, Levi and Harwerth 1977, Hess and Howell 1977, Hilz et al. 1977, Thomas 1978, Bradley and Freeman 1981, Selby and Woodehouse 1981).

Figure 3.6 shows the photopic CSFs of each eye of three amblyopes—one with strabismus (*A*), one with anisometropia (*B*), and one with both strabismus and anisometropia (*C*). Note that the amblyopic eye of each amblyope shows reduced contrast sensitivity, particularly at high spatial frequencies. To characterize the reduction in contrast sensitivity of the amblyopic eye, one can construct a *visuogram*, that is, a plot showing the ratio of the contrast sensitivities of the preferred to the amblyopic eyes. A visuogram is plotted below each of the three CSFs, and these show clearly that the two eyes of each amblyope are equal or nearly equal (ratios near 1) at low spatial frequencies but show marked losses in the sensitivity of the amblyopic eye at high spatial frequencies. Figure 3.7 shows visuograms for a larger group of amblyopes. Here, the plots are arranged to show the effects of different degrees of amblyopia, with the data of the mildest amblyopes (according to their Snellen acuity) at the bottom of each column and with increasing severity toward the top. There are several general points to be made.

First, the reduced contrast sensitivity found in most amblyopic eyes is most marked at high spatial frequencies, with a smaller or no loss at low spatial frequencies. Hess and Howell (1977) argued for two categories of loss in strabismics, that is, high spatial frequency only or both high and low spatial frequencies. It now appears likely that at least two sources can contribute to the low spatial frequency losses which they and other workers observed: (1) the use of small fields (Katz et al. 1984) and (2) magnification effects associated with anisometropia (Bradley and Freeman 1981). Katz et al. (1984) found that in amblyopic observers the magnitude of the loss of contrast sensitivity at low spatial frequencies depends on the size of the stimulus field. With large fields,

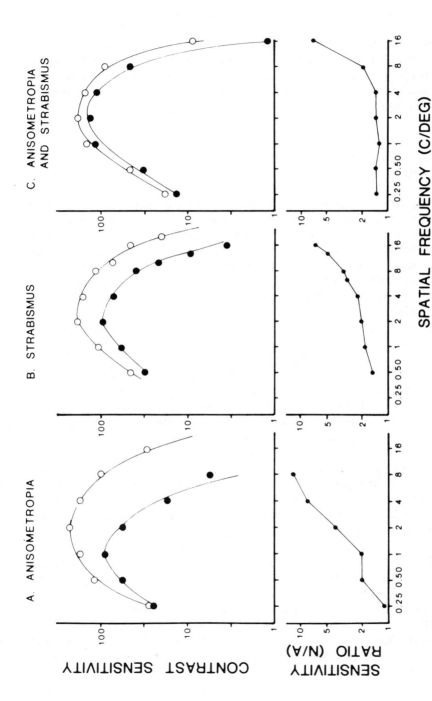

Figure 3.6 *Contrast sensitivity functions (above) and visuograms (below) for amblyopes with anisometropia (A), strabismus (B), and both (C). The data of the preferred eyes are shown by the open circles, data of the amblyopic eyes are shown by the filled circles.*

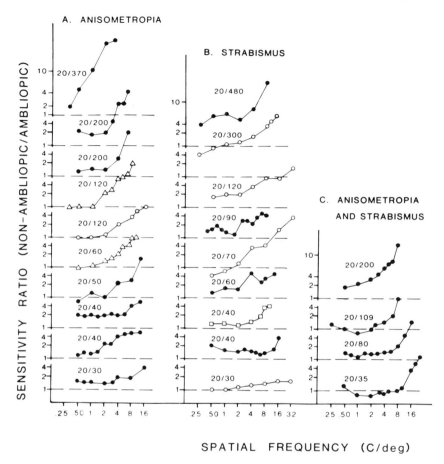

Figure 3.7 *Visuograms for 10 anisometropic, 9 strabismic, and 4 amblyopes with both strabismus and anisometropia from several laboratories. The filled circles represent data obtained by Levi and Harwerth, the open circles represent data from Hess et al. (1980), and the open triangles represent data from Selby and Woodehouse (1981).*

little or no loss was evident, while with small fields, there were substantial reductions in contrast sensitivity in the amblyopic eye at low spatial frequencies. This low spatial frequency loss with small fields may be related to edge effects, which extend over long distances in the amblyopic eye (discussed further later). In any event, the loss of contrast sensitivity is always greatest at high spatial frequencies.

Second, the loss of contrast sensitivity at high spatial frequencies increases with the severity of the amblyopia. The high spatial frequency cutoff (i.e., the highest spatial frequency that can be detected with 100% contrast) provides a measure of the resolution capacity of the eye. In normal foveal vision, the cutoff is around 40 to 50 cycles per degree (i.e., equivalent to normal Snellen acuity levels of about 20/15). In amblyopic eyes, the cutoff is also highly correlated with Snellen acuity. Correlation coefficients are often on the order of 0.9; however, high correlations do not imply perfect correspondence. Gstalder and Green (1971) first pointed out that the grating acuity of strabismic amblyopes was much better than their Snellen acuity. This finding has been confirmed by a number of investigators (Hess et al. 1978, Levi and Klein 1982a and b, Selenow et al. 1986). Figure 3.8 shows the grating acuity of 12 amblyopes plotted against their Snellen acuity. The circles represent data from the preferred eyes; the A's, S's, and B's are, respectively, the amblyopic eyes of anisometropes, strabismics, and amblyopes with both. On the log-log coordinates of this graph, a line with a slope of 1 indicates that the two acuity measures are affected in the same way by the amblyopic process. The results for the anisometropic amblyopes are consistent with a slope of 1; however, the data for the amblyopes with a constant strabismus (A's and B's) are not. In fact, for *strabismic amblyopes* (this term will be used for all amblyopes with constant strabismus), the slope of the best-fitting line is

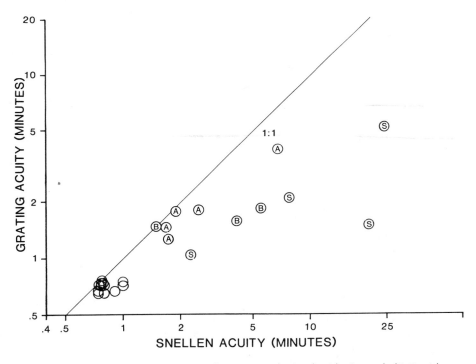

Figure 3.8 *Grating acuity versus Snellen acuity obtained with "crowded" Davidson-Eskridge charts. The circles represent the preferred eyes; circles with A's, S's, and B's represent eyes with amblyopia associated with anisometropia, strabismus, and both, respectively. (From Levi and Klein, 1982a.)*

approximately 0.5, showing that Snellen acuity is affected to a greater degree than grating acuity in strabismic amblyopes. In both cases, the correlation coefficients were high (> 0.9); however, the critical point is the slope of the line. This finding—that grating acuity underestimates the loss of Snellen acuity—highlights one of the drawbacks of the contrast sensitivity approach. Hess and colleagues (1978) reported on several strabismic amblyopes who showed abnormal Snellen acuity and almost normal contrast sensitivity. The results shown in Figure 3.8 also highlight an important difference in the behavior of strabismic and anisometropic amblyopes. The reduced Snellen acuity of anisometropes is proportional to their reduced resolution (and therefore to their contrast sensitivity).

Levi and Klein (1982b) noted that while the distribution of grating acuities was the same among strabismics and anisometropes, the strabismics had a preponderance of poor Snellen acuities. Thus they concluded that there is an extra loss (beyond simple resolution) in the visual system of strabismic amblyopes that contributes to their reduced Snellen acuity. Recently, Mayer (1986) has confirmed the finding that grating acuity underestimates Snellen acuity in young amblyopes; however, she found no difference in the slopes of the data of strabismic and anisometropic amblyopes. This discrepancy may be accounted for by the fact that Mayer used uncrowded Snellen optotypes, while Levi and Klein used charts that produced a constant, high degree of contour interaction. Detailed studies of the influence of contour interaction on the acuities of strabismic and anisometropic amblyopes are needed.

Despite the failure of the CSF to provide a complete account of the visual losses of strabismic amblyopes, it does provide a number of important insights into the functioning of the amblyopic visual system. First, the results just shown stress the spatial frequency–dependent nature of the losses that occur in amblyopia. These losses occur primarily at high spatial frequencies, and therefore, it is not surprising that studies using large stimuli (e.g., spots or slits) failed to find significant loss of function. Second, because of the steep slope of the high spatial frequency limb of the CSF, a small reduction in acuity is reflected by a large loss in contrast sensitivity. This can be seen in Figure 3.6C where the cutoff spatial frequencies of the two eyes differ by less than a factor of 2. However, there is almost a 10-fold reduction in the contrast sensitivity of the amblyopic eye at 16 cycles per degree. Thus measurements in the contrast domain (the vertical axis of the CSF) are inherently more sensitive than those in the acuity domain (the horizontal axis). Third, and perhaps most important, the reduced contrast sensitivity of the amblyopic eye does not result from optical factors (Fankhauser and Rohler 1967, Levi and Harwerth 1977, Hess and Smith 1977) or unsteady fixational eye movements (Higgins et al. 1982). Nor is it a result of eccentric fixation, since it occurs when the grating is sufficiently large to encompass the fovea. Thus the reduced CSF of the amblyopic eye represents a neural loss in foveal function. (Later we will take up questions related to whether this loss is confined to the central part of the visual field and its luminance dependence).

2D. Channels in Spatial Vision

One strong reason for the appeal of sine-wave gratings as a stimulus for studying spatial vision was the application of linear systems analysis to spatial vision. According to the Fourier theorem, any light distribution in the retinal image can be expressed as the sum of its sinusoidal components. Thus one can build up complex spatial waveforms by adding together a number of simple sinusoidal waveforms of different amplitudes, contrasts, and phases. For example, a square wave can be constructed by taking a simple sine wave and adding to it a third harmonic with one-third the amplitude and three times the frequency of the initial sine wave, plus a fifth harmonic, a seventh harmonic, and so on. Thus, according to linear systems theory, one can study how the visual system detects simple sinusoidal gratings of various spatial frequencies and attempt to understand how it might behave for more complex stimuli. It was, in fact, studies of contrast perception with simple and complex grating patterns that led Campbell and Robson (1968) to propose that the visual system possesses a number of separate neural *channels*, each tuned to detect a relatively narrow range of spatial frequencies (and orientations) and each with its own range of sensitivity to contrast.

The concept of channels specific to spatial frequency has received strong support from several lines of psychophysical investigation, such as selective adaptation, masking, and subthreshold summation studies. For reviews, see Braddick et al. (1978), Graham (1980), and Thomas (1986). These experiments have provided strong evidence for the existence of channels in human vision that are selectively tuned to spatial frequency and orientation. These channels in the human visual system may be organized in the same manner as single neurons found in the visual cortex of cats and monkeys (e.g., De Valois et al. 1982) that respond selectively to narrow bands of spatial frequencies and orientations. The notion of spatial frequency–selective mechanisms in human vision does not imply that the visual system performs Fourier analysis; rather, it suggests that there are cortical receptive fields (with a center-surround organization) of various sizes, shapes, and orientations at each point in the visual field. It is thought that the overall CSF simply reflects the upper envelope (i.e., the activity of the most sensitive) of each of the channels. This notion is illustrated schematically in Figure 3.9A.

Psychophysical studies of the response properties of channels are, by necessity, indirect, and the logic of such studies takes the following form: If stimuli A and B interact in their psychophysical effects (e.g., A makes B less visible, and A and C do not interact in this way), there must be some mechanism that is common to the processing of A and B; however, C is not processed in the same way by this mechanism. Thus the mechanism deals with only a subset of the possible stimuli along a given dimension (Braddick et al. 1978).

Could the reduced contrast sensitivity of the amblyopic eye result from either absent or abnormal spatial frequency channels? For example, the studies of Miller (1955), Grosvenor (1957), and Flynn (1967) all showed an increase in

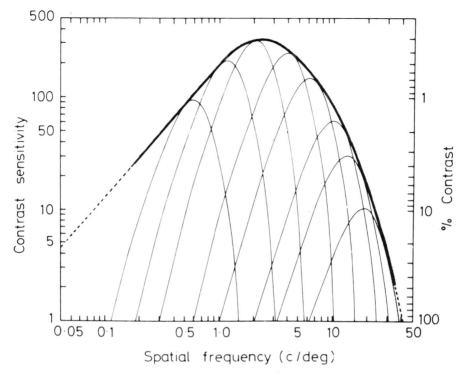

Figure 3.9(A) *Schematic representation of the contrast sensitivity function and the putative underlying filters. (From Lawden 1982.)*

spatial summation in the amblyopic eye, a finding that would be predicted from abnormal spatial frequency selectivity. Figure 3.9*B* shows the putative spatial frequency–selective mechanisms of each eye of a strabismic and anisometropic amblyope derived by masking. This figure shows the change in contrast threshold produced by masking gratings of 1, 2, 4, and 8 cycles per degree. In each case, the masking grating was 1 log unit above threshold. The ordinate is the log of the ratio of the masked to the unmasked thresholds. The open and filled symbols are the data of the preferred and amblyopic eyes, respectively. There are several points of note. First, the maximal change in contrast sensitivity coincided with each masking frequency tested. Second, each masking function is approximately one octave wide at half-height. Third, and most important, there is a striking similarity in the strength and specificity of the functions in the nonamblyopic and amblyopic eyes. These effects are most likely cortical, since similar spatial frequency–specific masking effects occur when the test grating is presented to one eye and the masking grating to the fellow eye, even in amblyopes (see section on binocular interactions). Moreover, the masking effects are orientation-specific (Levi et al. 1979). These results suggest that whereas amblyopes show reduced

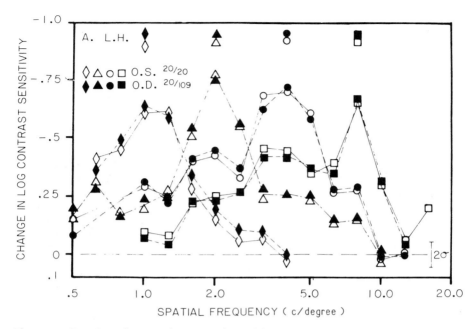

Figure 3.9(B)   *Spatial tuning functions derived from masking experiments for the preferred (open symbols) and amblyopic (filled symbols) eyes of a strabismic and anisometropic amblyope. (From Levi and Harwerth 1982.)*

contrast sensitivity, the specificity of the underlying mechanisms are similar in the two eyes (and similar to that found in normal observers). Thus the evidence from masking studies, as well as from studies of adaptation (Hess 1980; Rentschler et al. 1980), suggests that spatial frequency channels are present in the amblyopic visual system and are similar in their stimulus specificity to those found in normal vision. They differ from normal only in that they require higher contrast to be activated.

The findings just described imply that the organization of cortical receptive fields in the amblyopic visual system is normal. At first blush this appears to be at odds with earlier studies that suggested that there may be abnormal spatial summation and reduced lateral inhibition in the amblyopic eye (reviewed in the section on luminance increment thresholds). In each of these early studies, the stimuli were slits, spots, or edges (i.e., stimuli that may be considered broadband in their spatial frequency composition; a *broadband* stimulus is one that contains energy distributed over a wide spatial frequency range).

In an attempt to reconcile this apparent contradiction, Levi et al. (1981) investigated the spatial frequency response of the mechanisms used by each eye of amblyopes to detect an edge. This was done by determining the effect of adding subthreshold gratings of various spatial frequencies on the threshold for detecting an edge, that is, the method of subthreshold summation introduced by

Kulikowski and King-Smith (1973) and Shapley and Tolhurst (1973). The results of one amblyope (strabismic and anisometropic) are shown in Figure 3.10 *B*. The figure shows how gratings of different spatial frequencies facilitated detection of the edge. Open circles represent data for the nonamblyopic eye; filled circles represent the amblyopic eye. The curves for each eye show steep high- and low-frequency attenuation, and each displays a clear peak. For the preferred eye, this occurs at about 3 cycles per degree, in agreement with Shapley and Tolhurst's results in normal eyes. The curve of the amblyopic eye is similar in shape and bandwidth; however, the entire function, including the peak, is shifted to the left by about a factor of 2. Interestingly, the peak sensitivity of the "edge-detecting mechanism" for each eye coincides with the peak of the CSF for each eye (Figure 3.10*A*). This result is consistent with other evidence that edges are detected by mechanisms located at the peak of the CSF (Klein and Levi 1986). Because amblyopia reduces contrast sensitivity more for high than for low spatial frequencies, the peak contrast sensitivity of the amblyopic eye will be weighted toward lower spatial frequencies. This weighting will be reflected when the amblyopic eye views stimuli that are broadband. The linear size of these lower spatial frequency mechanisms is larger than the corresponding receptive field size used for detecting edges by the normal eye. Although the bandwidth of such mechanisms is normal in the frequency domain, the increased spatial extent of these receptive fields used in detecting broadband stimuli would account for the increased spatial summation that occurs in amblyopic eyes. The main point here is that it is not necessary to postulate alterations in the size or organization of receptive fields. Rather, each eye has a range of receptive field sizes—and uses the one with the highest contrast sensitivity to detect an edge (or any other broadband stimulus).

The loss of photopic contrast sensitivity at high spatial frequencies in central vision appears to be one of the defining characteristics of strabismic and anisometropic amblyopia and as such can be regarded as a necessary but not sufficient part of the description of the condition. The following sections will examine the extent of this loss across the visual field and its luminance dependence.

2E. Is Amblyopia Strictly a Loss of Foveal Function?

The classical view of amblyopia is that it represents an inhibition of visual acuity that is limited to the central field (Worth and Chevasse 1950) or a "loss of the physiologic superiority of the fovea" (Burian 1967). In fact, a number of studies have shown impaired foveal acuity in amblyopic eyes, with the acuity losses diminishing in peripheral vision. For example, Kirschen and Flom (1978) showed that by 10 degrees, Landolt ring acuity is similar in the two eyes. Other studies suggest that the extent of the visual acuity loss in peripheral vision is related to the degree of central loss—extending to greater eccentricities in more marked amblyopes (Levi et al. 1984). Sireteanu and Fronius (1981) reported

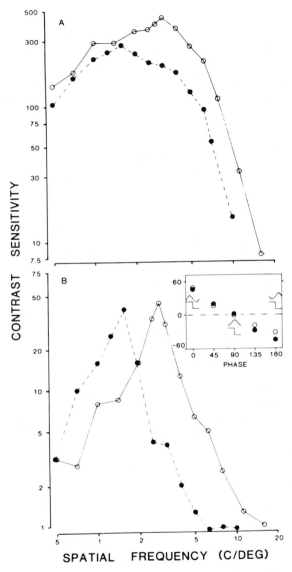

Figure 3.10 *A. Contrast sensitivity functions for each eye of a strabismic and anisome-tropic observer. Open circles represent data for the nonamblyopic eye; filled circles represent the amblyopic eye. B. This figure shows how gratings of different spatial frequencies facilitated detection of the edge. The subthreshold gratings were added to the edge in sine phase (0 degrees in the inset). Open circles represent data for the nonam-blyopic eye; filled circles represent the amblyopic eye. The curve of the amblyopic eye is similar in shape (and bandwidth); however, the entire function, including the peak, is shifted to the left by about a factor of 2. Interestingly, the peak sensitivity of the "edge-detecting mechanism" for each eye coincides with the peak of the CSF for each eye. (From Levi et al. 1981.)*

that the grating acuity deficits of strabismic amblyopes are frequently asymmetric, one hemifield being relatively spared, while those of anisometropic amblyopes are symmetrical and extend further into the peripheral field. While it has been suggested that the presence of asymmetries may depend on the specific method used to determine acuity (i.e., simple detection versus orientation discrimination; see Bedell 1982), recent studies of contrast sensitivity in the peripheral field of amblyopes suggest that these asymmetries, while common in strabismic amblyopes, depend on both the stimulus parameters and the depth of amblyopia (see below). This rather confusing state of affairs may be clarified by examining the loss in contrast sensitivity rather than acuity across the visual field.

2F. Extent of Reduced Contrast Sensitivity Across the Field

While it is clear that the visual acuity deficits of amblyopes are greatest in the central field, normal peripheral visual acuity is quite poor. There are several reasons for this. For example, in the normal periphery, there is a decrease in the density of retinal cones (Osterberg 1935, Coletta and Williams 1987) and ganglion cells (Perry and Cowey 1986), the sizes of both retinal and cortical receptive fields increase, and there is a dramatic reduction in the cortical magnification factor (i.e., the number of millimeters of cortex devoted to a degree of visual space) (Dow et al. 1981). Acuity measures reflect the limit of vision at each locus in the visual field; however, it is of theoretical interest to examine the loss of contrast sensitivity for a fixed spatial frequency across the visual field of amblyopes. Consider the hypothesis that the cause of visual loss in anisometropic amblyopia is defocus due to uncorrected refractive error. Since the optics of the eyes change little within the central 20 degrees or so (Jennings and Charman 1981), 2 diopters of defocus would have a more or less uniform effect at all eccentricities. Thus, if it results in reduced sensitivity for all spatial frequencies above, say, 4 cycles per degree in the fovea, it will have the same effect in the periphery. Since the range of visible spatial frequencies varies with eccentricity, any given spatial frequency that is affected by a blur in the fovea will also be affected in the periphery as long as it is within the visible range, and according to the blur hypothesis, acuity should "normalize" in the periphery when the window of visibility no longer includes spatial frequencies sensitive to the effects of the blur.

Several studies have investigated the contrast sensitivity of amblyopes as a function of retinal location (Thomas 1978, Katz et al. 1984, Bradley et al. 1985, Hess and Pointer 1985). Figure 3.11, from Hess and Pointer's extensive study, summarizes the two main findings: (1) within the binocular visual field, the contrast sensitivity deficit of anisometropic amblyopes (i.e., nonstrabismic) is essentially uniform, while (2) in strabismic amblyopes, the peripheral region of one or both hemifields is spared. The presence or absence of asymmetries depends on the depth of the strabismic amblyopia. Mild strabismic amblyopes

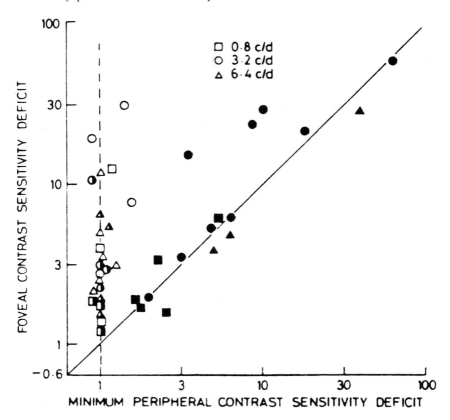

Figure 3.11   *This figure plots the ratio of the loss of foveal to the minimal peripheral contrast sensitivity. The peripheral point is taken at the locus where the loss in the amblyopic eye was minimal, within the central 30 degrees. (From Hess and Pointer 1985.)*

show marked asymmetries; severe cases tend to show more symmetric losses that are confined to the central 30 degrees.

The results for anisometropic but not strabismic amblyopes are consistent with the defocus hypothesis outlined above; however, it will be argued in a subsequent section that simple defocus is not a sufficient explanation because equal uncorrected refractive error in the two eyes does not result in marked amblyopia. Rather, it is the difference in retinal image clarity in the two eyes that is critical (Jampolsky et al. 1955). Thus it is likely that it is binocular competition induced by the monocular blur that results in the loss of contrast sensitivity in the amblyopic eye. Hess and Pointer provided an elegant test of this hypothesis by measuring contrast sensitivity in the monocular and binocular fields of the amblyopic eye. They found that the deficit in contrast sensitivity of the anisometropic amblyope that extends over 50 to 55 degrees of the binocular visual field disappears when the monocular field is tested. This result lends strong support to the notion that binocular competition plays an important role in amblyopia.

The marked difference between the results of strabismic and anisometropic amblyopes in the peripheral visual field is of particular interest. First, it suggests that the strabismic deficit is not explained by a simple defocus hypothesis. More important, it suggests that the pattern of binocular competition differs in strabismus and anisometropia. Thomas (1978) noted that his esotropic amblyopic observer showed the greatest loss of sensitivity in the temporal visual field (i.e., nasal retina) and suggested that this asymmetry in the CSF was a consequence of prolonged binocular suppression. Under binocular viewing conditions, the retinal image of the fixation target in the deviating eye of a strabismic will be imaged on the nasal retina in esotropia and on the temporal retina in exotropia. Thus Thomas's suggestion predicts a specific pattern of asymmetry in strabismus—a greater loss in the temporal field of esotropes and in the nasal field of exotropes. The results for the three exotropes and one esotrope of Hess and Pointer (1985) who showed marked asymmetries are consistent with this notion, as are the data for the esotropes tested by Katz et al. (1984) and by Bradley et al. (1985). These results are also consistent with the clinical picture of strabismic suppression (Jampolsky 1955). The relationship between strabismic suppression and strabismic amblyopia will be examined further in the section on binocular interactions.

Asymmetries in visual fields also occur in development. Lewis et al. (1984) have reported that the temporal visual field (nasal retina) develops sensitivity to visual stimuli earlier than the nasal field. Can the field-dependent losses of amblyopes be attributed to failure of development? This seems unlikely, because it would predict that losses would always occur in the nasal field. While such asymmetries do occur in monocularly deprived kittens (i.e., uncrossed projections from the temporal retina are more impaired than the crossed projections to the nasal retina; Bisti and Carmignoto 1986), esotropic amblyopes generally show more marked losses in the temporal field. Thus, at present, it seems likely that the asymmetric pattern of loss seen in strabismic amblyopes is related to binocular suppression.

2G. Luminance Dependence

Ammann (1921) first suggested that amblyopia could be distinguished from central retinal lesions and glaucoma based on the fact that the acuity of the amblyopic eye "normalized" when measured through neutral-density filters. The effects of adaptation level on the visual acuity of amblyopes have been examined in more detail by a number of investigators (von Noorden and Burian 1959a, b, Caloroso and Flom 1969, France 1984, Barbeito et al. 1987; see also Chapter 8).

Recently, Hess, Campbell, and Zimmern (1980) examined the contrast sensitivity of strabismic and anisometropic amblyopes under reduced illumination. Their results showed that for a particular grating spatial frequency, the contrast sensitivity loss of *strabismic* but not anisometropic amblyopes reduced with decreasing luminance. Von Noorden and Burian (1959a and b) suggested that the amblyopic deficit may be selective for the photopic pathways (i.e., cone vision). In other words, strabismic amblyopia may be *luminance-specific*. This would be a most surprising explanation, because rods and cones are thought to share the same ganglion cell pathways to the visual cortex (D'Zmura and Lennie 1986). An alternative explanation is that strabismic amblyopia may be selective for the central visual field, as suggested by Hess and coworkers (1980). In other words, strabismic amblyopia may be *locus-specific*. Thus, when contrast sensitivity is measured with an extended grating, the observer may detect the target with the abnormal central field under photopic conditions but use a "normal" region of the peripheral field of vision under scotopic conditions. Indirect evidence for the second hypothesis comes from the recent work of Hess and Pointer (1985), which suggests that strabismic but not anisometropic amblyopes show contrast sensitivity deficits that essentially normalize in the periphery.

In order to test these two hypotheses directly, Levi et al. (1989) measured resolution and separation discrimination thresholds of each eye of amblyopic observers using very localized stimuli presented in a region of the parafoveal retina where (1) the amblyopic deficit is evident at high luminance levels and (2) there is a reasonable concentration of both rods and cones. Figure 3.12 summarizes the separation discrimination data of the three observers for a fixed separation (between 15 and 25 minutes) at which each observer demonstrated a loss under photopic conditions by plotting the ratio of the thresholds of the amblyopic to nonamblyopic eyes. The amblyopic eyes of the three observers demonstrated elevated photopic thresholds at the fixation point, and it is interesting to note that the loss in precision of separation discrimination for a fixed separation persists at each eccentricity. At this separation, each of the observers demonstrates elevated separation discrimination thresholds at 2.5 degrees under photopic conditions, and this is also the case under scotopic conditions. Two observers (one with anisometropia, the other with both strabismus and anisometropia) showed a slightly diminished loss under scotopic conditions, while for the strabismic observer, the amblyopic loss actually increased slightly under scotopic conditions. Nonetheless, each of the amblyopes tested showed a loss in the precision of photopic separation discrimination at 2.5 degrees in the lower visual field that persisted under scotopic conditions. These results show that the amblyopic deficit persists under low luminance conditions and provides strong evidence against the luminance-specific hypothesis and support for the locus-specific hypothesis of Hess and coworkers.

2H. Orientation Dependence of the Amblyopic Deficit

Most early studies of contrast sensitivity in amblyopes used vertical sinusoidal gratings; however, Sireteanu and Singer (1980) reported an intriguing orientation dependence of the cutoff spatial frequency. They found that the grating

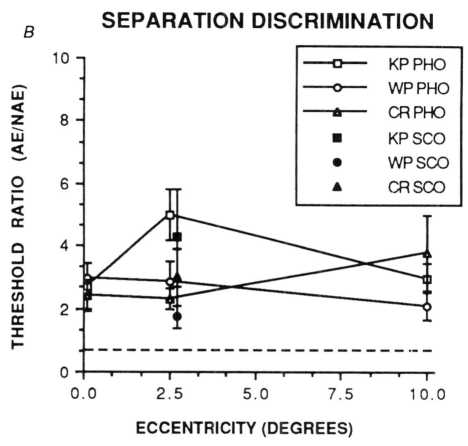

Figure 3.12 *This figure summarizes separation discrimination data of the three observers for a fixed (intermediate) separation at which each observer demonstrated a loss under photopic conditions (between 15 and 25 minutes) by plotting the ratio of the thresholds of the amblyopic to nonamblyopic eyes. The amblyopic eyes of the three observers demonstrated elevated photopic thresholds at the fixation point, and it is interesting to note that the loss in the precision of separation discrimination for a fixed separation persists at each eccentricity. At this separation, each of the observers demonstrates elevated separation discrimination thresholds at 2.5 degrees under photopic conditions (open symbols), and this is also the case under scotopic conditions (filled symbols). (From Levi et al. 1989.)*

acuity of strabismic amblyopes was poorer for vertical than for horizontal gratings. This result has been replicated in monkeys reared with surgically induced unilateral strabismus, which resulted in experimental amblyopia (Harwerth et al. 1983). Sireteanu and Singer suggested that this result was consistent with the physiologic results observed in the visual cortex of kittens reared with experimental amblyopia and could be attributed to a loss of neurons sensitive to horizontal binocular disparities. An alternative explanation is that the unsteady horizontal eye movements of strabismic amblyopes "smear" the contrast of vertical stimuli, thus reducing contrast sensitivity. On the other hand, horizontal stimuli would not be subject to this eye movement "smearing." Since the "vertical effect" was obtained with continuously viewed gratings, this explanation cannot be ruled out, and the nature of the vertical effect remains an important experimental question.

Summary

One of the defining characteristics of amblyopia is the reduction in photopic contrast sensitivity at high spatial frequencies in the central visual field. In anisometropic amblyopes, these deficits persist throughout the binocular field of vision, as might be expected if the deficit were a consequence of defocus. In strabismic amblyopes, the deficits disappear at low luminance levels and are often asymmetrically distributed across the visual field in a fashion that seems consistent with the pattern of binocular suppression found in strabismics. In both cases, the reduced contrast sensitivity reflects a neural deficit, since it cannot be explained on the basis of optical or oculomotor factors. Based on masking and adaptation studies, it seems unlikely that these deficits result from alterations in the size or organization of receptive fields of the amblyopic visual system.

The experiments reviewed in this section show that contrast detection is impaired in amblyopic vision. However, in normal everyday vision, stimuli have contrast levels well above threshold, and thus it is important to ask to what extent the threshold abnormalities impair amblyopes in performing suprathreshold tasks.

21. Suprathreshold Contrast Perception

Figure 3.13 from Loshin and Levi (1983), shows the results of a contrast matching experiment. Here, the subject adjusted the contrast of a grating seen by the amblyopic eye to match the perceived contrast of a standard grating presented for half a second to the nonamblyopic eye at various levels. The results are plotted so that if contrast matches between the two eyes are set to physical equality, the results will fall along the 1:1 line. Points above the line show that the amblyopic eye requires more contrast than the nonamblyopic eye. The filled symbols, which show the contrast thresholds for the two eyes, all fall above the 1:1 line, showing the contrast threshold deficit of the amblyopic eye. Note, however, that for each observer and at all spatial frequencies, at higher contrast levels, the reduced sensitivity of the amblyopic eye is much less marked and, at standard contrast levels of 30 to 40%, the amblyopic eye showed essentially veridical contrast perception (i.e., points on or even below the line). Loshin and Levi obtained identical results using magnitude estimation.

CONTRAST MATCHING

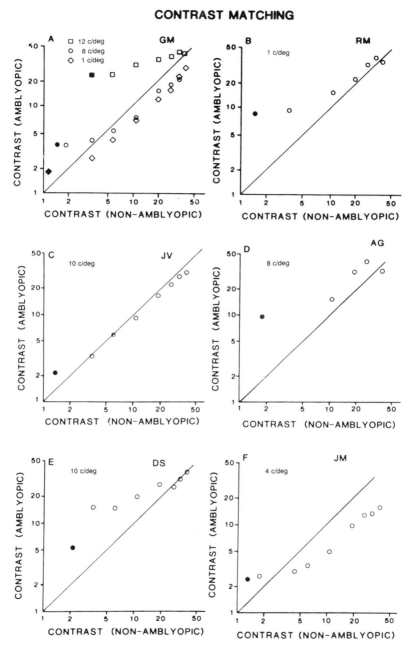

Figure 3.13 *The ordinate shows the contrast of a test grating presented to the amblyopic eye, which appeared to match that of a standard, whose contrast is shown on the abscissa, presented to the preferred eye. The 45 degree line represents equal perceived contrasts. The filled symbols represent the contrast thresholds of the two eyes. (From Loshin and Levi 1983.)*

Similar results were obtained by Hess and Bradley (1980), by Hess et al. (1983), and by Georgeson and Sullivan (1975) in meridional amblyopes showing that compensation for suprathreshold contrast perception occurs in the amblyopic eye (or in the amblyopic meridian). Moreover, compensation occurs under conditions of utrocular confusion (i.e., the experimental conditions were arranged so that the observer did not know which eye was being tested), thus ruling out response bias as an explanation (Loshin et al. 1983). The data in Figure 3.13 show substantial differences between subjects in the pattern of suprathreshold compensation. For anisometropic amblyopes D.S. and G.M. at high spatial frequencies, there is a range of contrasts (up to about a log unit) over which contrast perception is degraded in the amblyopic eye. Similar results were shown by R.M. (myopic anisometropia and constant exotropia). On the other hand, J.V. and J.M., both with constant esotropia (J.V. also has anisometropia), show compensation at very low contrast levels. Hess and Bradley (1980) suggested that for their sample of strabismic amblyopes, contrast perception was essentially veridical just slightly above threshold; however, their group of anisometropic amblyopes (associated with high degrees of unilateral myopia) showed a more gradual recovery of suprathreshold contrast perception (similar to the data for D.S. and G.M. in Figure 3.13). The results of the two studies are in general agreement, although there appear to be exceptions to the strict dichotomy both in the data of Loshin and Levi (e.g., strabismic amblyope A.G.) and in the data of Hess and Bradley (e.g. strabismic amblyope S.N.). Nonetheless, targets with reasonably high contrast will be perceived to have similar contrast in each eye of strabismic and anisometropic amblyopes, at least when viewed briefly. However, Ciuffreda (unpublished observations) has noted that both strabismic and anisometropic amblyopes report fading of target contrast during prolonged viewing with their amblyopic eyes.

How can the threshold and suprathreshold data be reconciled? Kaplan and Shapley (1982) have reported the existence of two distinct contrast-coding channels in the lateral geniculate nucleus of normal primates that respond to different contrast levels. Hess et al. (1983) suggested that in amblyopia the more sensitive channel (i.e., the one responding to low contrasts) may be selectively affected while the high contrast mechanism is spared. However, several other types of experiments suggest that contrast coding may indeed remain abnormal at suprathreshold levels. For example, VEP amplitudes of the amblyopic eye fail to show any suprathreshold compensation (Levi and Harwerth, 1978a and b; see also Chapter 4). Similarly, amblyopic eyes need more contrast to reach a criterion reaction time than do their fellow eyes. These results suggest an alternate interpretation to that of Hess et al. (1983). Contrast sensation, like color sensation, may be a quality. Once the stimulus is above threshold, its magnitude is known. However, reaction times and evoked potentials (as well as contrast thresholds) may all depend on pooling of information from many neurons. Thus there may simply be fewer responsive neurons that receive input through the amblyopic eye; if contrast sensation (or magnitude) does not depend on pooling of responses in the same way as reaction times and evoked potentials, then the discrepant results obtained with these methods are not so surprising. It is of interest to note that normal peripheral vision acts much like amblyopic vision in this regard (see section on periphery and amblyopia).

2J. Contrast Discrimination

An important aspect of visual processing of suprathreshold stimuli is the ability to discern variations in contrast. It is likely that contrast discrimination plays a critical role in making spatial discriminations (Badcock 1984; Klein and Levi 1985). In a recent study, Ciuffreda and Fisher (1987) compared contrast discrimination at several spatial frequencies in amblyopic and normal observers. Their results show that contrast discrimination is consistently impaired in amblyopic eyes and that the impairment increases with increasing spatial frequency.

The function relating contrast-increment threshold to background or pedestal contrast can be described as a "dipper" function, falling at low contrasts and rising at contrasts above the observer's detection threshold, typically following a power function. The shape of the contrast discrimination function appears to be invariant under a wide range of conditions in normal vision. For example, the shape of the function is similar when the spatial frequency, luminance, or eccentricity of the targets is varied (Bradley and Ozhawa 1986, Legge and Kersten 1987). Under each of these conditions, the functions superimpose when both the contrast-increment threshold and the contrast pedestal are specified in threshold units. Thus, as Legge and Kersten have pointed out, the entire contrast discrimination function can be specified simply by giving the contrast sensitivity for the stimulus. Figure 3.14 shows contrast discrimination data for each eye of a strabismic and anisometropic amblyope. Note that there is a large difference between the thresholds of the two eyes obtained with no background (i.e., the detection threshold is shown by the leftmost point), while there is only a small difference in contrast discrimination thresholds at high background contrast levels. Thus, while absolute contrast detection thresholds of the amblyopic eye are substantially elevated, contrast discrimination thresholds are only slightly elevated at high contrast levels. Bradley and Ohzawa (1986) and Hess et al. (1983) have reported similar data for their amblyopic observers. Figure 3.15 shows the contrast-increment threshold data of Figure 3.14 replotted with both the contrast-increment thresholds and pedestal contrasts specified in threshold units. This operation superimposes the curves of the two eyes and shows that the processes underlying contrast discrimination are essentially the same in normal and amblyopic vision. It also shows that the "scaling" factor for contrast discrimination of amblyopes, like that of the normal periphery (Legge and Kersten 1987), is the contrast threshold.

2K. Detection and Identification of Complex Stimuli

One of the strong appeals of sine-wave gratings is that to the extent the visual system approximates a linear system, its response to sine-wave gratings may be valuable in predicting the response to complex stimuli. Campbell and Robson (1968) first applied linear systems analysis to the detection and discrimination of complex gratings. Their results showed that over a wide range of spatial frequencies

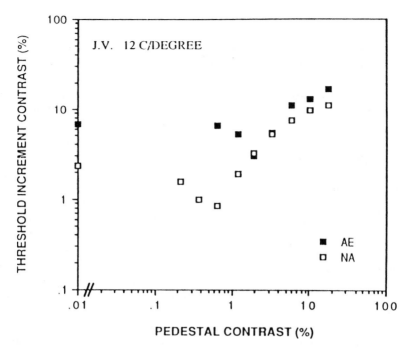

Figure 3.14 *Contrast-increment thresholds as a function of the pedestal contrast for both eyes of an amblyope with strabismus viewing a 12 cycle per degree grating. The open squares represent the preferred eye; filled squares represent the amblyopic eye. The leftmost point for each eye represents the absolute detection threshold.*

(> 1.0 cycle per degree), the contrast threshold of a complex grating is determined by the amplitude of the fundamental Fourier component of its waveform and that complex gratings can be distinguished from sine-wave gratings when the contrast of the relevant higher harmonics reach their independent contrast thresholds. These results were important because they provided strong evidence that the visual system responds independently to each spatial frequency component of the stimulus. Since any spatial pattern can be considered as the sum of a series of sinusoidal components, within limits, the response to a complex pattern may be predicted by considering the responses to the separate components. However, to specify a complex visual stimulus completely, information about the relative phase of the frequency components is also essential. Consider, for example, the ramp-wave grating shown in the inset of Figure 3.16. A ramp wave can be described by a series of harmonics (F + 2F + 3F + $\cdots$ + nF); however, only the fundamental and second harmonic are needed to identify the phase or polarity of the ramp wave (i.e., whether it is brighter on the left or right).

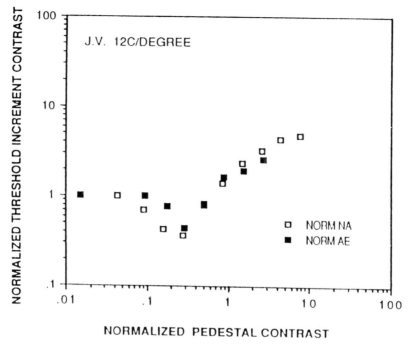

Figure 3.15 *The data from Figure 3.14 replotted with both the thresholds and the pedestal contrast specified in threshold units. This operation superimposes the curves of the two eyes.*

Pass and Levi (1982) compared the thresholds for detecting a ramp-wave grating, as well as for discriminating its polarity, to sine-wave thresholds. Normal observers detected ramp-wave gratings when the contrast of the fundamental spatial frequency was close to its independent threshold and correctly discriminated the polarity (phase) of the ramp when the second harmonic reached its independent threshold. For the amblyopic eyes, detection of the ramp also occurred when the contrast of the fundamental frequency was near its independent threshold. However, discrimination of the polarity (phase) of the ramp required contrast levels of 2 to 10 times greater than needed to detect the second harmonic. This difficulty in discriminating the phase of complex gratings was found to occur in both strabismic and anisometropic amblyopes. It is not a consequence of masking, and it has now been observed in several laboratories and under a variety of conditions (Lawden et al. 1982, Weiss et al. 1985, Mac Canna et al. 1986). This difficulty in discerning the relative phase of complex gratings cannot be attributed to the reduced contrast sensitivity of the amblyopic eye, because the discrimination ratios take into account the reduced contrast sensitivity of the amblyopic eye. In addition, Mac Canna et al. (1986) demonstrated abnormalities in phase discrimination even when the effective contrast of the two eyes was equated.

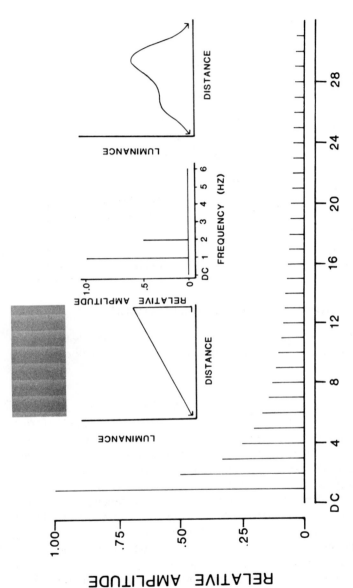

Figure 3.16   *A ramp wave (above) can be described by a series of harmonics (below). However, only the fundamental and second harmonic are needed to identify the phase or polarity of the ramp wave (i.e., whether it is brighter on the left or right-lower right). The left inset shows the luminance profile of a ramp. The center inset shows the power spectrum of a ramp that has been digitally filtered to limit the harmonic makeup to the fundamental and second harmonic. The right inset shows the luminance profile of such a digitally filtered ramp. Note that the phase of the resultant waveform is apparent. For normal eyes, the phase of the ramp can be identified when the second harmonic reaches its independent threshold. Amblyopic eyes require contrast 2 to 10 times above their thresholds for the second harmonic. (From Pass and Levi 1982.)*

Hess et al. (1978) initially suggested that the distorted appearance of suprathreshold gratings reported by some amblyopes may represent a phase-processing abnormality. At first glance, the experiments just described would appear to confirm this view; however, recent experiments suggest that phase discrimination is quite complex and relies on local contrast discrimination (Badcock 1984) and local edge blur discrimination (Hess and Pointer 1987). Moreover, recent experiments by Paul et al. (1986) suggest that there may be an even more fundamental phase abnormality in the amblyopic visual system. They found that normal observers are able to identify the polarity (i.e., black versus white) of a blurred bar (a Cauchy function) at the detection threshold, whereas at high spatial frequencies, the amblyopic eye of both strabismic and anisometropic amblyopes needs a good deal more contrast to identify the polarity of the target. This implies that the labeling of on and off channels thought to exist in normal vision may be scrambled in the amblyopic visual system. Nonetheless, it is clear from the work of Brettel et al. (1982) that scrambling of phase information can strongly influence the appearance of a scene (see Figure 3.17).

Summary

While amblyopes often demonstrate veridical contrast perception at suprathreshold contrast levels, they demonstrate several abnormalities of suprathreshold contrast processing. These include reduced contrast discrimination, reduced evoked potential gain, prolonged reaction times, and abnormalities in discerning the phase or polarity of a target. Moreover, some amblyopes report perceptual distortions of suprathreshold stimuli (see section on aberrations in spatial perception).

3. THE "SPATIAL SENSE"

While clinicians generally consider spatial vision in terms of Snellen acuity, with a limiting acuity of about 20/20 (i.e., critical detail of about 1 minute), the visual system is capable of making much finer spatial discriminations. For example, relative position, size, and orientation can be judged with an accuracy of 3 to 6 seconds of arc or better (Klein and Levi 1985). These low spatial thresholds are 5 to 10 times finer than either the cutoff spatial frequency or the intercone spacing. For this reason, Westheimer (1975) has coined the term *hyperacuity* to describe a variety of tasks that involve sensing the direction of spatial offset of a line or point relative to a reference.

This performance is remarkable considering that even the smallest foveal cones are separated by about 30 seconds and the point-spread function of the eye spreads the image over several cones. Moreover, Westheimer and McKee (1975) have shown that hyperacuity is robust to retinal image motion. Thus they

ZA ZP

1–4

2–8

4–16

8–32

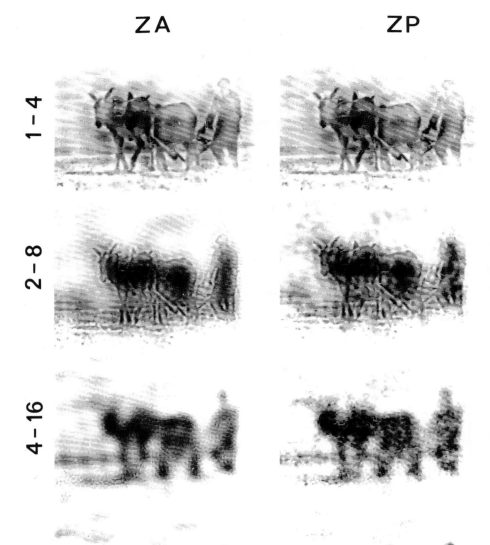

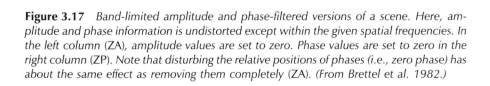

Figure 3.17 *Band-limited amplitude and phase-filtered versions of a scene. Here, amplitude and phase information is undistorted except within the given spatial frequencies. In the left column (ZA), amplitude values are set to zero. Phase values are set to zero in the right column (ZP). Note that disturbing the relative positions of phases (i.e., zero phase) has about the same effect as removing them completely (ZA). (From Brettel et al. 1982.)*

demonstrated that a Vernier target could be swept across about 100 cones in a 200-ms period without degrading performance.

Hyperacuity or positional acuity has been the focus of much recent research and modeling, both in normal and anomalous vision. There are several reasons for this. First, it is of basic interest to understand how the visual system achieves this high degree of accuracy, that is, how it solves the technical problem of "subpixel" resolution. Second, several lines of evidence suggest that performance on hyperacuity tasks reflects cortical processing (Levi et al. 1985, Klein and Levi 1987, McKee and Levi 1987). Third, it seems likely that the mechanisms underlying hyperacuity have the more general task of form and shape analysis (Marr 1982, Watt and Morgan 1985). Thus studying hyperacuity may provide a window into the operation of the cortical mechanisms of form perception. Not surprisingly, in amblyopia, which is considered to be an abnormality of the "form" sense, hyperacuity is markedly degraded. In hyperacuity tasks, several lines of evidence now suggest that the neural losses of strabismic and anisometropic amblyopes are fundamentally different.

3A. Hyperacuity, Snellen Acuity, and Grating Acuity

Figure 3.18 plots the Vernier acuity of a group of amblyopes against their Snellen acuity. These data, taken from several studies (Levi and Klein 1982a, b, 1985, Rentschler and Hilz 1985), show the close connection between the Snellen acuity and the position acuity of amblyopes. A similar relationship exists between bisection acuity and Snellen acuity (Levi and Klein 1983, 1986). The slope of the line drawn through the data of Figure 3.18 is unity, suggesting that Snellen acuity and position acuity are affected in the same way by the amblyopic process.

Figure 3.19 plots Vernier acuity (Figure 3.19*A*) and acuity for another position discrimination task, namely, bisection (Figure 3.19*B*), as a function of grating acuity. In each of these figures, the data of nonstrabismic anisometropic amblyopes are shown as A's, while those of strabismic amblyopes and those with both constant strabismus and anisometropia are shown as S's and B's, respectively. For both tasks, the A's fall along the straight line with unity slope, showing that grating resolution and positional acuity are similarly affected by the amblyopic process. However, the strabismic amblyopes show greater losses in accuracy for positional acuity than for grating resolution.

This result is similar to the decoupling of Snellen acuity and grating acuity in strabismic amblyopes described in the section on contrast sensitivity and again points to the close link between positional acuity and Snellen acuity. (This link will be examined in greater detail later.) Levi and Klein (1982b) showed that the reduced positional acuity of amblyopes could not be accounted for on the basis of eccentric fixation or faulty eye movements and thus represents a neural deficit or deficits in the amblyopic visual system. The nature of these deficits will be discussed later.

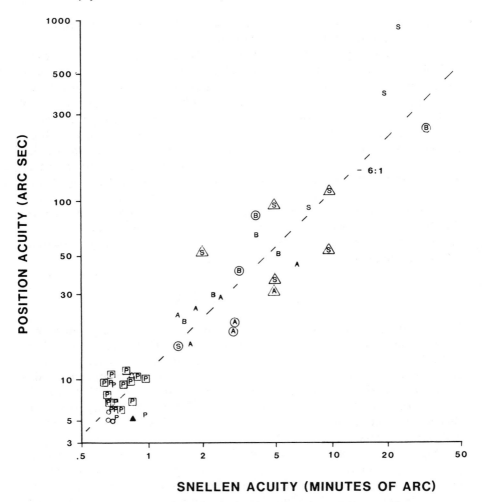

Figure 3.18 *Vernier acuity of a group of amblyopes is plotted against their Snellen acuity. These data are taken from several studies in our laboratory. Data of normal control observers are shown as open circles. Preferred eyes of strabismic amblyopes are shown as P's in boxes; those of anisometropic amblyopes are shown as P's. Data for the amblyopic eyes are shown as A's, S's, and B's for anisometropic and strabismic amblyopes and those with both. Also included are data for several subjects from Rentschler and Hilz (1985). The open triangle is the mean data for their normal observers; the filled triangle is the mean for the preferred eyes of their amblyopes. Letters in triangles show the amblyopic eyes of all but one of their observers.*

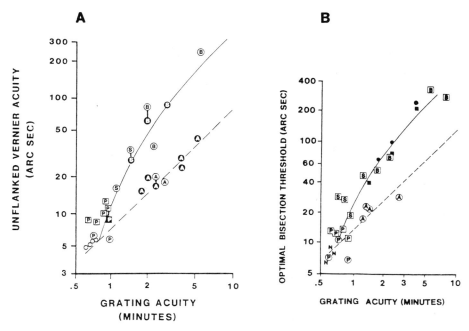

Figure 3.19 *Vernier acuity (A) and acuity for another position discrimination task, namely, bisection (B), as a function of grating acuity. In each of these figures, the data for nonstrabismic anisometropic amblyopes are shown as A's, while those for strabismic amblyopes and those with both constant strabismus and anisometropia are shown as S's and B's, respectively. For both tasks, the A's fall along the straight line with unity slope, showing that grating resolution and positional acuity are similarly affected by the amblyopic process. However, the strabismic amblyopes show greater losses in accuracy for positional acuity than for grating resolution. The data for the strabismic amblyopes fall close to the results obtained in the normal periphery (solid lines). (From Levi and Klein 1985, and Levi et al. 1987.)*

    The comparison of grating, position, and Snellen acuities in amblyopes raises an interesting question: Are the Snellen and Vernier acuities abnormally low in strabismic compared with anisometropic amblyopia, or is the grating acuity abnormally low in anisometropic amblyopes? A comparison of the population distributions of each acuity measure (from the sample of Levi and Klein 1982b) showed that the distribution of grating acuities was essentially identical in strabismic and anisometropic amblyopes. On the other hand, amblyopes with constant strabismus have a broader distribution of Vernier and Snellen acuities (see also section on visual acuity) owing to a preponderance of poorer Vernier and Snellen acuities. Thus Levi and Klein (1982b) concluded that strabismic amblyopes have an extra loss of spatial information needed for tasks involving spatial judgments (e.g., Vernier acuity) and for Snellen acuity. The inability of strabismic amblyopes to judge relative position is greatly exaggerated at high spatial frequencies (Levi and Klein 1982a and b). For normal eyes, and for the amblyopic eyes of anisometropic amblyopes, Vernier acuity was essentially independent of spatial frequency over a large range, increasing at spatial frequencies about one octave (a factor of 2) below the resolution limit. For strabismic amblyopes, on the other hand, the Vernier threshold doubled between two and three octaves below the resolution limit. This marked reduction in Vernier acuity when the interline spacing of the grating is small is an effect of spatial interference. In the following section it will be shown that interference with Vernier acuity scales is due to the Vernier threshold rather than to resolution (i.e., the size of the interference zone is proportional to the uncrowded Vernier threshold).

3B. Spatial Interference with Hyperacuity

Spatial interference or contour interaction effects are ubiquitous in spatial vision. Such effects occur for orientation discrimination (Westheimer et al. 1976), stereoacuity (Butler and Westheimer 1978), Vernier acuity (Westheimer and Hauske 1975, Levi et al. 1985), and Snellen acuity. Flom et al. (1963) measured the spatial extent of interference with acuity by placing flanking bars at various distances from a near-threshold Landolt C (see Chapter 8). They found that the linear extent of interference was far greater in the amblyopic than in the normal eyes, but that when scaled to the unflanked acuity (i.e., when the flank distance was expressed in multiples of the gap), the extent of interference was similar in normal and amblyopic eyes. Similar observations were reported by Hess and Jacobs (1979). (See section on acuity in Chapter 1.)

Vernier acuity is also markedly degraded when the target is flanked by a pair of optimally positioned flanks (Westheimer and Hauske 1975, Levi et al. 1985). This spatial interference with Vernier acuity is strongest when the flanks are 2 to 4 minutes from the target. It occurs even if the target is presented to one eye and the flanks to the other, suggesting that this effect is cortically mediated. Levi and Klein (1985) measured the extent of spatial interference with Vernier acuity in a group of amblyopic observers and compared this with the results of the normal fovea and periphery. Figure 3.20 shows the relationship between the Vernier threshold with no flanks and the distance at which the spatial interference was strongest. Shown in this figure are the results for control normal eyes (dots), preferred eyes of amblyopes (P's—these will be considered in more detail in a later section), amblyopic eyes (A's, B's, and S's), and the normal periphery (squares and circles). The solid line has a slope of 1 on these log-log coordinates. The slope of 1 would be expected if the distance of the flanks that gave the strongest masking scaled (i.e., was directly proportional) to the unflanked Vernier threshold. The data are compatible with this linear scaling (slope = 1.11 ± 0.18), suggesting that for the normal fovea, the periphery, and both eyes of amblyopes, the strongest spatial interference occurs with contours about 30 times the unflanked threshold distance from the target. Thus, if the unflanked threshold is 6 seconds (i.e., 0.1 minute), the strongest interference would be most marked at a distance of 3 minutes (30×0.1). In an

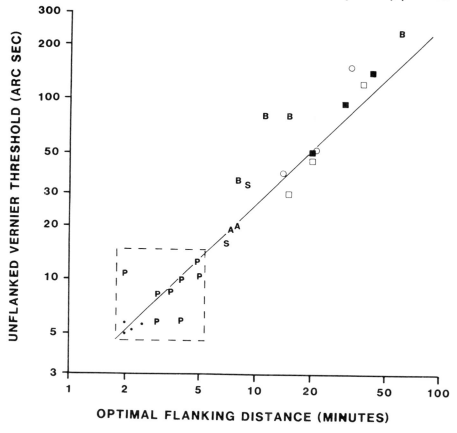

Figure 3.20 *The relationship between the Vernier threshold with no flanks and the distance at which the spatial interference was strongest. Shown in this figure are the results for control normal eyes (dots), preferred eyes of amblyopes (P's), amblyopic eyes (A's, B's, and S's), and the normal periphery (squares and circles). The solid line has a slope of 1 on these log-log coordinates; this linear relationship would be expected if the distance of the flanks that gave the strongest masking scaled to the unflanked Vernier threshold. The data are compatible with this linear scaling (slope = 1.11 ± 0.18), suggesting that for the normal fovea, the periphery, and both eyes of amblyopes, the strongest spatial interference occurs with contours about 30 times the unflanked threshold distance from the target. (From Levi and Klein 1985.)*

amblyopic eye with Vernier acuity five times poorer (0.5 minute), the interference would be strongest at 15 minutes (i.e., 30 × 0.5). In strabismic amblyopes, because Vernier acuity is often much more degraded than grating acuity, easily resolved targets may be subject to strong spatial interference, since the zone of interference is proportional to the Vernier acuity rather than to the grating acuity. Thus "crowding" would be expected to occur at spatial frequencies well below the cutoff in strabismic amblyopes.

3C. Cortical Modules for Spatial Processing

It has been suggested (Westheimer 1981b, Westheimer and McKee 1977, Levi et al. 1985) that position coding requires a processing zone of several minutes of arc in the normal fovea and correspondingly larger (in proportion to the threshold) in the periphery. When interfering contours are present within their zone, positional coding is degraded. Similar effects occur for orientation discrimination and letter acuity, suggesting that each may share a common basis.

Hubel and Wiesel (1974) first suggested that the striate cortex consists of a large number of repeating modules, each of which carries out a highly stereotyped analysis of the inputs from a small region of the visual field. Each module or *hypercolumn*, consists of a pair of ocular dominance columns (representing all possible orientations). Several new anatomic techniques have clarified and extended the notion that the visual cortex is organized in a modular fashion, and it now seems likely that there may be several types of modules (e.g., cytochrome oxidase blobs, hypercolumns) that may carry different information.

Barlow (1979, 1981) suggested the intriguing notion that the processing zone required for optimal hyperacuity has its anatomic basis in the modular organization of the visual cortex. The finding that the dimensions of this zone grow in peripheral vision in proportion to the cortical magnification factor (Levi et al. 1985), lends credence to this notion and suggests that spatial interference may reveal information about these modules in human vision. In the normal fovea, the psychophysical spatial processing module is 4 to 5 minutes of arc. This is approximately the spatial extent of a normal human ocular dominance column, which is about 1 mm (Hitchcock and Hickey 1980). It is interesting to note that this is also about the overall dimension of a threshold-level Snellen letter (20/20 letter = 5 minutes).

Figure 3.21 shows schematically the arrangement of these processing modules as a function of eccentricity. The heavily outlined boxes represent the normal visual system. Here, the vertical axis is in millimeters of cortex, each 1-mm module being about the size of a normal human ocular dominance column or a spatial processing module. The horizontal axis is eccentricity. The horizontal extent of each box represents the spatial extent of each 1-mm module, which was constructed to be approximately 4 minutes at 0 degrees eccentricity and to increase in proportion to the inverse of the cortical magnification factor. The stippled boxes represent the enlarged processing modules that are found in amblyopes. There are several possible reasons for the enlarged modules of the amblyopic eye. First, to achieve a high signal-to-noise ratio, a large fixed number of neurons may be required (Sakitt and Barlow 1982). The amblyopic loss of neurons in both strabismus and anisometropia would therefore necessitate a larger processing module. Second, the lack of fusion between the two eyes occurring in strabismus may cause an extra scattering of receptive fields in the deviating eye (Pettigrew 1974). Extending the zone of scattering by a constant (0.5 degree in Figure 3.21) would have the effect of increasing the relative size of the foveal processing module a lot, but it would have a proportionally smaller effect with increasing eccentricity.

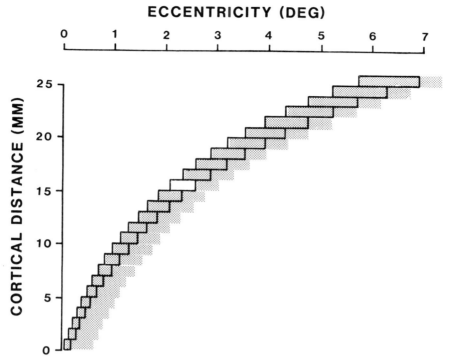

Figure 3.21 *Schematic illustration of the arrangement of the putative form-processing modules as a function of eccentricity. The heavily outlined boxes represent the normal visual system. Here, the vertical axis is in millimeters of cortex, each 1-mm module being about the size of a normal human ocular dominance column or a spatial processing module. The horizontal axis is eccentricity. The horizontal extent of each box represents the spatial extent of each 1-mm module, which was constructed to be approximately 4 minutes at 0 degrees eccentricity and to increase in proportion to the inverse of the cortical magnification factor. The stippled boxes represent the enlarged processing modules that are found in amblyopes. The modules were enlarged by extending the zone of scattering by a constant 0.5 degree. This has the effect of increasing the relative size of the foveal processing module, but it has a proportionally smaller effect with increasing eccentricity. (From Levi and Klein 1985.)*

This notion of processing modules may help to explain several other aspects of hyperacuity. Performance on hyperacuity tasks depends critically on the distances between the features that comprise the targets. For example, the precision of bisection depends critically on the separation of the lines. This is illustrated by the shaded regions in Figure 3.22, which shows the range of bisection thresholds of normal control observers. The N's in Figure 3.22 show bisection thresholds for the preferred eyes of two amblyopes, one with anisometropia (Figure 3.22*A*) and one with both strabismus and anisometropia (Figure 3.22*B*). The A's are the data for their amblyopic eyes. Note that for both

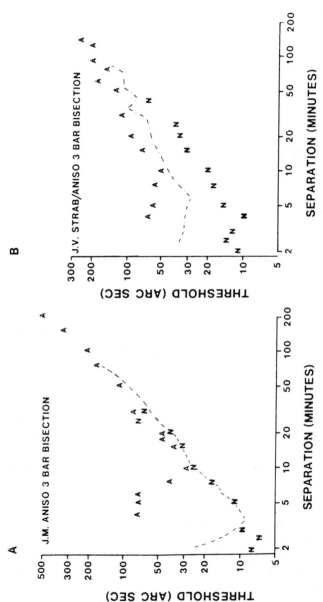

Figure 3.22 *Bisection thresholds as a function of separation. The N's show bisection thresholds for the preferred eyes of two amblyopes, one with anisometropia (A) and one with both strabismus and anisometropia (B). The A's are the data for their amblyopic eyes. The dot-dashed line in (B) shows the effect of shifting the data of the amblyopic eye down and to the right by a factor equal to the loss of grating acuity in the amblyopic eye. For the anisometropic amblyope, this scale factor shifts the entire curve to within normal range at all but the smallest separations. In contrast, this scale factor fails to superimpose adequately the curve of the strabismic amblyope within the normal range. (From Levi et al. 1987.)*

observers, the thresholds of the amblyopic eye are markedly elevated for small separations and are essentially normal for large separations. One possibility is that thresholds are markedly abnormal for stimuli whose features fall within a processing module of the amblyopic eye but are more or less normal when comparing stimuli whose features fall within separate modules. For J.M., a "module" would be about 10 minutes (30 times the optimum threshold of about 20 seconds), while for J.V., a module would be approximately 25 minutes (30 × 50 seconds). For both observers, thresholds are normal for larger separations (i.e., features in separate modules) and abnormal for smaller separations. This notion also could account for the finding that amblyopes can accurately discriminate the orientation of long but not short lines (Vandenbussche et al. 1986) and of low but not high spatial frequency gratings (Skotton et al. 1986), to be described in more detail later.

The dot-dashed line in Figure 3.22*B* shows the effect of shifting the data for the amblyopic eye down and to the right by a factor equal to the loss of grating acuity in the amblyopic eye. For the anisometropic amblyope, this scale factor shifts the entire curve to within normal range at all but the smallest separations. In contrast, this scale factor fails to adequately superimpose the curve of the strabismic amblyope within the normal range. Thus, as with Vernier acuity, the loss of precision for bisection acuity of anisometropes is approximately proportional to the resolution loss, whereas in strabismic amblyopes there appears to be an extra loss of positional information.

3D. Aberrations in Spatial Perception

Pugh (1958) first reported that amblyopes may have perceptual distortions and see ghost images of the letters on an acuity chart. This and related observations of perceptual distortion also have been made by Selenow and Ciuffreda (1986) and are illustrated in Figure 3.23. Hess et al. (1978) have described reports by some amblyopes of perceptual distortions for grating patterns. These introspective reports of distorted perception take the form of fading of part of the grating, nonuniform bar widths, or added spurious lines and are shown in Figure 3.24. These perceptual distortions are not reported by all amblyopes, and it is difficult at present to assess their role in the performance of the amblyopic eye (Bradley and Freeman 1985a).

The preceding section focused on the *precision* of spatial judgments in amblyopic eyes. Precision refers to the threshold, or just-noticeable change in position, obtained from the slope of the psychometric function. The data from a number of laboratories now strongly suggest that the precision of the spatial judgments with an amblyopic eye is reduced, particularly under conditions where normal eyes perform most precisely. In this section we examine the *veridicality* of spatial judgments in amblyopia (i.e., how well subjective judgments of alignment agree with physical measures of alignment). There are many anecdotal

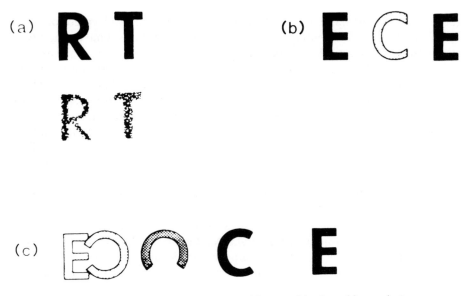

Figure 3.23 *Appearance of optotypes reported by a strabismic amblyope during monocular viewing: (a) sharp contours during foveal fixation (above) and diffuse contours during eccentric fixation (below), (b) reduced perceived contrast of the fixated letter C (possibly due to contour interaction), and (c) perceived contrast gradient and spatial asymmetry when fixating the reversed C with the eccentric point. (From Selenow and Ciuffreda 1986.)*

reports that strabismic amblyopes mislocalize targets; for example, Irvine (1948) reported that some amblyopes made errors in assessing the direction of an ophthalmoscope beam imaged between the macula and optic disk. Following an observation by Schor (1972) that a strabismic amblyope made large errors in partitioning experiments, Bedell and Flom (1981, 1983) had amblyopes judge whether a thin line appeared aligned between two large triangles spaced approximately 1 degree apart (this is a Vernier-like task). They noted that strabismic but not anisometropic amblyopes frequently made large constant errors. These constant errors can be thought of as spatial mislocalizations. Figure 3.25 shows the stimulus used by Bedell and Flom. The position of the test line corresponds to a condition judged by some amblyopic observers to be aligned. Bedell and Flom interpreted these constant errors in terms of local compressions and expansions of space, (i.e., monocular spatial distortions) resulting from abnormal binocular interactions. However, the notion of compressions and expansions of space predicts shifts in the perceived locations of targets (constant errors) with *no* net loss in precision (i.e., precision may be decreased in compressed regions, but it should be increased in expanded regions).

Large constant errors also occur in peripheral vision (see section on periphery as a model for strabismic amblyopia). In performing bisection experiments in the periphery, observers frequently mislocalize a bisecting target in the direction

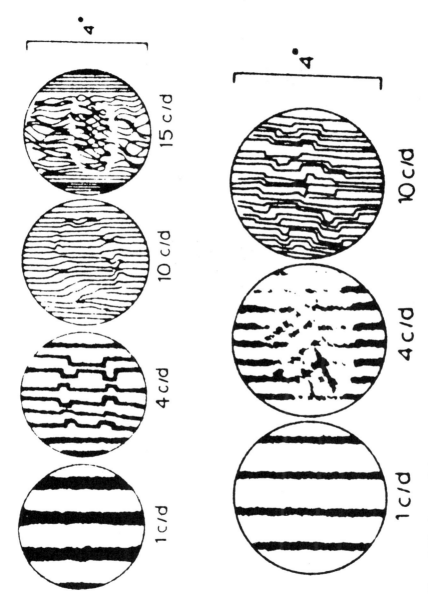

Figure 3.24 *Perceptual distortions for grating patterns. These introspective reports of distorted perception made by an amblyope take the form of fading of part of the grating, nonuniform bar widths, or added spurious lines. (From Hess et al. 1978.)*

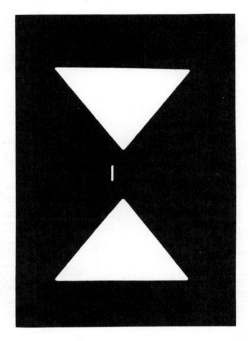

Figure 3.25   *Bedell and Flom had amblyopes judge whether a thin line appeared aligned between two large triangles spaced approximately 1 degree apart (this is a Vernier-like task). They noted that strabismic but not anisometropic amblyopes frequently made large constant errors. The position of the test line corresponds to a condition judged by some amblyopic observers to be aligned.*

of the fovea. A simple explanation for such mislocalizations is that the observer takes the geometric mean of the positions of the reference targets, which are weighted by the cortical magnification factor. Thus a reference target close to the fovea will have a higher weighting than one that is distant. This is analogous to performing bisection in *cortical* rather than retinal space. A similar explanation could account for the mislocalizations of strabismic amblyopes (who frequently have eccentric fixation).However, this explanation raises the intriguing possibility that cortical magnification in the amblyopic eye of at least some amblyopes may be highest at a non-foveal location. This is an area that clearly needs further study.

In a recent study, Bedell et al. (1985) compared both the precision and the accuracy of spatial localization judgments with visual acuity. All 23 of their strabismic amblyopes demonstrated marked spatial imprecision (elevated thresholds, outside the normal range), and two-thirds of them also showed marked inaccuracies in spatial location. Their results showed a higher correlation of visual acuity with precision (threshold) than with accuracy (constant error), suggesting that it is the precision of spatial information that is critically important in visual acuity.

3E. Orientation Discrimination

Orientation or tilt discrimination is closely related to Vernier acuity. In fact, two- or three-dot Vernier alignment tasks may be a special case of relative orientation discrimination (Sullivan et al. 1972). Figure 3.26 shows the data for two amblyopes (one with anisometropia, the other with strabismus and anisometropia) for three-dot Vernier alignment. The threshold offset (in seconds of arc) is plotted as a function of the horizontal separation between the dots for the amblyopic eye. The shaded region shows the range of normal thresholds. Note that for small separations, the thresholds of the amblyopic eye are markedly elevated; however, for larger separations, the amblyopic eye is normal or near normal. The dot-dashed line shows the results for the amblyopic eye when scaled by the resolution deficit (as applied in the bisection studies described earlier). For the anisometropic amblyope, this scaling works well at all but the smallest separations; however, for the strabismic amblyope, it fails.

It is of interest to note that at large gaps, threshold is proportional to the gap. One interpretation of this proportionality is that Vernier thresholds for well-separated targets represent a constant orientation (i.e., the angular tilt implied by the just-visible offset of the center dot) (see Sullivan et al. 1972, Watt et al. 1983). For the data shown here, the normal observers could detect a change in orientation of about 1 degree for all separations exceeding about 5 minutes. For the amblyopic eyes at small separations, the orientation threshold was markedly elevated; however, at large separations, the orientation threshold was essentially normal. These results imply that amblyopes should have little difficulty in judging the tilt of a long line but will have difficulty in making such judgments for short lines. This is precisely the result obtained by Venverloh (1983) and more recently by Vandenbussche et al. (1986). In a related study, Skottun et al. (1986) found that strabismic amblyopes had little difficulty in judging the orientation of low spatial frequency gratings but had marked difficulty with high spatial frequencies. The line-length and spatial frequency results may be closely linked. Cortical mechanisms tuned to orientation show a strong relationship between the heights and widths of their receptive fields (i.e., a more or less fixed aspect ratio). Thus low spatial frequency (large) mechanisms will respond best to long lines, while high spatial frequency (small) mechanisms will respond best to short lines. The results of these experiments in amblyopes are compatible with the more general finding that small (high spatial frequency) mechanisms are most susceptible to the effects of amblyopia.

How can the losses of positional information in amblyopic eyes be understood? A review of models for positional acuity is beyond the scope of this chapter, but there are now several models that attempt to account for the high precision of foveal positional acuity on the basis of the spatial filtering and spatial sampling properties of the visual system (e.g., Watt and Morgan 1985, Klein and Levi 1985, Wilson 1986a, Levi 1988). In the following section we consider several factors that could account for the losses that occur in the amblyopic visual system and their implications.

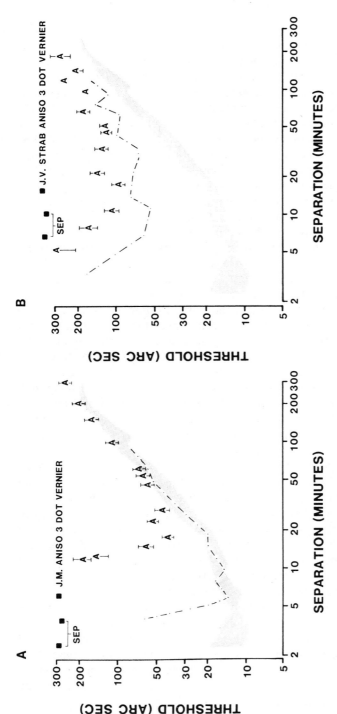

Figure 3.26   *Three-dot Vernier alignment data for two amblyopes, one with anisometropia (A), the other with both strabismus and anisometropia (B). The threshold offset (in seconds of arc) is plotted as a function of the horizontal separation between the dots for the amblyopic eye. The shaded region shows the range of normal thresholds. Note that for small separations, the thresholds of the amblyopic eye are markedly elevated; however, for larger separations, the amblyopic eye is normal or near normal. The dot-dashed line shows the results of the amblyopic eye when scaled by the resolution deficit (as applied in the bisection studies shown in Figure 3.22). For the anisometropic amblyope, this scaling works well at all but the smallest separations; however, for the strabismic amblyope, it fails. (Unpublished data from Levi and Klein.)*

3F. Factors That May Contribute to the Amblyopic Loss
of Positional Information

A number of factors have been suggested that could potentially limit spatial processing. These include

1. The contrast sensitivity of the mechanisms (receptive fields)
2. The spatial sampling density
3. The collection of spatial samples
4. Disorder of the topographic mapping of visual space

Contrast Sensitivity of Mechanisms

A key feature of several recent models for position discrimination is the contrast sensitivity and suprathreshold contrast-response function of the putative spatial filters or receptive fields (Watt and Morgan 1985, Klein and Levi 1985, Wilson 1986a). In amblyopes, there is ample evidence for reduced contrast sensitivity, and thus it is plausible that reduced contrast sensitivity or signal-to-noise ratio of the filters may result in reduced positional sensitivity. The clear implication of this notion is that there should be a proportional reduction in position sensitivity, that is, a single scale factor should account for the loss of contrast sensitivity/resolution and position acuity. In anisometropic amblyopes, this appears to be the case (Bradley and Freeman 1985a, Levi and Klein 1982a and b, 1983, 1985); however, in strabismic amblyopes, there appears to be an additional loss of positional acuity.

If indeed the reduced positional acuity of anisometropic amblyopes is attributed to reduced contrast sensitivity, it is reasonable to ask whether the amblyope uses larger mechanisms (with better contrast sensitivity but poorer positional sensitivity) or the same-size mechanism as the normal eye but with lower sensitivity. Watt and Hess (1987) have recently examined this question by measuring Vernier acuity in the presence of one-dimensional Gaussian blur (i.e., the luminance profile of the target lines is a Gaussian whose spread is defined as the standard deviation of the Gaussian). Their results show that for both eyes of anisometropic amblyopes, Vernier thresholds were degraded when the standard deviation of the Gaussian blur exceeded about 3 minutes. These results imply that the two eyes use the same size filters for the Vernier task. Bradley and Freeman (1985a) showed that the poor positional acuity of the amblyopic eye could be mimicked by reducing the contrast of the stimulus. Taken together, these findings suggest that at least to a first-order approximation, the position losses of anisometropic amblyopes for a variety of conditions (Vernier versus spatial frequency, bisection versus separation) can be understood in terms of a reduced contrast sensitivity (signal-to-noise ratio) of the filters of the amblyopic eye. This notion has physiologic support from the studies of Eggers and Blakemore (1978), who showed that neurons in the cortex of kittens with experimental anisometropia have reduced contrast sensitivity. Similar results have recently been reported in monkeys reared with one eye blurred (Movshon et al. 1987).

Spatial Sampling Density

An important consideration for positional acuity is the sampling density of the mechanisms (i.e., the degree of overlap of receptive fields of a particular class). Little is known about how visual information is actually sampled by the two-dimensional array of cortical receptive fields. There is clearly a tradeoff between the need for adequate representation of various sizes, orientations, and so on and the requirement for efficiency (since there are a finite number of neurons).

A disproportionate loss or aberrant position labeling of the cortical neurons would result in critical local cues for position discrimination being missed. Thus a sparse cortical sampling grain would be expected to result in a greater loss of position acuity than grating acuity or contrast sensitivity as occurs in strabismic amblyopia. If the sampling losses were nonuniform, local spatial distortions may occur (Hess et al. 1978, Bedell and Flom 1983). Moreover, sparse sampling in the absence of changes in the sensitivity of the filters could result in losses in position sensitivity with little loss in resolution or contrast sensitivity. Figure 3.27 illustrates schematically one way in which a sparse cortical sampling grain could occur. The top row shows an array of "Mexican hat" filters with a peak spatial frequency of 15 cycles per degree, a cutoff spatial frequency of 30 cycles per degree, and a spatial sampling interval of 2 minutes. The second row shows the same filters, but they are sampled at, on average, 4-minute intervals. An image viewed through this second array would be sparsely sampled in comparison with the first array. Moreover, the spacing is inconsistent, so there may be a good deal of spatial uncertainty (as indicated by the question marks in the figure). The perceptual distortions for grating patterns illustrated in Figure 3.24 could be a consequence of the aliasing that might be expected to occur in a visual system with sparse sampling (Bradley and Thibos 1988).

An alternative scheme is one suggested recently by Blasdel (personal communication). In the normal visual cortex, repeating processing modules contain information from each eye (i.e., a left plus right ocular dominance column) and all orientations. If, as seems likely, binocular competition in strabismus leads to shrinkage of the inputs from the deviated eye, then in any given module particular orientations may not be represented. This notion makes several specific predictions that seem to be borne out by the data. First, grating acuity or contrast sensitivity should be less affected than Snellen acuity, which requires local information at all the orientations represented in the letter. Second, Vernier acuity should be markedly degraded because it relies on very localized relative orientation and position information. Third, positional acuity may be especially poor with short lines and should benefit from the addition of samples because the noise between samples along the length of lines would be uncorrelated.

A

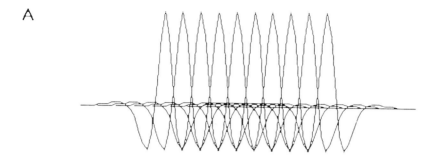

B

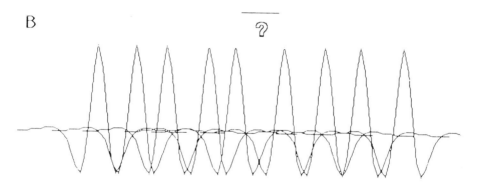

Figure 3.27 *Schematic illustration of one way in which a sparse cortical sampling grain could occur. A. Shows an array of "Mexican hat" filters with a peak spatial frequency of 15 cycles per degree, a cutoff spatial frequency of 30 cycles per degree, and a spatial sampling interval of 2 minutes. B. Shows the same filters, but now they are sampled at, on average, 4-minute intervals, and the spacing is irregular. An image viewed through this array would be sparsely sampled, and, as illustrated by the question mark, would be subject to a high degree of positional uncertainty. (Adapted from Levi 1988.)*

The Collection of Spatial Samples

In foveal vision, the image of a stimulus is spread by the optical blur function of the eye over several cones and is highly magnified in the cortex. Thus, in foveal vision, even a single dot will be sampled by many overlapping cortical receptive fields, so sparse sampling is never present. Adding samples will have little effect on the accuracy of positional information. On the other hand, in a sparsely sampled visual system, positional uncertainty should be high with a single stimulus sample, and adding samples would be expected to reduce positional uncertainty in proportion to the square root of the number of samples. Figure 3.28 shows the results of an experiment performed to examine this question. Levi and Klein (1986) measured bisection thresholds for stimuli comprised of discrete

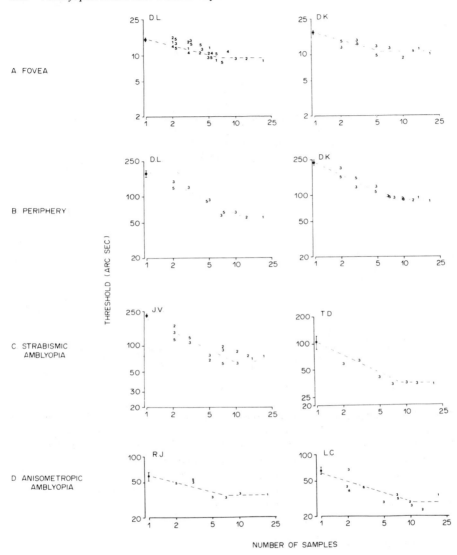

Figure 3.28 *Bisection thresholds for stimuli comprised of discrete samples (dots) are plotted as a function of the number of samples (resolvable dots) comprising the stimulus. For the normal fovea (A) and for anisometropic amblyopes (D), adding samples (up to about 5) resulted in only a small improvement in thresholds. However, for strabismic amblyopes (C), thresholds were very high with 1 sample (showing marked intrinsic positional uncertainty in the absence of spatial and temporal averaging), and adding samples (up to about 10) resulted in a marked improvement in performance in proportion to the square root of the number of samples. Similar data were obtained at 2.5 degrees in the normal periphery. (From Levi et al. 1987.)*

samples (dots). For the normal fovea (*A*) and for anisometropic amblyopes (*D*), adding samples (up to about 5) resulted in only a small improvement in thresholds. However, for strabismic amblyopes (*C*), thresholds were very high with 1 sample (showing marked intrinsic positional uncertainty in the absence of spatial and temporal averaging), and adding samples (up to about 10) resulted in a marked improvement in performance in proportion to the square root of the number of samples. Very similar results were obtained in the normal periphery (*B*) (Levi, Klein, and Yap 1987).

Disorder of the Topographic Mapping of Visual Space

In the normal mammalian visual system, visual space is topographically mapped in a highly ordered manner at a number of levels along the visual pathway. Disorder of the spatial metric would be expected to exert a profound influence on visual processing of positional information. This notion has been suggested by Hess (1982). Scrambling of the spatial metric would likely have a marked effect on positional acuity and Snellen acuity (where local spatial relationships are critical) but should have less influence on resolution or contrast sensitivity. It is quite likely that disorder of the spatial metric may be a consequence of abnormal spatial sampling. Recently, Wilson (1986b) has attempted to model the hyperacuity of amblyopes. He found that the data for strabismic amblyopes could be quantitatively modeled by assuming both spatial undersampling and positional uncertainty, while that for anisometropic amblyopes was modeled by a reduced gain of the small cortical receptive fields.

 ## Summary

Amblyopia is characterized by marked spatial uncertainty (inprecision). The inability of amblyopes to judge relative position, width, and orientation is most marked under conditions where normal observers perform best, that is, when the features are close together. In anisometropic amblyopia, the loss of positional information is commensurate with the reduced resolution and contrast sensitivity of the amblyopic eye. In contrast, strabismic amblyopes show an extra loss in positional acuity, often accompanied by aberrations of space perception. The losses in the precision of spatial judgments are closely linked with the amblyopes' Snellen acuity.

It is likely that the high precision of spatial judgments in normal foveal vision is the outcome of mechanisms that have the more general task of form/pattern discrimination. Thus the studies described earlier provide a psychophysical window into the neural mechanisms of form perception in amblyopia.

In anisometropic amblyopes, it is hypothesized that the reduced positional acuity and resolution share a common basis, that is, the reduced contrast sensitivity (signal-to-noise ratio) of the spatial filters of the amblyopic eye. In strabismic amblyopia, a more tenable hypothesis is that sparse spatial sampling due to loss of neurons or scrambling of their signals may account for the high degree of intrinsic positional uncertainty.

4. AMBLYOPIA AND PERIPHERAL VISION

Analogies between the performance of the normal periphery and the central field of amblyopes appear frequently in the literature. For example, acuity is degraded in both visual systems, and contour interaction extends over greater distances (Flom et al. 1963). Spatial summation of contrast extends over larger distances (Miller 1955, Grosvenor 1957, Flynn 1967), and contrast detection (Katz et al. 1984) and discrimination (Bradley and Ozhawa 1986) are similarly reduced in both visual systems.

There is now considerable evidence that for a variety of detection and resolution tasks, central and peripheral vision are similar when the stimulus dimensions are appropriately scaled (Koenderink et al. 1978, Rovamo et al. 1978, Limb and Rubenstein 1977, Swanson and Wilson 1985). This notion is illustrated schematically in Figure 3.29*A*, which shows idealized contrast sensitivity functions obtained in central and peripheral vision with appropriate scaling. The important point here is that the peak contrast sensitivity is similar at both loci, and a single scale factor (shown by the arrows) suffices to superimpose both curves (and the underlying filters). Data such as these have been reported by a number of investigators, and the scale factor needed to superimpose curves obtained at the fovea and at 7.5 degrees is estimated to be between 2 and 4 (Swanson and Wilson 1985). This scale factor is similar to the variation in cone separation (within the central 10 degrees) with eccentricity.

Figure 3.29*B* shows the contrast sensitivity function for each eye of a strabismic and anisometropic amblyope. For testing the amblyopic eye, the field size was scaled in proportion to the observers cutoff spatial frequency. The data for the amblyopic eye are similar to the schematic shown in Figure 3.29*A* for the normal periphery. In particular, the peak sensitivities of the two eyes are equal, and second, a single scale factor (1.5) suffices to superimpose the two curves.

Similarly, Vernier acuity and its associated crowding effects are similar in central and peripheral vision when scaled according to the cortical magnification factor (i.e., the number of millimeters of cortex devoted to each degree of visual space; the cortical magnification factor specifies the cortical sampling grain). It should be noted, however, that the scale factor for position acuity is quite different from that for contrast sensitivity/grating acuity. Figure 3.30 from Levi et al. (1985) illustrates that not all functions fall off at the same rate with eccentricity. It is only when comparing performance on two tasks with *different*

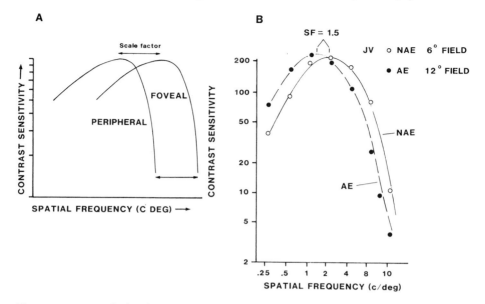

Figure 3.29   (A) *Idealized contrast sensitivity functions obtained in central and peripheral vision with appropriate scaling. The important point here is that the peak contrast sensitivity is similar at both loci, and a single scale factor (arrows) suffices to superimpose both curves (and the underlying filters). (B) The contrast sensitivity function for each eye of a strabismic and anisometropic amblyope is shown. For testing the amblyopic eye, the field size was scaled in proportion to the observers cutoff spatial frequency. The data for the amblyopic eye are similar to the schematic shown in (A) for the normal periphery. First, the peak sensitivities of the two eyes are equal, and second, a single scale factor (1.5) suffices to superimpose the two curves. (From Levi et al. 1987.)*

scales (e.g., position acuity and grating acuity) that one can clearly distinguish central and peripheral vision.

In comparing grating acuity versus position acuity in amblyopes (Figure 22), it can now be seen that the data for strabismic amblyopes are similar to the normal periphery (the *solid lines* are data for the periphery), while the results for anisometropic amblyopes are not.

What is the link between strabismic amblyopia and peripheral vision? In strabismic amblyopia and in the normal periphery, positional acuity is worse than would be predicted from the reduced resolution, contrast sensitivity, or suprathreshold contrast response and cannot be simply mimicked by optical blurring (Bedell et al. 1985). Moreover, both the normal periphery and strabismic amblyopes show similar spatial benefit from the addition of samples (Figure 3.28), suggesting that both these visual systems may be sparsely sampled. In the normal periphery, sparse sampling has its basis in the reduction of cone density and cortical magnification with eccentricity. In strabismic amblyopia, similar functional

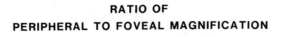

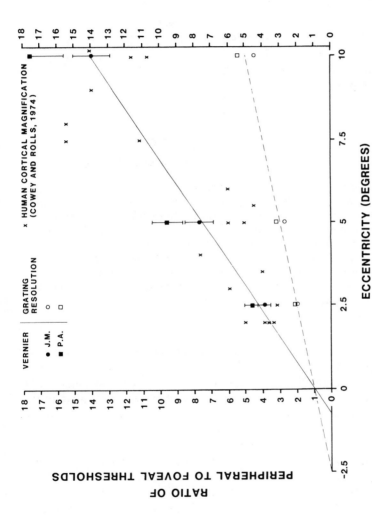

Figure 3.30   *This figure illustrates schematically that not all functions fall off at the same rate with eccentricity. Plotted here are the ratio of peripheral to foveal thresholds for grating acuity (open symbols) and Vernier acuity (filled symbols) against eccentricity. In each case, the foveal thresholds have been normalized to a value of 1. The dashed line, which provides a reasonable fit to the grating acuity data, shows the variation in cone separation (Rolls and Cowey 1970), while the solid line shows the variation in the inverse cortical magnification factor (reanalyzed from the data of Dow et al. 1981). (From Levi et al. 1985.)*

losses may result from a loss of cortical neurons and/or a scrambling of their connections as a consequence of abnormal binocular interaction.

5. TEMPORAL PROCESSING IN THE AMBLYOPIC VISUAL SYSTEM

While amblyopia is typically characterized as an anomaly of spatial vision, a large number of studies have addressed the question of temporal processing in amblyopia. In this section several aspects of the temporal processing of amblyopic eyes will be discussed.

5A. Temporal Resolution

Many early studies were concerned with the *critical fusion frequency* (CFF) of the amblyopic eye, that is, the highest flicker rate at which an intermittent stimulus appears to just flicker. The results of these studies are somewhat contradictory. For example, Feinberg (1956) found a significant and consistent reduction in the CFF of his subjects. Alpern et al. (1960) found rather smaller losses, and Miles (1949) actually found CFF to be superior in the amblyopic eye of about half his sample. Thus CFF is sometimes but not always reduced in amblyopic eyes, and the losses are generally quite small. This is not really surprising, considering that the stimuli used for measuring CFF generally have a lot of low spatial frequency information. Although CFF represents one limit of temporal resolution, it is in many respects analogous to the measurement of visual acuity in the spatial domain.

5B. Temporal Contrast Sensitivity

A more complete description of temporal processing may be obtained by measuring the *temporal contrast sensitivity function* (de Lange function), that is, 1 over the threshold contrast needed to detect temporal variations in a uniform field over a wide range of temporal frequencies (de Lange 1958). Since the stimulus is temporally modulated about a constant mean luminance level, adaptation level is easily controlled.

The temporal contrast sensitivity of amblyopic eyes also shows considerable between-subject variation. For example, substantial losses in the temporal contrast sensitivity function of the amblyopic eye, particularly at low temporal frequencies, were observed in some studies (e.g., Wesson and Loop 1982, Spekreijse et al. 1972), while little or no loss was evident in other studies. For example, Manny and Levi (1982a) found small losses in about half their population. These losses were most prominent at low temporal frequencies and were found to depend on both the adaptation level (they normalize at low luminance levels) and the field size.

Bradley and Freeman (1985b) have addressed the question of field size in more detail. Figure 3.31, from Bradley and Freeman (1985b), shows their analysis of data from seven studies of flicker sensitivity. Plotted here is the amblyopic deficit (a ratio of 1 shows no deficit; a ratio of 2 shows a twofold loss) versus field size. The results clearly show an inverse relationship between the stimulus size and the observed deficits. Small deficits in CFF (open symbols) and temporal contrast sensitivity (filled symbols) were found with large stimuli (e.g., Manny and Levi 1982a), while large deficits in CFF (e.g., Feinberg 1956) or temporal contrast sensitivity (Wesson and Loop 1982) were found with small targets. The results shown in Figure 3.31 represent the mean data, averaged across subjects, from each of the studies and therefore do not reveal marked individual variations. However, the results make it clear that much of the deficit in "temporal" processing of amblyopes revealed by uniform field flicker studies is a consequence of the spatial parameters of the stimulus. Thus a more informative approach is to examine spatiotemporal processing in the amblyopic visual system.

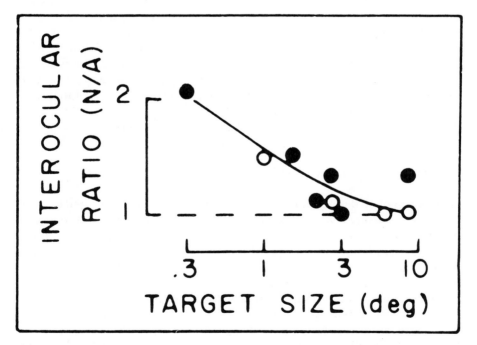

Figure 3.31 *Interocular ratios are given for temporal contrast sensitivity (filled circles) and CFF (open circles). Ratios are plotted against field size (a ratio of 1 shows no deficit; a ratio of 2 shows a twofold loss). The results from seven studies of flicker sensitivity clearly show an inverse relationship between the stimulus size and the observed deficits. (From Bradley and Freeman 1985b.)*

5C. Spatiotemporal Contrast Sensitivity in Amblyopia

One method for examining spatiotemporal processing in amblyopic vision is to determine contrast thresholds for detecting sine-wave gratings that are either flickering or drifting at different rates. If the loss is critically dependent on only the spatial parameters of the stimulus, then variations in temporal frequency should have little or no effect on the degree of loss. The results from several such studies (Manny and Levi 1982b, Schor and Levi 1980a, Bradley and Freeman 1985b) are summarized schematically in Figure 3.32, which shows how the contrast sensitivity deficit varies with both spatial and temporal frequency. This figure represents a spatiotemporal visuogram and illustrates schematically the two patterns of loss that have been observed. For some amblyopes, the contrast sensitivity deficit depends only on spatial frequency (for example, in Manny and Levi's population, all the anisometropic amblyopes and one strabismic amblyope showed this pattern of

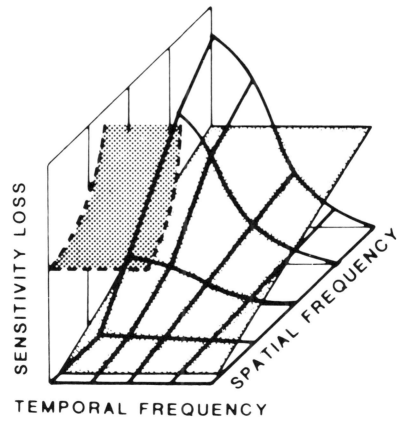

Figure 3.32   *Schematic representation of the loss in sensitivity as a function of spatial and temporal frequency for various amblyopes. (From Manny and Levi 1982b.)*

loss), illustrated by the shaded surface. For other amblyopes, the pattern of loss is highly dependent on both spatial and temporal frequency, illustrated by the unshaded surface. For these amblyopes, the deficits are most marked at high spatial frequencies and low temporal frequencies. This result suggests that for some amblyopes there is a distinct spatiotemporal pattern of loss. How can the temporal frequency specificity of this pattern be explained? One hypothesis is that the apparent temporal frequency specificity is due to the abnormal fixational eye movements of amblyopes. For example, Bradley and Freeman (1985b) have argued that the rapid drifts transiently reduce the temporal modulation on the retina, thereby enhancing sensitivity at low temporal frequencies. Schor and Levi (1980a and b) and Manny and Levi (1982b) recorded eye movements in several subjects while viewing such stimuli and concluded that abnormal eye movements could not account for the temporal frequency–dependent pattern of loss (i.e., some subjects with quite steady fixation demonstrated substantial losses of temporal contrast sensitivity). An alternative explanation is based on the findings that in normal vision, temporal processing is subserved by more than one mechanism. While spatial contrast sensitivity is determined by the responses of many, relatively narrowly tuned mechanisms, temporal sensitivity appears to be subserved by a small number of mechanisms with broad temporal bandwidths (Watson and Robson 1981). For stimuli with spatial frequencies above about 1 cycle per degree, there may be only two mechanisms, while for lower spatial frequencies there may be an additional high temporal frequency mechanism. Thus, it is plausible that there could be a selective loss of one temporal frequency mechanism in amblyopia. There is indirect evidence that these mechanisms develop at different rates. Based on developmental changes in the visually evoked potential, Orel-Bixler and Norcia (personal communication) have suggested that the higher temporal frequency mechanisms develop early, while the lower temporal frequency mechanisms (which have better spatial resolution) develop later. This idea is also consistent with the rapid development of CFF in infants (Regal 1981). Thus selective losses at high spatial and low temporal frequencies may indeed reflect neural deficits that depend on the age of onset of the amblyopic condition. Below we argue that processing of time and space are inseparable and that the high spatial/low temporal frequency loss reflects a loss of slow-velocity motion-sensitive mechanisms.

A selective loss of low temporal frequency sensitivity could account for several aspects of spatiotemporal processing in amblyopic eyes. For example, this pattern is consistent with the finding of normal or near normal CFF with reduced sensitivity to low rates of temporal modulation or drift. Moreover, amblyopes frequently report difficulty in discerning the temporal change (flicker or apparent motion) in drifting or counterphase gratings at high spatial and low temporal frequencies (Manny and Levi 1982b; Schor and Levi 1980a).

5D. Temporal Hyperacuity

Simultaneity Detection

If two closely spaced lines are presented with a temporal onset asynchrony of just a few milliseconds, normal observers can easily detect that they were not simultaneous and can tell which line was presented first (i.e., they can discriminate the temporal order). Since the temporal asynchrony thresholds obtained are smaller than would be predicted by the temporal resolution of the visual system (i.e., the CFF), this represents a temporal hyperacuity, by analogy to spatial hyperacuity. The cue in this simultaneity task is the direction of apparent motion of the lines, and this may be equivalent to detecting a fast velocity of motion. Thus, to the extent that this simultaneity task involves mechanisms that respond to fast velocities, amblyopes should show little difficulty in performing the task. Recently, Steinman et al. (1988) tested the simultaneity discrimination of amblyopes. Their results showed that strabismic and anisometropic amblyopes have little or no difficulty in performing these tasks with either eye as long as the lines are separated by about three times their resolution limit (similar to the results of normal subjects).

Asynchrony Discrimination

If two lines are presented with a fixed "reference" asynchrony of 30 to 50 ms, normal observers can accurately judge whether a second line pair had a longer or shorter asynchrony. In normal foveal vision, the threshold for asynchrony discrimination under these conditions is also a temporal hyperacuity, yielding thresholds as low as 3 ms (McKee and Taylor 1984). This task differs from the simultaneity task described earlier in that it likely involves slow-velocity mechanisms. Thus, to the extent that asynchrony discrimination is analogous to slow velocity discrimination, amblyopes would be expected to perform poorly when viewing with their amblyopic eyes. This is exactly the pattern that Steinman et al. (1988) observed. Amblyopes show little or no loss for detection of simultaneity but substantial loss in discriminating asynchronies of 30 to 50 ms. Moreover, Steinman et al. (1988) found that amblyopes can accurately discriminate between two fast velocities (> 10 degrees per second) with their amblyopic eye. For the amblyopic eye, like that of the normal, $\Delta V/V$ (the Weber fraction for velocity discrimination) is about 5%. On the other hand, the ability to discriminate slow velocities (< 5 degrees per second) is markedly impaired in the amblyopic eye. Steinman et al. found that the optimal temporal asynchrony threshold of the amblyopic eye was directly and *linearly* (i.e., a slope of 1 on log-log coordinates) related to the observers' resolution limit. Amblyopic eyes demonstrate increased horizontal drift during attempted fixation, and the magnitude of the drift is correlated with visual acuity (Ciuffreda et al. 1980). Thus one possible reason for the abnormal velocity discrimination is that there is summation between the amblyopic eye's drift velocity (about 0.5 to 1.5 degrees per second) and the stimulus velocity. This would have a large effect at slow, but not at fast velocities. This seems unlikely to account for the results found by Steinman et al., since similar losses occurred for both nasalward and temporalward motion, as well as for upward and downward motion. Moreover, the losses occurred with stimulus durations too brief for tracking eye movements. Therefore, Steinman et al. (1988) suggested a sensory explanation for the deficit. Specifically, they argued that the processing of space and time are inseparably linked in the human visual system by velocity-sensitive mechanisms and that temporal thresholds simply reflect the activity of these motion-detecting mechanisms. Thus the degradation of temporal processing is a consequence of the effect of abnormal visual experience on motion or velocity processing mechanisms. In normal vision, slow velocities depend on mechanisms with small receptive fields (Koenderink et al. 1985, McKee et al. 1986). Only the normal fovea is sensitive to slow velocities (Koenderink et al. 1985, Steinman et al. 1988). The amblyopic eye is characterized by reduced spatial resolution, presumably resulting from a loss of small receptive fields. This reduced contribution of small receptive fields in the amblyopic fovea would be expected to result in the loss of sensitivity to low velocities. Thus temporal and motion thresholds *indirectly* reflect the spatial resolution of the amblyopic eyes of *both* strabismic and anisometropic amblyopes. Apparently, the spatial distortions and undersampling evident in the strabismic amblyopes' positional judgments do not produce further motion deficits in strabismic amblyopes. This conclusion is further supported by the results of Levi et al. (1984), who measured instantaneous motion (displacement) thresholds. Their results, shown in Figure 3.33, also show the 1:1 correspondence between motion-displacement thresholds of strabismic and anisometropic amblyopes and their grating acuity. It would be interesting to know to what extent the poor tracking eye movements of amblyopes found at slow target velocities (see Chapter 5) may be, at least in part, a consequence of a reduced sensitivity to slow velocities.

6. RESPONSE LATENCY AND SPATIOTEMPORAL INTERACTION

6A. Simple ReactionTime

Both eye-hand (Mackensen 1958, von Noorden 1961) and saccadic (Ciuffreda et al. 1978) reaction times (RTs) can be prolonged in the amblyopic eye. More recently, Hamasaki and Flynn (1981) showed a correlation between the delay in reaction time to an annulus of light and the reduction in visual acuity in the amblyopic eye. Amblyopes with the poorest acuity were most likely to show prolonged RTs. These experiments and studies of "perceptual blanking" in amblyopic eyes (von Noorden and Burian 1960) have been frequently interpreted in terms of increased latency of neural mechanisms in the amblyopic retina (Hamasaki and Flynn 1981) or cortex (von Noorden 1980). Since the finding of prolonged neural latencies may be important for an understanding of amblyopia, Levi et al. (1979) examined reaction time to grating patterns. The circles in Figure 3.34 show how RT for each eye of an anisometropic amblyope

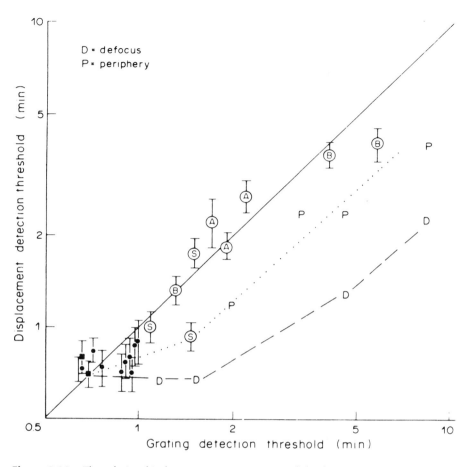

Figure 3.33 *The relationship between grating acuity and displacement detection thresholds for normal observers (squares), preferred eyes of amblyopes (circles), and amblyopic eyes of observers with strabismus (S), anisometropia (A) and both (B).*

depends on the spatial frequency of a high-contrast (44%) grating. At low spatial frequencies RTs are similar in the two eyes; at higher spatial frequencies (8 cycles per degree and greater) the difference in RT of the two eyes approaches 100 msec. A similar trend is also seen in the VEP latency (increased phase lag) of the two eyes, as shown by the diamonds in Figure 3.34. Figure 3.35, from Loshin and Levi (1983), shows how RT for a fixed spatial frequency depends on grating contrast. The results of three amblyopes, one with strabismus and anisometropia (J.V.), one with anisometropia (D.S.), and one with strabismus (J.M.) are shown. For each eye of both observers, RT decreases as stimulus contrast increases. At low contrast levels, the curves for the two eyes diverge, showing differences in RT of several hundred milliseconds, while at higher

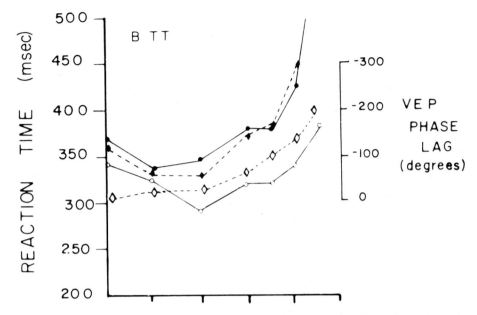

Figure 3.34   *The circles show that RT for each eye of an anisometropic amblyope depends on the spatial frequency of a high-contrast (44%) grating. Open and filled symbols are for the preferred and amblyopic eyes, respectively. At low spatial frequencies, RTs are similar in the two eyes; at higher spatial frequencies (8 cycles per degree and greater), the difference in RT of the two eyes approaches 100 msec. A similar trend is also seen in the VEP latency (increased phase lag) of the two eyes, as shown by the diamonds. (From Levi et al. 1979.)*

contrast levels, the RTs of the two eyes are quite similar. As was the case for contrast discrimination (Figures 3.14 and 3.15), expressing the contrast in threshold rather than stimulus units more or less equates the curves of the two eyes. Taken together, these results suggest that the increased reaction time found in amblyopic eyes does not reflect a fixed neural delay, but rather reflects the contrast-threshold deficit of the amblyopic eye. Stimuli with equal effective contrast (i.e., the same number of units above threshold) give equal RTs in the amblyopic and preferred eyes. This explanation also helps clarify the relationship between the acuity deficit and the RT delay found by Hamasaki and Flynn (1981). Amblyopes with the poorest acuity will show the most marked losses in contrast sensitivity and therefore the most prolonged RTs.

The RT results also provide evidence for a failure of suprathreshold contrast compensation in amblyopic eyes. The "effective" contrast of the stimuli (in terms of providing equal RTs in the two eyes) is related to the threshold for each eye. This is consistent with data from evoked potentials and contrast discrimination (discussed in the section on suprathreshold contrast perception) and may be understood in terms of current RT models (e.g., Luce and Green 1972;

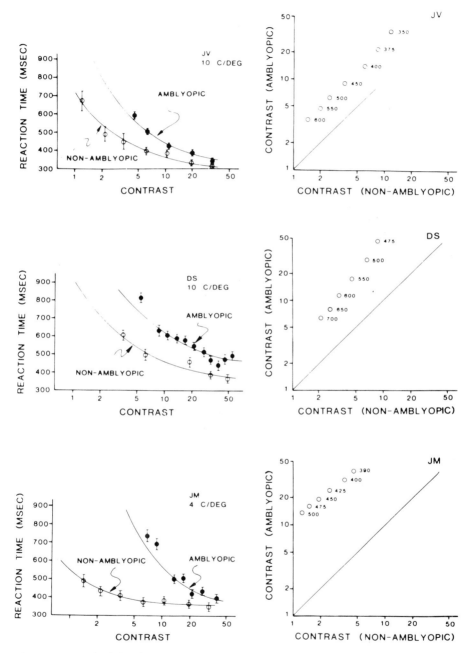

Figure 3.35   *The left column shows mean RT versus contrast for both the nonamblyopic (open circles) and amblyopic (filled circles) eyes of three observers. The right column shows the contrast required by each eye (amblyopic, ordinate; nonamblyopic, abscissa) to produce equal-criterion RTs (shown beside the data). (From Loshin and Levi 1983.)*

McGill 1963). In these models, sensory events lead to the accumulation of inputs at a "decision center," and when some criterion number of inputs is exceeded, a response is triggered. In an amblyopic eye, a reduced number of inputs to the decision center (due to fewer effective neurons driven through the amblyopic eye) would result in prolonged RT, particularly at low contrast levels.

Summary

Amblyopes show abnormalities in spatiotemporal processing that can be largely understood in terms of the reduced spatial contrast sensitivity of the amblyopic eye. Thus amblyopes show either small or no losses for large uniform fields or low spatial frequency gratings flickering rapidly. However, they do show reduced sensitivity for small fields and for high spatial frequencies, and these losses are most pronounced at low temporal frequencies. Whether this temporal dependence is a result of abnormal eye movements or a selective loss of slow mechanisms is still a matter of controversy. In addition, amblyopes show normal velocity discrimination for high velocities but poor velocity discrimination for slow velocities, a finding that may bear on their reduced ability to track slowly drifting targets.

REFERENCES

Alpern M, Flitman DB, Joseph RH. (1960) Centrally fixed flicker thresholds in amblyopia. *Am. J. Ophthalmol.* 49:1194–1202.

Amman E. (1921) Einige Beobachtunger bei den Funktionsprufungen in der Sprechstunde: "Zentrales" Sehen-Sehen der Glaukomatosen-Sehen der Amblyopen. *Klin. Monatsbl. Augenheilkd.* 66:564–73.

Badcock DR. (1984) How do we discriminate relative spatial phase? *Vision Res.* 24:1847–57.

Barbeito R, Bedell HE, Flom MC, Simpson TL. (1987) Effects of luminance on the visual acuity of strabismic and anisometropic amblyopes and optically blurred normals. *Vision Res.* 27:1543–9.

Barlow HB. (1979) Reconstructing the visual image in space and time. *Nature* 279:189–90.

Barlow HB. (1981) Critical limiting factors in the design of the eye and visual cortex. *Proc. R. Soc. Lond. [Biol.]* 212:1–34.

Bedell HE. (1980) Central and peripheral retinal photoreceptor orientation in amblyopic eyes as assessed by the psychophysical Stiles-Crawford effect. *Invest. Ophthalmol. Vis. Sci.* 19:49–59.

Bedell HE. (1982) Symmetry of acuity profiles in esotropic amblyopic eyes. *Hum. Neurobiol.* 1:221–4.

Bedell HE, Flom MC. (1981) Monocular spatial distortion in strabismic amblyopia. *Invest. Ophthalmol. Vis. Sci.* 20:26–8.

Bedell HE, Flom MC. (1983) Normal and abnormal space perception. *Am. J. Optom. Physiol. Opt.* 60:426–35.

Bedell HE, Flom MC, Barbeito R. (1985) Spatial aberrations and acuity in strabismus and amblyopia. *Invest. Ophthalmol. Vis. Sci.* 26:909–16.

Bisti S, Carmignoto G. (1986) Monocular deprivation in kittens differentially affects crossed and uncrossed visual pathways. *Vision Res.* 26:875–84.

Bjerrum J. (1884) Untersuchungen uber den Lichtsinn und den Raumsinn bei verschiedenen Augenkrankheiten. *Arch. Ophthalmol.* 30:201.

Braddick O, Campbell FW, Atkinson J. (1978) Channels in Vision: Basic Aspects. In Held R, Leibowitz HW, Teuber HL (Eds.), *Handbook of Sensory Physiology*, Vol. 7: *Perception*, pp. 3–38. New York: Springer-Verlag.

Bradley A, Freeman RD. (1981) Contrast sensitivity in anisometropic amblyopia. *Invest. Ophthalmol. Vis. Sci.* 21:467–76.

Bradley A, Freeman RD. (1985a) Is reduced Vernier acuity in amblyopia due to position, contrast or fixation deficits? *Vision Res.* 25:55–66.

Bradley A, Freeman RD. (1985b) Temporal sensitivity in amblyopia: An explanation of conflicting reports. *Vision Res.* 25:39–46.

Bradley A, Ozhawa I. (1986) A comparison of contrast detection and discrimination. *Vision Res.* 26:991–8.

Bradley A, Thibos L. (1988) Perceptual aliasing in human amblyopia. *Invest. Ophthalmol. Vis. Sci.* 27:1404–9.

Bradley A, Dahlman C, Switkes E, De Valois K. (1986) A comparison of color and luminance discrimination in amblyopia. *Invest. Ophthalmol. Vis. Sci.* 29(Suppl.):76.

Bradley A, Freeman RD, Appelgate R. (1985) Is amblyopia spatial frequency specific or retinal locus specific? *Vision Res.* 25:47–54.

Brettel H, Caelli T, Hilz R, Rentschler I. (1982) Modeling perceptual distortion: Amplitude and phase transmission in the human visual system. *Hum. Neurobiol.* 1:61–7.

Burian HM. (1967) The behavior of the amblyopic eye under reduced illumination and the theory of functional amblyopia. *Doc. Ophthalmol.* 23:189–202.

Butler T, Westheimer G. (1978) Interference with stereoscopic acuity: Spatial, temporal, and disparity tuning. *Vision Res.* 18:1387–92.

Caloroso E, Flom MC. (1969) Visual acuity in amblyopia: Influence of luminance on visual acuity in amblyopia. *Am. J. Optom. Physiol. Opt.* 46:189–95.

Campbell FW, Green DG. (1965) Optical and retinal factors affecting visual resolution. *J. Physiol. (Lond.)* 181:576–93.

Campbell FW, Gregory AH. (1960) The spatial resolving power of the human retina with oblique incidence (Letter). *J. Opt. Soc. Am.* 50:831.

Campbell FW, Robson JG. (1968) Application of Fourier analysis to the visibility of gratings. *J. Physiol. (Lond.)* 197:551–66.

Ciuffreda KJ, Fisher SK. (1987) Impairment of contrast discrimination in amblyopic eyes. *Ophthalmic. Physiol. Opt.* 7:461–7.

Ciuffreda KJ, Kenyon RV, Stark L. (1978) Increased saccadic latencies in amblyopic eyes. *Invest. Ophthalmol. Vis. Sci.* 17:697–702.

Ciuffreda KJ, Kenyon RV, Stark L. (1980) Increased drift in amblyopic eyes. *Br. J. Ophthalmol.* 64:7–14.

Coletta NJ, Williams DR. (1987) Psychophysical estimate of extrafoveal cone spacing. *J. Opt. Soc. Am. [A]* 4:1503–13.

De Lange H. (1958) Research into the dynamic nature of the human fovea-cortex systems with intermittent and modulated light: I. Attenuation characteristics with white and modulated light. *J. Opt. Soc. Am.* 48:777–84.

De Valois RL, Albrecht DG, Thorell LG. (1982) Spatial frequency selectivity of cells in macaque visual cortex. *Vision Res.* 22:545–59.

Dow BM, Snyder RG, Vautin RG, Bauer R. (1981) Magnification factor and receptive field size in foveal striate cortex of the monkey. *Exp. Brain Res.* 44:213–28.

D'Zmura M, Lennie P. (1986) Shared pathways for rod and cone vision. *Vision Res.* 26:1273–80.

Eggers HM, Blakemore C. (1978) Physiological basis of anisometropic amblyopia. *Science* 201:262–67.

Enoch JM. (1957) Amblyopia and the Stiles-Crawford effect. *Am. J. Optom.* 34:298–309.

Enoch JM. (1967) The current status of receptor amblyopia. *Doc. Ophthalmol.* 23:130–148.

Fankhauser F, Rohler R. (1967) The physical stimulus, the quality of the retinal image and foveal brightness discrimination in one amblyopic and two normal eyes. *Doc. Ophthalmol.* 23:149–84.

Feinberg I. (1956) Critical flicker frequency in amblyopia ex anopsia. *Am. J. Ophthalmol.* 42:473–81.

Flom MC, Weymouth FW, Kahnemann D. (1963) Visual resolution and contour interaction. *J. Opt. Soc. Am.* 53:1026–32.

Flynn JT. (1967) Spatial summation in amblyopia. *Arch. Ophthalmol.* 78:470–4.

France TD. (1984) Amblyopia update: Diagnosis and therapy. *Am. J. Orthopt.* 34:4–12.

Francois J, Verriest G. (1967) La discrimination chromatique dans l'amblyopie strabique. *Doc. Ophthalmol.* 23:318.

Georgeson M, Sullivan GD. (1975) Contrast constancy: Deblurring in human vision by spatial frequency channels. *J. Physiol. (Lond.)* 252:627–56.

Graham N. (1980) Spatial Frequency Channels in Human Vision: Detecting Edges without Edge Detectors. In Harris C (Ed.), *Visual Coding and Adaptability*, pp. 215–62. Hillsdale, N.J.: Erlbaum Press.

Green DG. (1986) The search for the site of visual adaptation. *Vision Res.* 26:1417–29.

Grosvenor T. (1957) The effects of duration and background luminance upon the brightness discrimination of an amblyope. *Am. J. Optom. Physiol. Opt.* 34:634–63.

Gstalder RJ, Green DG. (1971) Laser interferometric acuity in amblyopia. *J. Pediatr. Ophthalmol.* 8:251–6.

Hamasaki DI, Flynn JT. (1981) Amblyopic eyes have longer reaction times. *Invest. Ophthalmol. Vis. Sci.* 21:846–53.

Harwerth RS, Levi DM. (1977) Increment threshold sensitivity in anisometropic amblyopia. *Vision Res.* 17:585–90.

Harwerth RS, Levi DM. (1978) A sensory mechanism for amblyopia: Psychophysical studies. *Am. J. Optom. Physiol. Opt.* 55:151–62.

Harwerth RS, Smith EL, Okundaye OJ. (1983) Oblique, vertical and meridional amblyopia in monkeys. *Exp. Brain Res.* 53:142–50.

Hecht S, Mintz EU. (1939) The visibility of single lines of various illuminations and the retinal basis of visual resolution. *J. Gen. Physiol.* 22:593–612.

Hess RF. (1980) A preliminary investigation of neural function and dysfunction in amblyopia: I. Size-selective channels. *Vision Res.* 20:749–54.

Hess RF. (1982) Developmental sensory impairment: Amblyopia or tarachopia? *Hum. Neurobiol.* 1:17–29.

Hess RF, Bradley A. (1980) Contrast perception above threshold is only minimally impaired in human amblyopia. *Nature* 287:463–4.

Hess RF, Howell ER. (1977) The threshold contrast sensitivity function in strabismic amblyopia: Evidence for a two-type classification. *Vision Res.* 17:1049–55.

Hess RF, Jacobs RJ. (1979) A preliminary report of acuity and contour interactions across the amblyope's visual field. *Vision Res.* 19:1403–8.

Hess RF, Pointer JS. (1985) Differences in the neural basis of human amblyopias: The distribution of the anomaly across the visual field. *Vision Res.* 25:1577–94.

Hess RF, Pointer JS. (1987) Evidence for spatially local computations underlying discriminations of periodic patterns in fovea and periphery. *Vision Res.* 27:1343–60.

Hess RF, Smith G. (1977) Do optical aberrations contribute to visual loss in strabismic amblyopia? *Am. J. Optom. Physiol. Opt.* 54:627–33.

Hess RF, Bradley A, Piotrowski L. (1983) Contrast coding in amblyopia: I: Differences in the neural basis of human amblyopia. *Proc. R. Soc. Lond. [Biol.]* 217:309–30.

Hess RF, Campbell FW, Greenhalgh T. (1978) On the nature of the neural abnormality in human amblyopia: Neural aberrations and neural sensitivity loss. *Pflugers Arch.* 377:201–7.

Hess RF, Campbell FW, Zimmern R. (1980) Differences in the neural basis of human amblyopias: the effects of mean luminance. *Vision Res.* 20:295–305.

Higgins KE, Daugmann JG, Mansfield RJW. (1982) Amblyopic contrast sensitivity: Insensitivity to unsteady fixation. *Invest. Ophthalmol. Vis. Sci.* 23:113–20.

Hilz R, Rentschler I, Brettel H. (1977) Myopia and strabismic amblyopia: Substantial differences in human visual development. *Exp. Brain Res.* 30:445–6.

Hitchcock B, Hickey T. (1980) Ocular dominance columns: Evidence for their presence in humans. *Brain Res.* 182:176–9.

Hubel DH, Wiesel TN. (1974) Uniformity of monkey striate cortex: A parallel relationship between field size, scatter, and magnification factor. *J. Comp. Neurol.* 158:295–306.

Irvine SR. (1948) Amblyopia-exanopsia: Observations on retinal inhibition, scotoma, projection, light difference discrimination and visual acuity. *Trans. Am. Ophthalmol. Soc.* 46:527–75.

Jampolsky A. (1955) Characteristics of suppression in strabismus. *Arch. Ophthalmol.* 54:683–96.

Jampolsky A, Flom BC, Weymouth FW, Moses LE. (1955) Unequal corrected visual acuity as related to anisometropia. *Arch. Ophthalmol.* 54:893–905.

Jennings JAM, Charman WN. (1981) Off-axis image quality in the human eye. *Vision Res.* 21:445–55.

Kaplan E, Shapley RM. (1982) X and Y cells in the lateral geniculate nucleus of macaque monkeys. *J. Physiol. (Lond.)* 330:125–43.

Katz LM, Levi DM, Bedell HE. (1984) Central and peripheral contrast sensitivity in amblyopia with varying field size. *Doc. Ophthalmol.* 58:351–73.

Kirschen DA, Flom MC. (1978) Visual acuity at different retinal loci of eccentrically fixating functional amblyopes. *Am. J. Optom. Physiol. Opt.* 55:144–50.

Klein SA, Levi DM. (1985) Hyperacuity thresholds of 1 second: Quantitative predictions and empirical validation. *J. Opt. Soc. Am. [A]* 2:1170–90.

Klein SA, Levi DM. (1986) Local multipoles for measuring contrast and phase sensitivity. *Invest. Ophthalmol. Vis. Sci.* 27(Suppl.):225.

Klein SA, Levi DM. (1987) Position sense of the peripheral retina. *J. Opt. Soc. Am. [A]* 4:1543–53.

Koenderink JJ, Bouman MA, Bueno de Mesquita AE, Slappendel S. (1978) Perimetry of contrast detection thresholds of moving sine wave patterns. *J. Opt. Soc. Am. [A]* 68:845–65.

Koenderink JJ, van Doorn AJ, van de Grind WA. (1985) Spatial and temporal parameters of motion detection in the peripheral visual field. *J. Opt. Soc. Am. [A]* 2:252–9.

Kulikowski JJ, King-Smith PE. (1973) Spatial arrangement of line, edge and grating detectors as revealed by subthreshold summation. *Vision Res.* 13:1455–78.

Lawden MC. (1982) The analysis of spatial phase in amblyopia. *Hum. Neurobiol.* 1:55–60.

Lawden MC, Hess RF, Campbell FW. (1982) The discriminability of spatial phase relationships in amblyopia. *Vision Res.* 22:1005–16.

Lawwill T, Burian HM. (1966) Luminance, contrast function and visual acuity in functional amblyopia. *Am. J. Ophthalmol.* 62:511–20.

Legge GE, Kersten D. (1987) Contrast discrimination in peripheral vision. *J. Opt. Soc. Am. [A]* 4:1594–8.

Levi DM. (1988) The "spatial grain" of the amblyopic visual system. *Am. J. Optom. Physiol. Opt.* 65:767–86.

Levi DM, Harwerth RS. (1974) Brightness contrast in amblyopia. *Am. J. Optom. Physiol. Opt.* 51:371–81.

Levi DM, Harwerth RS. (1977) Spatiotemporal interactions in anisometropic and strabismic amblyopia. *Invest. Ophthalmol. Vis. Sci.* 16:90–5.

Levi DM, Harwerth RS. (1978a) Contrast evoked potentials in amblyopia. *Invest. Ophthalmol. Vis. Sci.* 17:571–5.

Levi DM, Harwerth RS. (1978b) A sensory mechanism for amblyopia: Electrophysiological studies. *Am. J. Optom. Physiol. Opt.* 55:163–71.

Levi DM, Harwerth RS. (1982) Psychophysical mechanisms in humans with amblyopia. *Am. J. Optom. Physiol. Opt.* 59:936–51.

Levi DM, Klein SA. (1982a) Hyperacuity and amblyopia. *Nature* 298:268–70.

Levi DM, Klein SA. (1982b) Differences in Vernier discrimination for gratings between strabismic and anisometropic amblyopes. *Invest. Ophthalmol. Vis. Sci.* 23:398–407.

Levi DM, Klein SA. (1983) Spatial localization in normal and amblyopic vision. *Vision Res.* 23:1005–17.

Levi DM, Klein SA. (1985) Vernier acuity, crowding and amblyopia. *Vision Res.* 25:979–91.

Levi DM, Klein SA. (1986) Sampling in spatial vision. *Nature* 320:360–2.

Levi DM, Harwerth RS, Smith EL. (1979) Humans deprived of normal binocular vision have binocular interactions tuned to size and spatial frequency. *Science* 206:852–4.

Levi DM, Klein SA, Aitsebaomo AP. (1984) Detection and discrimination of the direction of motion in central and peripheral vision of normal and amblyopic observers. *Vision Res.* 24:789–800.

Levi DM, Klein SA, Aitsebaomo AP. (1985) Vernier acuity, crowding and cortical magnification. *Vision Res.* 25:963–77.

Levi DM, Klein SA, Yap YL. (1987) Positional uncertainty in peripheral and amblyopic vision. *Vision Res.* 27:581–97.

Levi DM, Yap YL, Greenlee M. (1989) Is amblyopia an anomaly of photopic vision? *Clin. Vis. Sci.* 3:243–54.

Levi DM, Harwerth RS, Pass AF, Venverloh J. (1981) Edge-sensitive mechanisms in humans with abnormal visual experience. *Exp. Brain Res.* 43:270–80.

Lewis TL, Maurer D, Brent HP. (1984) Experience influences the development of detection in the nasal visual field of humans. *Invest. Ophthalmol. Vis. Sci.* 25(Suppl.):220.

Limb JO, Rubenstein CB. (1977) A model of threshold vision incorporating inhomogeneity of the visual field. *Vision Res.* 17:571–84.

Loshin DS, Levi DM. (1983) Suprathreshold contrast perception in functional amblyopia. *Doc. Ophthalmol.* 55:213–36.

Loshin DS, White J. (1984) Contrast sensitivity: The visual rehabilitation of the patient with macular degeneration. *Arch. Ophthalmol.* 102:1303–6.

Loshin DS, Levi DM, Klein SA. (1983) Utrocular contrast discrimination: A signal detection approach. *Invest. Ophthalmol. Vis. Sci.* 24(Suppl.):96.

Luce RD, Green DM. (1972) A neural timing theory for response times and the psychophysics of intensity. *Psychoanal. Rev.* 59:936–51.

Mac Canna F, Cuthbert A, Lovegrove W. (1986) Contrast and phase processing in amblyopia. *Vision Res.* 26:781–90.

Mackensen G. (1958) Reaktionszeitmessungen bei Amblyopie. *Arch. Ophthalmol.* 159:636–42.

Manny RE, Levi DM. (1982a) Psychophysical investigations of the temporal modulation sensitivity function in amblyopia: Uniform field flicker. *Invest. Ophthalmol. Vis. Sci.* 22:515–24.

Manny RE, Levi DM. (1982b) Psychophysical investigations of the temporal modulation function in amblyopia: Spatiotemporal interactions. *Invest. Ophthalmol. Vis. Sci.* 22:525–34.

Maraini G, Cordella M. (1961) Il comportamento dell'occhio ambliopico strabico dopo abbagliamento maculare. *Rass. Ital. Ottalmol.* 30:122–24.

Marr D. (1982) *Vision.* San Francisco: Freeman.

Marshall RL, Flom MC. (1970) Amblyopia, eccentric fixation, and the Stiles-Crawford effect. *Am. J. Optom. Physiol. Opt.* 42:81–90.

Mayer DL. (1986) Acuity of amblyopic children for small field gratings and recognition stimuli. *Invest. Ophthalmol. Vis. Sci.* 27:1148–53.

McGill WJ. (1963) Stochastic Latency Mechanisms. In Luce RD, Buch RR, Galanter E (Eds.), *Handbook of Mathematical Psychology*, Vol. 1, pp. 309–60. New York: Wiley.

McKee SP, Levi DM. (1987) Dichoptic hyperacuity: The precision of nonius alignment. *J. Opt. Soc. Am. [A]* 4:1104–8.

McKee SP, Taylor DM. (1984) Discrimination of time: Comparison of foveal and peripheral sensitivity. *J. Opt. Soc. Am. [A]* 1:620–7.

McKee SP, Silverman GH, Nakayama K. (1986) Precise velocity discrimination despite variations in temporal frequency and contrast. *Vision Res.* 26:609–19.

Miles WP. (1949) Flicker fusion frequency in amblyopia ex anopsia. *Am. J. Ophthalmol.* 32:225–31.

Miller EF II. (1955) The nature and cause of impaired visual acuity in amblyopia. *Am. J. Optom.* 32:10–8.

Movshon JA, Eggers HM, Gizzi MS, Hendrickson A, Kiorpes L, Boothe RG. (1987) Effects of early unilateral blur on the macaque's visual system: III. Physiological observations. *J. Neurosci.* 7:1340–51.

Oppel O. (1960) Uber unsere gegenwartigen Vorstellungen vom Wesen der funktionellen Schwachsichtigkeit. *Klin. Monatsbl. Augenheilkd.* 136:1–20.

Oppel O, Kranke D. (1958) Vergleichende Untersuchunger uber das Verhalten der Dunkeladaption normaler und schielamblyopen Augen. *Arch. Ophthalmol.* 159:486–501.

Osterberg G. (1935) Topography of the layer of rods and cones in the human retina. *Acta Ophthalmol [Suppl.] (Copenh.)* 65:1–102.

Pass AF, Levi DM. (1982) Spatial processing of complex stimuli in the amblyopic visual system. *Invest. Ophthalmol. Vis. Sci.* 23:780–6.

Paul A, Levi DM, Klein SA. (1986) A fundamental phase anomaly in amblyopia. *Invest. Ophthalmol. Vis. Sci.* 27(Suppl.):3.

Perry VH, Cowey A. (1985) The ganglion cell and cone distributions in the monkey retina: Implications for central magnification factors. *Vision Res.* 25:1795–1810.

Pettigrew JD. (1974) The effect of visual experience on the development of stimulus specificity by kitten cortical neurones. *J. Physiol. (Lond.)* 237:49–74.

Pokorny J, Smith VC, Verriest G, Pinckers AJLG (Eds.). (1979) *Congenital and Acquired Color Vision Defects.* New York: Grune & Stratton.

Pugh M. (1958) Visual distortion in amblyopia. *Br. J. Ophthalmol.* 42:449–60.

Regal DM. (1981) Development of critical flicker frequency in human infants. *Vision Res.* 21:549–55.

Rentschler I, Hilz R. (1985) Amblyopic processing of positional information: I. Vernier acuity. *Exp. Brain Res.* 60:270–8.

Rentschler I, Hilz R, Brettel H. (1980) Spatial tuning properties of human amblyopia cannot explain the loss of optotype acuity. *Behav. Brain Res.* 1:433–43.

Rovamo J, Virsu V, Nasanen R. (1978) Cortical magnification factor predicts the photopic contrast sensitivity of peripheral vision. *Nature* 271:54–6.

Sakitt B, Barlow HB. (1982) A model for the economical encoding of the visual image in the cerebral cortex. *Biol. Cybernet.* 43:97–108.

Schor CM. (1972) Oculomotor and Neurosensory Analysis of Amblyopia. Doctoral dissertation, University of California, Berkeley.

Schor CM, Levi DM. (1980a) Direction selectivity for perceived motion in strabismic and anisometropic amblyopia. *Invest. Ophthalmol. Vis. Sci.* 19:1094–1104.

Schor CM, Levi DM. (1980b) Disturbances of small field horizontal and vertical optokinetic nystagmus in amblyopia. *Invest. Ophthalmol. Vis. Sci.* 19:668–83.

Selby SA, Woodhouse JM. (1981) The spatial frequency dependence of interocular transfer in amblyopes. *Vision Res.* 21:1401–8.

Selenow A, Ciuffreda KJ. (1986) Vision function recovery during orthoptic therapy in an adult esotropic amblyope. *J. Am. Optom. Assoc.* 57:132–40.

Selenow A, Ciuffreda KJ, Mozlin R, Rumpf D. (1986) Prognostic value of laser interferometric visual acuity in amblyopia therapy. *Invest. Ophthalmol. Vis. Sci.* 27:273–7.

Shapley RM. (1986) The importance of contrast for the activity of single neurons, the VEP and perception. *Vision Res.* 26:45–61.

Shapley RM, Tolhurst DJ. (1973) Edge detectors in human vision. *J. Physiol. (Lond.)* 229:165–83.

Sireteanu R, Fronius M. (1981) Nasotemporal asymmetries in human amblyopia: Consequences of long-term interocular suppression. *Vision Res.* 21:1055-63.

Sireteanu R, Singer W. (1980) The "vertical effect" in human squint amblyopia. *Exp. Brain Res.* 40:568-72.

Skottun BC, Bradley A, Freeman RD. (1986) Orientation discrimination in amblyopia. *Invest. Ophthalmol. Vis. Sci.* 27:532-7.

Spekreijse H, Khoe LH, van der Tweel LH. (1972) A Case of Amblyopia, Electrophysiology and Psychophysics of Luminance and Contrast. In Arden GB (Ed.), *The Visual System: Proceedings of the 9th ISCERG Symposium*, p. 141. New York: Plenum.

Sperling HG, Harwerth RS. (1971) Red-green interactions in the increment-threshold spectral sensitivity of primates. *Science* 172:180-4.

Steinman SB, Levi DM, Mckee SP. (1988) Discrimination of time and velocity in the amblyopic visual system. *Clin. Vis. Sci.* 2:265-76.

Sullivan GO, Oatley K, Sutherland NS. (1972) Vernier acuity as affected by target length and separation. *Percep. Psychophys.* 12:438-44.

Swanson WH, Wilson HR. (1985) Eccentricity dependence of contrast matching and oblique masking. *Vision Res.* 25:1285-96.

Thomas J. (1978) Normal and amblyopic contrast sensitivity functions in central and peripheral retinae. *Invest. Ophthalmol. Vis. Sci.* 17:746-53.

Thomas JP. (1986) Spatial vision then and now. *Vision Res.* 26:1523-32.

Vandenbussche E, Vogels R, Orban GA. (1986) Human orientation discrimination: Changes with eccentricity in normal and amblyopic vision. *Invest. Ophthalmol. Vis. Sci.* 27:237-45.

Venverloh JR. (1983) Quantitative Measures of Orientation Discrimination in and Perceptual Errors for Line and Dot Stimuli in Functional Amblyopes. Master's thesis, University of Houston.

von Noorden GK. (1961) Reaction time in normal and amblyopic eyes. *Arch. Ophthalmol.* 66:695-701.

von Noorden GK. (1967) Classification of amblyopia. *Am. J. Ophthalmol.* 63:238-44.

von Noorden GK. (1980) *Burian–von Noorden's Binocular Vision and Ocular Motility.* St. Louis: Mosby.

von Noorden GK, Burian HM. (1959a) Visual acuity in normal and amblyopic patients under reduced illumination: I. Behavior of visual acuity with and without neutral density filters. *Arch. Ophthalmol.* 61:437-44.

von Noorden GK, Burian HM. (1959b) Visual acuity in normal and amblyopic patients under reduced illumination: II. The visual acuity at various levels of illumination. *Arch. Ophthalmol.* 62:396-9.

von Noorden GK, Burian HM. (1960) Perceptual blanking in normal and amblyopic eyes. *Arch. Ophthalmol.* 64:817-22.

Wald G, Burian HM. (1944) The dissociation of form vision and light perception in strabismic amblyopia. *Am. J. Ophthalmol.* 27:950-63.

Watson AB, Robson JG. (1981) Discrimination at threshold: Labeled detectors in human vision. *Vision Res.* 21:1115-22.

Watt RJ, Hess RF. (1987) Spatial information and uncertainty in anisometropic amblyopia. *Vision Res.* 27:661-74.

Watt RJ, Morgan MJ. (1985) A theory of the primitive spatial code in human vision. *Vision Res.* 25:1661-74.

Watt RJ, Morgan MJ, Ward RM. (1983) The use of different cues in Vernier acuity. *Vision Res.* 23:991–5.

Weiss C, Rentschler I, Caelli T. (1985) Amblyopic processing of positional information: II. Sensitivity to phase distortion. *Exp. Brain Res.* 60:279–88.

Wesson MD, Loop MS. (1982) Temporal contrast sensitivity in amblyopia. *Invest. Ophthalmol. Vis. Sci.* 22:98–102.

Westheimer G. (1975) Visual acuity and hyperacuity. *Invest. Ophthalmol. Vis. Sci.* 14:570–2.

Westheimer G. (1981a) Visual Acuity. In Moses RA (Ed.), *Adler's Physiology of the Eye*, pp. 530–44. St. Louis: C.V. Mosby.

Westheimer G. (1981b) Visual hyperacuity. *Prog. Sensory Physiol.* 1:1–30.

Westheimer G, Hauske G. (1975) Temporal and spatial interference with Vernier acuity. *Vision Res.* 15:1137–41.

Westheimer G, Mckee SP. (1975) Visual acuity in the presence of retinal image motion. *J. Opt. Soc. Am.* 65:847–50.

Westheimer G, Mckee SP. (1977) Integration regions for visual hyperacuity. *Vision Res.* 17:89–93.

Westheimer G, Shimamura K, Mckee SP. (1976) Interference with line-orientation sensitivity. *J. Opt. Soc. Am.* 66:332–8.

Wilson HR. (1986a) Responses of spatial mechanisms can explain hyperacuity. *Vision Res.* 26:453–70.

Wilson HR. (1986b) Model of peripheral and amblyopic hyperacuity. *Invest. Ophthalmol. Vis. Sci.* 27(Suppl.):95.

Worth CA, Chevasse FB. (1950) *Squint: Its Causes, Pathology and Treatment*, 8th Ed. Philadelphia: Blakiston.

Chapter 4

Effects of the Amblyopic Process on Different Levels of the Geniculostriate Pathway

In this chapter we consider the anatomic and physiologic effects the amblyopic process may have on various levels of the visual pathway both in humans with naturally occuring amblyopia and in animals with experimental amblyopia. Because the visual systems of humans and monkeys are so similar, the emphasis on animal models in this chapter is limited largely to studies of primates (for an excellent review of the experimental work on cats with experimental amblyopia, see Mitchell and Timney 1984). Specifically, we shall consider what alterations may occur at (1) the retina, (2) the lateral geniculate nucleus (LGN), and (3) the striate cortex.

RETINA

One of the most controversial issues is the question of retinal involvement accompanying strabismic and/or anisometropic amblyopia. The controversy revolves around two fundamental issues that will be examined in this section. First is the claim that the spatial resolution of retinal ganglion cells in the deviating eye of strabismic kittens is reduced. The second relates to reports of abnormal electroretinograms (ERGs) elicited by patterned stimuli in humans with strabismic amblyopia. In this section we argue that if indeed retinal anomalies exist in strabismic and anisometropic amblyopia, they (1) are secondary to cortical anomalies, probably as a consequence of retrograde degeneration, (2) are not a general property of the amblyopic syndrome and therefore do not occur in all amblyopes, and (3) do not account for the functional deficits observed in the psychophysical studies described in Chapter 3.

Anatomy and Physiology

To date, there have been no studies of either the anatomic or physiologic properties of the retina in monkeys reared with experimental amblyopia due to strabismus or anisometropia. Ikeda and Tremain (1979) reported that kittens reared with experimental esotropia showed deficits in the spatial resolution (cutoff spatial frequency) of retinal ganglion cells in the area centralis of the deviating eye. This is a surprising result, considering that more radical forms of deprivation, such as lid suture, do not result in reduced ganglion cell resolution (Cleland et al. 1980). Moreover, this surprising result occurred only in kittens made esotropic by rather radical surgical procedures (i.e., removal of one or two extraocular muscles). Less radical surgery can still result in amblyopia, but with no deficit in the resolution of the ganglion cells (Cleland et al. 1982). Thus it is likely that the ganglion cell deficits are a consequence of the specific surgical technique used by Ikeda and Tremain and not a general property of amblyopia. In fact, the presence of a ganglion-cell deficit in strabismic animals would be quite surprising in light of the normal resolution of retinal ganglion cells in cats and monkeys reared with one eyelid sutured, a far more severe form of deprivation. It should be noted that the effect of lid suture is much more likely to influence retinal processing than strabismus or anisometropia, since lid suture results in highly degraded retinal pattern stimulation and reduced light stimulation (about 1 log unit). In fact, the only reported abnormalities in primate retina occur in monkeys that have been lid-sutured for very extended periods (24 months, equivalent to about 8 human years). In these animals, prolonged lid suture produces a decrease in the size and density of parafoveal retinal ganglion cells (von Noorden et al. 1977); lid suture for shorter periods does not result in alterations in the size or density of ganglion cells or in the number of retinal synapses (von Noorden 1973). The long time course for alterations in retinal ganglion-cell size and density is strongly suggestive of a process of retrograde degeneration secondary to cortical alterations that occur following even very brief periods of monocular deprivation. Clearly, there is an urgent need for anatomic studies of the retinae of humans with well-documented amblyopia.

The Electroretinogram in Amblyopia

In humans with amblyopia, the electroretinogram (ERG) provides the only direct measure of retinal processing. Most early studies of retinal responses in amblyopes used unpatterned flashing lights to elicit electrical responses from the retina. The results were quite mixed, with some investigators reporting mild abnormalities and others reporting none (Nawratski et al. 1966, Spekreijse et al. 1972, Burian and Lawwill 1966). Figure 4.1 shows ERGs elicited by modulating a uniform field using a pseudorandom binary sequence (Levi and Manny 1982) for each eye of a strabismic amblyope. Despite a marked acuity loss, this observer shows no difference in the amplitude or latency of the *a* and *b* waves in the impulse response of the luminance ERG of the two eyes. This result suggests that the retinal responses to luminance stimuli are normal in amblyopia due to strabismus and/or anisometropia. This is not surprising, since the major anomaly in amblyopia appears to be in processing of spatial or form information rather than in the "light sense." Moreover, the ERG elicited by flashing lights is a mass response, reflecting activity that is largely dominated primarily by rods in the parafovea and periphery.

More recent studies have attempted to deal with these difficulties by utilizing patterned stimuli to elicit retinal responses. There is considerable controversy surrounding the origin of these "pattern" ERGs; nonetheless, several investigators, starting with Tuttle (1973), have measured the ERG to patterned stimuli in amblyopic eyes. While several investigators have reported abnormalities in the pattern ERG of amblyopic eyes (Sokol and Nadler 1979, Arden et al. 1980), they do not appear to be either general or correlated with the psychophysical deficits (Hess and Baker 1984). The normal pattern ERG is very small when compared with the flash or luminance ERG and is very susceptible to degradation by inappropriate refraction or unsteady fixation. In the most careful study of pattern ERGs undertaken in amblyopic observers, Hess and Baker (1984) very carefully controlled fixation and refracted their subjects for the test situation. Their results in deep amblyopes showed either no or only minimal pattern ERG abnormalities that could not be linked with their psychophysical

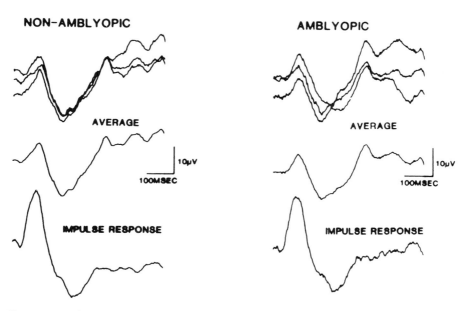

Figure 4.1 *Three ERGs obtained in response to pseudorandom modulation of a uniform field in a strabismic/anisometropic amblyope. The average of these traces is shown in the middle row, while the lower trace shows the impulse response. Note the close similarity between the data of the two eyes. (From Levi and Manny 1982).*

anomalies (Hess and Baker 1984). Thus, while some strabismic and anisometropic amblyopes may show idiosyncratic retinal anomalies, they do not appear to be a general feature of amblyopia and cannot be related to their psychophysical abnormalities. One might speculate that what retinal abnormalities may exist in amblyopes result from retrograde degeneration in long-standing cases of amblyopia. However, they are not a general finding. These results and the anatomic and physiologic studies reviewed earlier raise strong doubts regarding a primary retinal abnormality in amblyopia.

LATERAL GENICULATE NUCLEUS

Von Noorden et al. (1983) were able to conduct a postmortem examination of the dorsal lateral geniculate nucleus of a human anisometropic amblyope. They found a shrinkage of cells in the parvocellular layers with input from the amblyopic eye. Similar cell shrinkage occurs in monkeys reared with lid suture (von Noorden and Crawford 1977), chronic atropinization (Hendrickson et al. 1987), and surgical strabismus (von Noorden 1973, Crawford and von Noorden 1979). No such shrinkage occurs in monkeys reared with prisms (i.e., concomitant strabismus), presumably because these animals alternate fixation and thus do not become amblyopic. Although these anatomic effects on the LGN have been clearly established, the functional effects are less clear. In primates, at least, even lid suture from birth apparently causes little or no change in the functional properties of LGN neurons (Blakemore and Vital-Durand 1979).

STRIATE CORTEX

The most profound and consistent effects of the amblyopic process are found in striate cortex. Both surgical strabismus and prism rearing lead to a massive loss (around 80% of more) of binocular neurons (Baker et al. 1974, Crawford and von Noorden 1979, 1980). However, in surgical (nonconcomitant) strabismus, there is a marked shift in ocular dominance, such that most cells are driven through the nondeviated eye. Similar effects occur in animals reared with monocular deprivation, as noted in Figure 4.2. The effects of monocular deprivation are most profound early in life (Figure 4.2*A* through *D*), resulting in few cells driven by the deprived eye and few binocular cells, while deprivation from 1 to 2 years has a less marked effect (Figure 4.2*E*). Deprivation even for 1.5 years starting at the age of 6 has no effect on the distribution of ocular dominance (Figure 4.2*F*). This age-dependent effect of deprivation was discussed at length in Chapter 2 and also occurs in animals reared with surgical strabismus (Baker et al. 1974).

The effects of concomitant strabismus induced by prism rearing are illustrated in Figure 4.3. Crawford and von Noorden (1980) have suggested that the loss of binocular cells is associated with the loss of functional binocularity (and

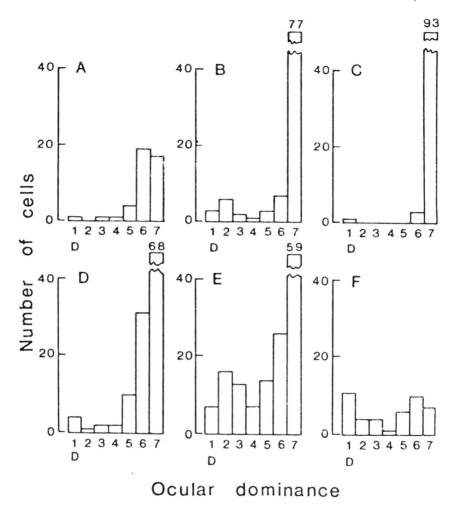

Figure 4.2   *Distribution of ocular dominance among samples of visual cortical cells recorded in each of six monkeys subjected to a period of monocular deprivation at progressively later ages. Periods of eyelid closure were from (A) day 2 to 24, (B) day 21 to day 36, (C) 5.5 weeks to 16 months, (D) 10 weeks to 16 months, (E) 1 year to 2 years, and (F) 6 years to 7.5 years. Letter D indicates group completely dominated by the deprived eye. (Adapted from LeVay et al. 1980, by Mitchell and Timney 1984).*

stereopsis), while the shift in ocular dominance is associated with visual acuity loss. While it is tempting to speculate that the massive loss of functional input from the deviated (or deprived) eye to the visual cortex is the source of spatial undersampling evident in the psychophysical performance of strabismic amblyopes, to date there have been no quantitative studies of spatial resolution in the cortex of strabismic monkeys.

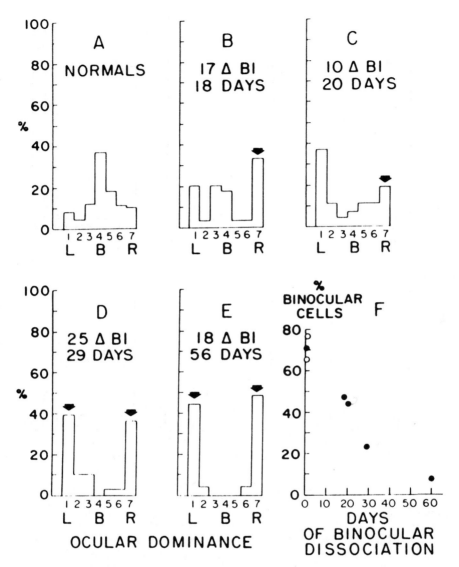

Figure 4.3   *Ocular dominance histograms of striate cortex neurons from rhesus monkeys. (A) Composite histogram from normal control monkeys. (B–E) Individual histograms from monkeys that had increasing periods of binocular dissociation. (F) Summary of the decrease in binocular neurons as a function of the duration of binocular dissociation. (From Crawford and von Noorden 1980.)*

It should be noted that caution must be exercised in evaluating animal models for human strabismic amblyopia. For one thing, human amblyopes generally have concomitant strabismus, while some investigators have had difficulty in producing amblyopia in primates with concomitant strabismus. Moreover, the specific effects of radical surgery are not known. Perhaps the most interesting question is why all human concomitant strabismics do not adopt a strategy of alternating fixation and thus avoid amblyopia. This point was discussed at greater length in Chapter 2. The recent discovery of naturally occurring strabismic monkeys may provide invaluable insights into the neural processes of amblyopia (Kiorpes and Boothe, 1981).

The effects of form deprivation shown in Figure 4.2 are as extreme as they are presumably because of the profound nature of the deprivation, which essentially eliminates form perception. Thus it is not clear to what extent it can be applied to the most common type of amblyopia in humans, anisometropic amblyopia, where the deprivation is selective for high spatial frequencies. Successful animal models of anisometropic amblyopia have been developed both in monkeys (Smith et al. 1985) and in kittens (Eggers and Blakemore 1978) that were reared with goggles with a high minus lens before one eye. While no physiologic recordings have yet been reported in monkeys with anisometropic amblyopia induced by goggle-rearing, Eggers and Blakemore have studied the contrast sensitivity of neurons in kittens. They discovered that neurons driven through the amblyopic eye showed reduced contrast sensitivity, particularly at high spatial frequencies. Their electrophysiologic contrast sensitivity function (CSF) shows reduced contrast sensitivity in the "amblyopic" eye, much like that seen in humans. Similar results also have been obtained in monkeys reared with chronic atropinization (Kiorpes et al. 1987, Hendrickson et al. 1987, Movshon et al. 1987) along with shrinkage of ocular dominance columns of the treated eye. While atropinization only results in blur at near distances, the behavioral consequences of early rearing with chronic atropinization of one eye are remarkably similar to the results seen in human anisometropic amblyopia. As can be seen in Figure 4.4, the CFSs of these animals are quite similar to those seen in humans with anisometropic amblyopia (e.g., Levi and Harwerth 1977, Bradley and Freeman 1981). The results suggest that the selective deprivation of high spatial frequencies in the retinal image produced by monocular defocus is reflected in the behavioral deficits. More important, these investigators also studied the anatomy (Hendrickson et al. 1987) and physiology (Movshon et al. 1987) of the retina, LGN, and cortex in the same animals. These studies provide strong support for the notion that the primary effects of monocular blur on the developing visual nervous system are cortical. These investigators found that the retina and all other eye tissues were normal. Cells in the parvocellular layer of the LGN were slightly smaller in the deprived than in the nondeprived laminae, but with normal physiologic properties of visual resolution. However, monocular blur produced marked effects on the spatial properties of neurons in striate cortex. Neurons driven by the defocused eye tended to have lower optimal spatial frequencies, poorer spatial resolution, and lower contrast sensitivity than neurons driven by the untreated eye. Rearing with monocular blur also reduced the degree of binocular interaction in striate cortical neurons and shifted eye dominance toward the treated eye. Perhaps one of the most interesting findings

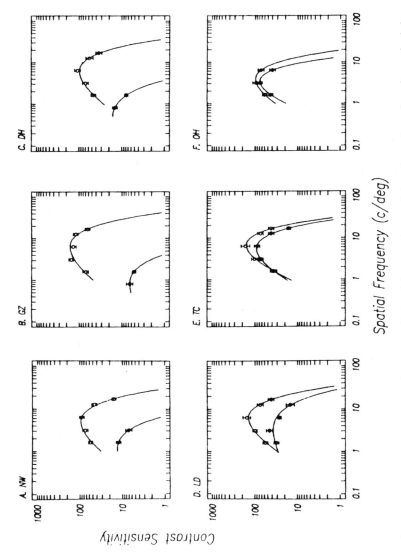

Figure 4.4 *Contrast sensitivity functions obtained from each experimental monkey after the end of the atropine rearing period. Open circles represent the untreated eye viewing; filled circles represent the treated eye. (From Kiorpes et al. 1987).*

concerns the spatial tuning of binocular neurons encountered in the cortices of these animals. Figure 4.5 illustrates these tuning functions. It is clear that for cells preferring relatively low spatial frequencies (Figure 4.5*A*), the interocular differences are quite small, while for cells preferring high spatial frequencies (Figure 4.5*C* and *D*), the interocular differences are large. This finding, in turn, suggests that anisometropic amblyopes may demonstrate normal binocular interactions when tested with low spatial frequency stimuli but abnormal binocular interactions at high spatial frequencies, in line with the psychophysical findings of Holopigian et al. (1986). As suggested in Chapter 3, the functional changes in the physiology of animals reared with monocular blur are a loss of spatial resolution and contrast sensitivity, primarily at high spatial frequencies. Similar quantitative studies of strabismic animals are sorely needed.

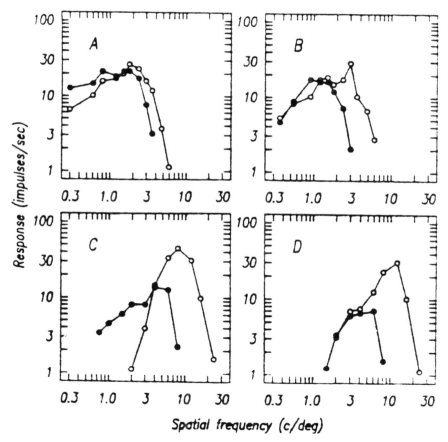

Figure 4.5 *Spatial frequency tuning characteristics for four binocular neurons tested separately through each eye. Data for the treated eye are represented by filled symbols; for the untreated eye, as open symbols. (From Movshon et al. 1987).*

Visual Evoked Potentials (VEPs)

In humans with naturally occurring amblyopia, the VEP is generally the only direct method available for studying cortical responses to visual stimuli. The VEP may provide a valuable tool for the assessment of visual function in amblyopia for several reasons: (1) it provides an objective measure of function that may be useful in infants and nonverbal patients; (2) it may aid in localizing function and dysfunction; (3) it could be valuable in assessing prognosis (however, its value in this domain is as yet unproven) and in monitoring therapy; and (4) it may be helpful in bridging the gap between psychophysics and physiology. The use of patterned stimuli for eliciting VEPs of amblyopes has proven quite useful in the diagnosis of amblyopia and in monitoring treatment in infants and young children (Arden et al. 1974, Sokol 1977). More recently, the application of rapid techniques (e.g., the spatial frequency "sweep" technique) in conjunction with zero-voltage extrapolation have allowed a more quantitative approach to the measurement of visual acuity and the assessment of treatment in amblyopes (Regan 1977, Tyler et al. 1979). The VEP also has provided useful information regarding the mechanisms of amblyopia. VEP studies are consistent with the notion originally suggested by Wald and Burian (1944) that amblyopia represents primarily an abnormality of the "form sense" that is present at or prior to primary visual cortex.

Uniform Field Stimulation

As might be expected from the psychophysics (see Chapter 3), strabismic and anisometropic amblyopes show little or no deficit in VEPs elicited by large homogeneous flashes of light or flickering stimuli (Fishman and Copenhaver 1967, Spekreijse et al. 1972, Levi 1975, Levi and Manny 1982), but they show marked losses for spatially structured stimuli (Lombroso et al. 1969, Spekreijse et al. 1972, Arden et al. 1974, Levi 1975, Sokol 1977, Levi and Harwerth 1978a and b, Levi and Manny 1982, Regan 1977, Apkarian et al. 1981). These losses, like the psychophysical losses, depend on the pattern size or spatial frequency and retinal location. They are most profound for small stimuli and within the central part of the visual field (Levi and Walters 1977). Figure 4.6*A* and *B* shows that the response of the amblyopic eye to spatial contrast is abnormal over a wide range of contrast values. This figure shows examples of VEP amplitude (expressed here in terms of signal-to-noise ratio) versus the contrast of a 4 cycle per degree sine wave grating for two strabismic amblyopes. For both nonamblyopic and amblyopic eyes, the relationship between the logarithm of the stimulus contrast and the VEP amplitude is approximately linear over some range of contrast values (Campbell and Maffei 1974, Levi and Harwerth 1978a and b). Characteristically, the data of the amblyopic eyes showed a lower slope than those of the fellow eyes, particularly at high spatial frequencies. The lower slope of the contrast function of the amblyopic eye is not explained on the basis of

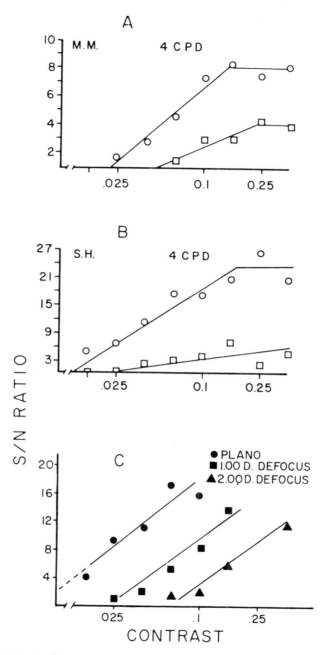

Figure 4.6 *VEP signal-to-noise ratio as a function of the contrast of a 4 cycle per degree sine-wave grating for two amblyopic observers (A and B). The open circles represent data for the preferred eyes; open squares represent data for the amblyopic eyes. (C) The effects of optical defocus on 0.0 diopter (filled circles), 1.0 diopter (filled squares), and 2.0 diopters (filled triangles) on the VEP of a normal observer.*

optical blur, since the effect of blur is to lower the effective contrast of the stimulus. Thus optical blur should shift the line to the right without altering its slope, as shown in Figure 4.6C. The lower slope of the VEP contrast response function of the amblyopic eye is reminiscent of the effect of orthogonal masks on the VEP of adults (Morrone and Burr 1986). In adults, a masking grating with its orientation orthogonal to the test stimulus produces a reduction in the slope of the VEP amplitude versus contrast function (with no change in the threshold). This is due to a multiplicative alteration produced by the mask. Interestingly, Morrone and Burr found that this effect did not occur in infants younger than about 6 months of age. They have suggested the intriguing notion that the multiplicative alteration is linked to the development of cortical inhibition.

In the VEP of the amblyopic eye, there are two notable effects. First, there is a threshold effect (i.e., the line fit to the data of the amblyopic eye extrapolates to a signal-to-noise ratio of 1 at higher contrast levels than the preferred eye), probably due to fewer and/or less sensitive neurons. Second, there is the suggestion of a recurrent multiplicative response alteration due to excessive cortical inhibition. While there is presently no psychophysical evidence for this notion, tonic cortical inhibition has long been invoked in the etiology of amblyopia (e.g., Worth and Chevasse 1950). Moreover, this idea leads to the prediction that amblyopia may not develop prior to age 6 months in humans when tonic inhibition is first evident (see Chapter 2).

Summary

A survey of anatomic and physiologic studies of the visual pathways of animals and humans with amblyopia provides a clear picture of markedly disturbed cortical function. Specifically implicated here are the contrast sensitivity of cortical neurons (in anisometropic amblyopia) and the dramatic loss of cortical connections of the amblyopic eye (strabismic amblyopia). The LGN also shows anatomic effects of amblyopia, and it is likely that the shrinkage of cells seen in the deprived layers is secondary to the cortical alterations. The most controversial claim is that of retinal deficits. At least in humans with amblyopia, the weight of ERG studies suggests that retinal abnormalities are not a fundamental characteristic of amblyopia and that if they exist, they do not underlie the more marked psychophysical abnormalities.

INADEQUATE STIMULATION
OR BINOCULAR COMPETITION?

One of the long-standing issues in amblyopia is whether the anatomic, physiologic, and behavioral effects result from inadequate or inappropriate stimulation of the amblyopic eye or binocular competitive interactions between the two eyes.

Inadequate Stimulation

Some of the earliest notions regarding amblyopia grew out of the idea that the reduced vision was a consequence of inadequate stimulation. Thus, in earlier texts, the term *amblyopia ex anopsia* (amblyopia through disuse) was frequently used. Von Noorden (1967) and others have argued that this is a misnomer, since the amblyopic eye receives light and form stimulation, moves conjugately with the fellow eye, and has consensual accommodation, thus receiving a clear retinal image much of the time. However, the notion of inappropriate stimulation has received considerable attention from Ikeda and her colleagues. Ikeda and Wright (1974) proposed that defocused images provide inappropriate stimulation for the development of sustained ganglion cells of the central retina. In the absence of clear retinal imagery, these cells would fail to develop normal properties. This, in turn, would result in abnormal development of geniculate and cortical receptive fields. Ikeda and Wright suggested that this could provide a common mechanism for amblyopia due to early unilateral cataract, anisometropia, and strabismus. In cataract and anisometropia, it is quite obvious that the amblyopic eye's image would be defocused. In cataract, the image is also diffused. Ikeda and Wright suggested that a similar effect occurs in unilateral esotropia. Because accommodation is determined by the normally fixing eye, the fovea of the squinting eye may receive blurred images of objects at different distances from the fixation point. This notion implies that the degree of amblyopia should be related to the magnitude of the strabismus, which it is not.

It now appears unlikely that poorly focused images result in retinal changes (e.g., Cleland et al. 1982). Furthermore, given consensual accommodation, it is likely that the strabismic's eye's image would be sharply focused much of the time. On the other hand, defocused images could provide inadequate stimulation for the development of normal cortical receptive field properties. An alternative hypothesis is that the amblyopic deficit results not simply from inappropriate stimulation, but from binocular competition.

Binocular Competition

Wiesel and Hubel (1965) first noticed that lid suturing one eye of a kitten (monocular deprivation) resulted in much more severe effects on visual cortical functioning than suturing both eyes (binocular deprivation). This difference is even more marked in primates. Regal et al. (1976) showed that binocularly deprived infant monkeys recover good visual acuity within a month, while monkeys monocularly deprived for the same time may show no recovery (von Noorden 1973). These observations led Wiesel and Hubel to hypothesize that the afferent connections from the two eyes compete for control of cortical neurons. Thus, in unilateral cataract, the fellow eye would be at a competitive advantage and would thus capture target neurons to the detriment of the cataractous eye. This concept has strong implications for a variety of conditions in which there is an imbalance in the sensory input through the two eyes, including anisometropia and strabismus.

There are two lines of evidence to support the concept of binocular competition. First, it is consistent with the differential effects of monocular versus binocular deprivation. Second, it is consistent with the observation that monocular deprivation produces more striking anatomic effects in the binocular segments of the LGN than in the monocular segments (Guillery and Stelzner 1970). Moreover, Guillery and Stelzner showed that a circumscribed retinal lesion in the nondeprived eye of a monocularly deprived kitten prevented cell shrinkage in the LGN laminae of the deprived eye in a corresponding segment of the visual field. This is also evidence for binocular competition in human amblyopia. For example, Hess and Pointer (1985) demonstrated that the amblyopic eye of anisometropic amblyopes had reduced contrast sensitivity across the binocular visual field but normal contrast sensitivity in the monocular segment of the visual field.

A striking feature of the normal mature primate striate cortex is the alternative pattern of ocular dominance columns revealed by autoradiographic techniques (Figure 4.7A). While the formation of ocular dominance columns begins in utero (Rakic 1977), at birth afferents from the two eyes are intermingled in layer IV and the organization of the cortex into ocular dominance columns is incomplete. Hubel et al. (1977) have argued that binocular competition plays a key role in the formation of ocular dominance columns by causing retraction of inappropriate connections. As the process of normal segregation proceeds, binocular competition is reduced, thus decreasing the susceptibility of layer IV to the effects of monocular deprivation.

If one eye has a competitive advantage prior to the completion of segregation into ocular dominance columns (e.g., because the fellow has a degraded retinal image), only the afferents of the deprived eye will retract. Thus the nondeprived eye "captures" neural territory that it would normally relinquish, while the deprived eye loses connections that it would normally maintain (LeVay et al. 1980). It is this process of binocular competition that leads to the expansion of cortical territory subserving the nondeprived eye and the shrinkage of the ocular dominance columns of the deprived eye (Figure 4.7B).

Binocular Inhibition (Suppression)

A somewhat different notion of binocular competition is evident in the clinical literature, that is, one involving a continuously active (tonic) inhibition. In some of the earlier literature, the term *suppression amblyopia* was used to reflect this idea. Thus interocular suppression mechanisms have been widely assumed to play an important role in the development of amblyopia and may exert a strong influence on the vision of the amblyopic eye well beyond the so-called "sensitive" period (see Chapter 10). One line of evidence for such tonic suppression is the observation that patients with strabismic amblyopia often show considerable recovery of visual acuity if their preferred eye is lost as a consequence of injury or disease (von Noorden and Crawford 1979, Burian 1969, Vereecken and Brabant 1984, Rabin 1984; see also Ciuffreda 1986 for a detailed review). Recently, Harwerth and colleagues have demonstrated marked recovery of visual

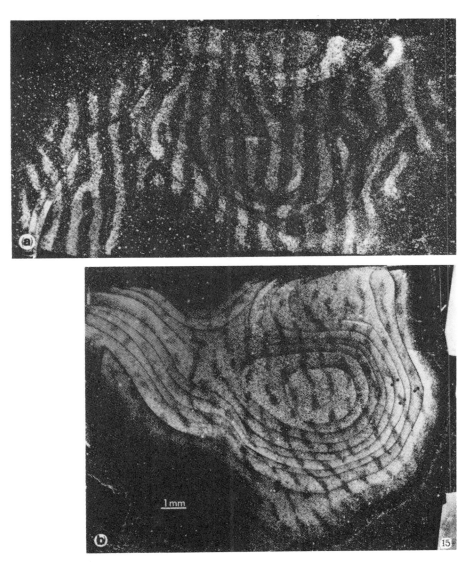

Figure 4.7 *Autoradiographic montages showing labeling of ocular dominance columns of layer IVc of normal (A) and monocularly deprived (B) monkeys. (A) Pattern of labeling in normal adult monkey. (B) Labeling pattern in a monocularly deprived monkey (right eye sutured shut at 2 weeks; left eye injected at 18 months). Note the expansion of labeled columns of the open eye at the expense of the deprived eye. (From Hubel and Wiesel 1977 and LeVay et al. 1980.)*

resolution in the amblyopic eye of strabismic monkeys following enucleation of the fellow eye (Harwerth et al. 1986). In monocularly deprived cats, enucleation of the nondeprived eye can result in an immediate increase in the number of cells that can be driven through the deprived eye (e.g., Kratz and Spear 1976, but see also Blakemore and Hillman 1977). However, neither the behavioral nor the physiologic effects have been consistent across animals or laboratories. Singer (1977) has provided further physiologic evidence for interocular suppression on the basis of electrical stimulation of the optic nerve. His work suggests that intracortical inhibitory pathways are less susceptible to the effects of monocular deprivation than are the excitatory pathways. This finding has an analogue in the psychophysical finding that human amblyopes show potent inhibitory binocular interactions but little or no excitatory interaction (Levi et al. 1979).

Perhaps the most dramatic evidence for binocular suppression comes from studies of the effects of bicuculline, which acts as an antagonist to the inhibitory neurotransmitter 8-aminobutyne acid (GABA). Duffy et al. (1976) demonstrated that following intravenous administration of bicuculline, a number of previously unresponsive neurons in the striate cortex of monocularly deprived kittens could be driven. Sillito et al. (1981) found that roughly one-third of the cells initially dominated by the nondeprived eye of monocularly deprived kittens responded to visual stimulation of the deprived eye during the application of bicuculline. Sillito and colleagues also noted that the application of bicuculline results in even more marked alterations in ocular dominance in the normal visual cortex, suggesting that GABA-mediated intracortical inhibition plays an important role in normal vision. It is likely that the clinical effects of orthoptic treatment act on suppression.

Summary

Three factors—inappropriate stimulation, binocular competition, and binocular inhibition—have all been implicated in the development of amblyopia. Evidence for the effects of inappropriate stimulation is primarily from effects of deprivation on the monocular segments of the LGN. It is not clear to what extent these monocular effects occur in the more common forms of amblyopia in humans. Abnormal binocular interaction does appear to be a common feature of amblyopia, and both binocular competition and binocular inhibition are likely to play a strong role in the development of amblyopia and in recovery of function during treatment or following loss of the fixing eye. In unilateral cataract or anisometropia, one eye has a clear competitive advantage and is thus likely to control more cortical connections. The role of binocular competition in strabismic amblyopia is as yet less clear. If indeed strabismus precedes the development of amblyopia, what gives one eye a competitive advantage? To state the question differently, why do some strabismics develop amblyopia while others adopt a strategy of alternating fixation and thus retain normal visual acuity in each eye? One possibility is in fact that those strabismics who become amblyopes have unequal refractive errors early in life providing the more nearly emmetropic eye with a competitive advantage. About 30% of amblyopes have both strabismus and anisometropia. However, about one-third of amblyopes have strabismus with no significant anisometropia. An alternative hypothesis for these amblyopes is that one eye achieves a competitive advantage because its afferents reach target neurons in the LGN or cortex first. Thus both the strabismus and the amblyopia may result from a common cause.

REFERENCES

Apkarian P, Levi DM, Tyler CW. (1981) Binocular facilitation in the visual evoked potential of strabismic amblyopes. *Am. J. Optom. Physiol. Opt.* 58:820-30.

Arden GB, Barnard WM, Mushin AS. (1974) Visually evoked responses in amblyopia. *Br. J. Ophthalmol.* 58:183-192.

Arden GB, Carter RM, Hogg CR, Powell DJ, Vaegan. (1980) Reduced pattern electroretinograms suggest a preganglionic basis for nontreatable human amblyopia. *J. Physiol. (Lond.)* 308:82P-83P.

Baker FH, Grigg P, von Noorden GK. (1974) Effects of visual deprivation and strabismus on the responses of neurons in the visual cortex of the monkey, including studies on the striate and prestriate cortex in the normal animal. *Brain Res.* 66:185-208.

Blakemore C, Hillman P. (1977) An attempt to assess the effects of monocular deprivation and strabismus on synaptic efficiency in the kitten's visual cortex. *Exp. Brain Res.* 30:187-202.

Blakemore C, Vital-Durand F. (1979) Development of the neural basis of visual acuity in monkeys: Speculations on the origin of deprivation amblyopia. *Trans. Ophthalmol. Soc. U.K.* 99:363-8.

Boothe RG, Kiorpes L, Hendrickson A. (1982) Anisometric amblyopia in *Macaca nemestrina* monkeys produced by atropinization of one eye during development. *Invest. Ophthalmol. Vis. Sci.* 22:228-33.

Bradley A, Freeman RD. (1981) Contrast sensitivity in anisometropic amblyopia. *Invest Ophthalmol. Vis. Sci.* 21:467-76.

Burian HM, Lawwill T. (1966) Electroretinographic studies in strabismic amblyopia. *Amer. J. Ophthalmol.* 61:422-30.

Campbell FW, Maffei L. (1974) Contrast and spatial frequency. *Sci. Am.* 231:106-14.

Ciuffreda KJ. (1986) Visual System Plasticity in Human Amblyopia. In Hilfer SR, Sheffield JB (Eds.), *Cell and Development Biology of the Eye: Development of Order in the Visual System*, pp. 211-244. New York: Springer-Verlag.

Cleland BG, Crewther DP, Crewther SG, Mitchell DE. (1982) Normality of spatial resolution of retinal ganglion cells in cats with strabismic amblyopia. *J. Physiol. (Lond.)* 236:235-49.

Cleland BG, Mitchell DE, Crewther SG, Crewther DP. (1980) Visual resolution of retinal ganglion cells in monocularly-deprived cats. *Brain Res.* 192:261-6.

Crawford MLJ, von Noorden GK. (1979) The effects of short-term experimental strabismus on the visual system in *Macaca mulatta*. *Invest. Ophthalmol. Vis. Sci.* 18:496-505.

Crawford MJL, von Noorden GK. (1980) Optically induced concomitant strabismus in monkeys. *Invest. Ophthalmol. Vis. Sci.* 19:1105-9.

Duffy FH, Snodgrass SR, Burchfield JL, Conway JL. (1976) Bicuculline reversal of deprivation amblyopia in the cat. *Nature* 260:256-7.

Eggers HM, Blakemore C. (1978) Physiological basis of anisometropic amblyopia. *Science* 201:262-7.

Fishman RS, Copenhaver RM. (1967) Macular disease and amblyopia: The visual evoked response. *Arch. Ophthalmol.* 77:718-25.

Guillery RW, Stelzner DJ. (1970) The differential effects of unilateral lid closure upon the monocular and binocular segments of the dorsal lateral geniculate nucleus in the cat. *J. Comp. Neurol.* 139:413-22.

Harwerth RS, Smith EL, Duncan GC, Crawford MJL, von Noorden GK. (1986) Multiple sensitive periods in the development of the primate visual system. *Science* 232:235-238.

Hendrickson A, Movshon JA, Boothe RG, Eggers H, Gizzi M, Kiorpes L. (1987) Effects of early unilateral blur on the macaque's visual system: II. Anatomical observations. *J. Neurosci.* 7:1327-39.

Hess RF, Baker CL. (1984) Assessment of retinal function in severely amblyopic individuals. *Vision Res.* 24:1367-76.

Hess RF, Pointer JS. (1985) Differences in the neural basis of human amblyopias: The distribution of the anomaly across the visual field. *Vision Res.* 25:1577-94.

Hubel DH, Wiesel TN, Levay S. (1977) Plasticity of ocular dominance columns monkey striate cortex. *Philos. Trans. R. Soc. London [Biol.]* 278:377-409.

Holopigian K, Blake R, Greenwald MJ. (1986) Selective losses in binocular vision in anisometropic amblyopes. *Vision Res.* 26:621-30.

Ikeda H, Tremain KE. (1979) Amblyopia occurs in retinal ganglion cells in cats reared with convergent squint without alternating fixation. *Exp. Brain Res.* 35:559-82.

Ikeda H, Wright MJ. (1974) Is amblyopia due to inappropriate stimulation of "sustained" visual pathways during development? *Br. J. Ophthalmol.* 58:165-75.

Kiorpes L, Boothe RG. (1981) Naturally occurring strabismus in monkeys (*Macaca nemestrina*). *Invest. Ophthalmol. Vis. Sci.* 20:257-63.

Kiorpes L, Boothe RG, Hendrickson A, Movshon JA, Eggers HM, Gizzi MS. (1987) Effects of early unilateral blur on the macaque's visual system: I. Behavioral observations. *J. Neurosci.* 7:1318-26.

Kratz KE, Spear PD. (1976) Effects of visual deprivation and alterations in binocular competition on responses of striate cortex neurons in the cat. *J. Comp. Neurol.* 170:141-52.

Levay S, Wiesel TN, Hubel DH. (1980) The development of ocular dominance columns in normal and visually deprived monkeys. *J. Comp. Neurol.* 191:1-51.

Levi DM. (1975) Patterned and unpatterned visual evoked response in strabismic and anisometropic amblyopia. *Am. J. Optom. Physiol. Opt.* 52:445-64.

Levi DM, Harwerth RS. (1977) Spatiotemporal interactions in anisometropic and strabismic amblyopia. *Invest. Ophthalmol. Vis. Sci.* 16:90-5.

Levi DM, Harwerth RS. (1978a) Contrast evoked potentials in amblyopia. *Invest. Ophthalmol. Vis. Sci.* 17:571-5.

Levi DM, Harwerth RS. (1978b) A sensory mechanism for amblyopia: Electrophysiological studies. *Am. J. Optom. Physiol. Opt.* 55:163-71.

Levi DM, Manny RE. (1982) The pathophysiology of amblyopia: Electrophysiological studies. *Ann. N.Y. Acad. Sci.* 388:243-63.

Levi DM, Walters JW. (1977) Visual evoked responses in strabismic and anisometric amblyopia: Effects of check size and retinal locus. *Am. J. Optom. Physiol. Opt.* 54:691-8.

Levi DM, Harwerth RS, Smith EL. (1979) Humans deprived of normal binocular vision have binocular interactions tuned to size and spatial frequency. *Science* 206:852-4.

Lombroso CT, Duffy FH, Robb RM. (1969) Selective suppression of cerebral evoked potentials to patterned light in amblyopia ex anopsia. *Electroencephalog. Clin. Neurophysiol.* 27:238-47.

Mitchell DE, Timney B. (1984) Postnatal Development of Function in the Mamallian Visual System. In *American Physiological Society Handbook of Physiology,* Section 1: *The Nervous System,* Vol. 3: Darian-Smith I. (Ed.), *Sensory Processes.* Part 1. Bethesda, MD: American Physiological Society.

Morrone C, Burr DC. (1986) Evidence for the existence and development of visual inhibition in humans. *Nature* 321:235-7.

Movshon JA, Eggers HM, Gizzi MS, Hendrickson A, Kiorpes L, Boothe RG. (1987) Effects of early unilateral blur on the macaque's visual system: III. Physiological observations. *J. Neurosci.* 7:1340-51.

Nawratzki I, Auerbach E, Rowe H. (1966) Amblyopia ex anopsia: The electrical response in retina and occipital cortex following photic stimulation of normal and amblyopic eyes. *Am. J. Ophthalmol.* 61:430-5.

Rabin J. (1984) Visual improvement in amblyopia after visual loss in the dominant eye. *Am. J. Optom. Physiol. Opt.* 61:334.

Rakic P. (1977) Prenatal development of the visual system in rhesus monkey. *Philos. Trans. R. Soc. Lond. [Biol.]* B278:245-60.

Regal DM, Booth R, Teller DY, Sackett GB. (1976) Visual acuity and visual responsiveness in dark-reared monkeys (*Macaca nemistrina*). *Vision Res.* 16:523-30.

Regan D. (1977) Rapid Methods for Refracting the Eye and for Assessing Visual Acuity in Amblyopia, Using Steady-State Visual Evoked Potentials. In Desmedt JE (Ed.), *Visual Evoked Potentials in Man: New Developments,* p. 418. Oxford, England: Clarendon Press.

Sillito AM, Kemp JA, Blakemore C. (1981) The role of GABAergic inhibition in the cortical effects of monocular deprivation. *Nature* 291:318-20.

Singer W. (1977) Effects of monocular deprivation on excitatory and inhibitory pathways in cat striate cortex. *Brain Res.* 30:25-41.

Sireteanu R, Fronius M. (1981) Nasotemporal asymmetries in human amblyopia: Consequences of long-term interocular suppression. *Vision Res.* 21:1055-63.

Smith EL, Harwerth RS, Crawford MLJ. (1985) Spatial contrast sensitivity deficits in monkeys produced by optically induced anisometropia. *Invest. Ophthalmol. Vis. Sci.* 26:330-42.

Sokol S. (1977) Visual Evoked Potentials in Checkerboard Pattern Stimuli in Strabismic Amblyopia. In Desmedt JE (Ed.), *Visual Evoked Potentials in Man: New Developments,* p. 410. Oxford, England: Clarendon Press.

Sokol S, Nadler D. (1979) Simultaneous electroretinograms and visually evoked potentials from adult amblyopes in response to pattern stimulus. *Invest. Ophthalmol. Vis. Sci.* 18:848-55.

Spekreijse H, Khoe LH, van der Tweel LH. (1972) A Case of Amblyopia, Electrophysiology and Psychophysics of Luminance and Contrast. In Arden GB (Ed.), *The Visual System: Proceedings of the 9th ISCERG Symposium,* p. 141. New York: Plenum.

Tuttle DR. (1973) Electrophysiological Studies of Functional Amblyopia Utilizing Pattern Reversal Techniques. Ph.D. Thesis, University of Louisville.

Tyler CW, Apkarian P, Levi DM, Nakayama K. (1979) Rapid assessment of visual function: An electronic sweep technique for the pattern visual evoked potential. *Invest. Ophthalmol. Vis. Sci.* 18:703–13.

Vereecken EP, Brabant P. (1984) Prognosis for vision in amblyopia after loss of the good eye. *Arch. Ophthalmol.* 102:220–4.

von Noorden GK. (1967) Classification of amblyopia. *Am. J. Ophthalmol.* 63:238–44.

von Noorden GK. (1973) Histological studies of the visual system in monkeys with experimental amblyopia. *Invest. Ophthalmol.* 12:727–38.

von Noorden GK, Crawford MLJ. (1977) Form vision deprivation without light deprivation produces the visual deprivation syndrome in *Macaca mulatta*. *Brain Res.* 129:37–44.

von Noorden GK, Crawford MLJ. (1979) The sensitive period. *Trans. Ophthalmol. Soc. U.K.* 99:1422–60.

von Noorden GK, Crawford MLJ, Levacy RA. (1983) The lateral geniculate nucleus in human anisometropic amblyopia. *Invest. Ophthalmol. Vis. Sci.* 24:788–9.

Wald G, Burian HM. (1944) The dissociation of form vision and light perception in strabismic amblyopia. *Am. J. Ophthalmol.* 27:950–63.

Weisel TN, Hubel DH. (1965) Comparison of the effects of unilateral and bilateral eye closure on cortical unit responses in kittens. *J. Neurophysiol.* 28:1029–40.

Worth CA, Chevasse FB. (1950) *Squint: Its Causes, Pathology and Treatment*, 8th Ed. Philadelphia: Blakiston.

Chapter 5

Eye Movements

The two primary purposes of the human eye movement system are to provide for accurate tracking and retinal-image stabilization of objects in the visual field (Leigh and Zee 1983). This allows for the image of the object to be maintained within the central foveal area, thus providing for fine localization and high resolution of details in the scene. Objects moving with simple lateral motion are tracked by versional (conjugate) eye movements, whereas when a depth component is added, vergence (disjunctive) movements are invoked. Generally, both eye movement systems are cojointly activated for fixating and following during our everyday activities. However, if one has had a period of early abnormal visual experience, such as that caused by a habitually defocused or suppressed retinal image in one eye leading to the development of functional amblyopia, this might affect the sensory processing and motor control of eye movements. In this chapter the adverse effects on the various oculomotor control subsystems in human amblyopia will be reviewed (Figure 5.1).

FIXATIONAL EYE MOVEMENTS

During attempted steady monocular fixation, the eye does not remain perfectly motionless. It moves over a small region of space forming a normal bivariate distribution of fixation points, usually less than 10 minutes of arc in extent (Ratliff and Riggs 1950). These fixational movements are of three varieties: microsaccades, drift, and tremor.

The *high-velocity microsaccades* have a mean amplitude of 5 minutes of arc, ranging from 2 to 25 minutes of arc, but rarely exceeding 10 minutes of arc (Ratliff and Riggs 1950), and they occur with a frequency of 1 to 3 per second (Adler and Fliegelman 1934, Steinman et al. 1973). These movements are always synchronous, are conjugate with respect to direction, and are highly correlated in amplitude, thus suggesting nonindependent controllers for the two eyes. The microsaccades are probably controlled by the same physiologic mechanism as used for larger voluntary saccades (Zuber et al. 1965). One of their

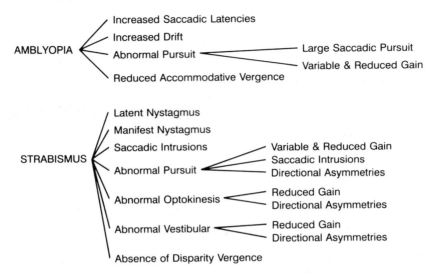

Figure 5.1 *Overview of eye movement abnormalities in amblyopia and strabismus.*

functions is to correct drift-induced fixational errors (Adler and Fliegelman 1934, Cornsweet 1957, Nachmias 1959, Krauskopf et al. 1960).

In contrast to these fast microsaccades, there are *slow drifts*. They have amplitudes of up to 5 minutes of arc (Adler and Fliegelman 1934, Ratliff and Riggs 1950) and are uncorrelated between the two eyes (Krauskopf et al. 1960). While they have generally been regarded as noise in the fixational system (Cornsweet 1957), more recent investigations have clearly demonstrated that drifts can function to reduce as well as produce the fixational error (Nachmias 1959, Steinman et al. 1967, St. Cyr and Fender 1969, Skavenski and Steinman 1970, St. Cyr 1973). This point was dramatically demonstrated by Skavenski and Steinman (1970) and Steinman et al. (1967, 1973), where during monocular fixation with concurrent voluntary microsaccade suppression, eye position could be maintained reasonably steadily, suggesting that drift can indeed serve in a corrective capacity. However, drift, in contrast to microsaccades, required visual feedback to operate in this mode. Nachmias (1959) suggested, based on an analysis of his two-dimensional fixational data, that in those meridians in which microsaccades were not effective in reducing the fixational error, corrective drifts might be employed.

The third type of movement is *tremor*. Ratliff and Riggs (1950) reported a median amplitude of 17.5 seconds of arc, with movements as large as 2 minutes of arc occurring. The frequency-amplitude relationship has been clearly provided by Riggs et al. (1954), with extreme values ranging from approximately 5 seconds of arc at a frequency of 40 Hz to 20 seconds of arc at a frequency of 105 Hz in one subject. These values are in good agreement with other reports (Adler and Fliegelman 1934, Ratliff and Riggs 1950, Riggs and Ratliff 1951, Riggs et al. 1954). The movements are reported to be independent in the two eyes (Riggs and Ratliff 1951). Cogan (1956) believed tremor to be a manifestation of the tonic activity of the lateral and medial recti emanating for the abducens and oculomotor nuclei in the brainstem. Its precise origin and function remain somewhat elusive.

Besides their role in eye position maintenance, all three types of movements are effective in preventing adaptation of the retinal receptors, which, if allowed to occur, would result in fading of the retinal image. Thus the fixational movements serve in an anti-image stabilization capacity, continually allowing "fresh" retina to receive the impinging light distributions.

For the remainder of this section we will review and discuss several clinical and laboratory studies of fixational eye movements in amblyopia. In many of the earlier studies, a description and/or documentation of the "fixation instability" was usually provided, without further segregation into its component parts. Later work began to do so, with more quantitative descriptions, aided by improved eye movement recording techniques of the three major anomalous fixational movements: (1) increased drift, (2) saccadic intrusions, and (3) latent and manifest jerk nystagmus.

Selected Early Studies

An early study by Wald and Burian (1944), while not directly investigating eye movements in patients with strabismus amblyopia, but rather dark adaptation and spectral sensitivity, set the stage for a most controversial aspect of eye movement control in these patients. Based on the similarity of the psychophysical results between the normal and amblyopic eye during these most difficult fixation tasks, they concluded that the amblyopic eye must have maintained accurate central fixation during the experimental sessions; furthermore, they concluded that light perception capabilities between the normal and amblyopic eye were comparable. These results suggested the association of amblyopia with photopic vision and the dissociation of light perception and form vision in these patients.

Von Noorden and Burian (1958), apparently influenced by the earlier Wald-Burian results, investigated fixational eye movements in both the light- and dark-adapted state in nine patients with strabismus (constant esotropia) amblyopia (6/12 to 6/60), with fixation behavior determined clinically and varying from central fixation to unsteady eccentric fixation. Midline fixation, as well as fixation 25 degrees to the left and right of midline, was assessed by the electro-oculographic technique. All patients exhibited unsteady fixation, with the amblyopic eye fixating in the light-adapted state. The fellow eye exhibited a normal fixation pattern under similar testing conditions. Most interestingly, under dark-adapted conditions, the fixation behavior of the amblyopic eye was now comparable with that of the normal eye. These researchers regarded these data as suggestive of a return of the photopically suppressed function of the fovea under low levels of illumination. Unfortunately, their data are difficult to interpret owing to the constant shift in baseline inherent in the alternating current (AC), versus the direct current (DC), recording technique, as well as their use of data obtained from young children in most of the eye movement records presented.

The question of fixation behavior as a function of retinal adaptation level was investigated further by Lawwill (1966). Fixational movements in 20 patients with strabismus amblyopia, generally with eccentric fixation, were observed under three levels of illumination. With either normal room illumination or total room darkness, the fixation pattern was observed with a specially designed infrared ophthalmoscope. In addition, fixation was studied using a hand-held ophthalmoscope with a target centered in the red-free filter. Lawwill noted no difference in the amblyopic eye fixation pattern under either normal room illumination or in darkness during infrared ophthalmoscopy; however, he observed an increased frequency, amplitude, and apparent "randomness" of the oscillatory movements with the bright hand-held ophthalmoscopic method of assessing fixation. He concluded that the increased fixation instability in this latter case reflected difficulty (for the subject) in seeing the target owing to reduced contrast produced by the bright ("dazzling") light of the ophthalmoscope. Unfortunately, objective eye movement recordings were not performed during these tests, which would have clearly defined and quantified the types of changes in fixation behavior under these three important conditions.

This difference in fixational eye movements, noted between traditional ophthalmoscopic observation and other methods such as infrared ophthalmoscopy and electro-oculography, had been observed earlier by Mackensen (1957a), who found, in some cases, a difference in electro-oculographic versus ophthalmoscopic estimation of the magnitude of these abnormal fixational movements, thus advocating the incorporation of complementary techniques in estimating fixation behavior. He suggested that the ophthalmoscope be used to estimate fixation locus (i.e., eccentric fixation) and the electro-oculogram to register fine dynamic details of the movements. Using electro-oculography, he noted random saccadic movements and jerk nystagmus having amplitudes of up to 10 degrees during fixation in his patients. However, a detailed quantitative analysis of the results was not performed. Unsteady fixation of the amblyopic eye was later verified with electro-oculography by von Noorden and Mackensen (1962a). While a direct relationship between visual acuity and magnitude of eccentric fixation was not established in their study, they did observe an increase in the estimated total area of fixation as the magnitude of eccentric fixation increased using fundus photography (von Noorden et al. 1959). However, only a gross quantitative analysis of the data was performed.

Using a limbal mirror reflection technique and cinematography, Hayashi (1961) studied two-dimensional fixational eye movements in subjects with deep (20/200 to 20/2000) amblyopia and eccentric fixation (Figure 5.2). From his measurements, an estimate of the amount of change in the site of fixation per fixational movement can be roughly calculated; this averaged 0.8, 1.4, and 2.0

degrees, respectively, for the subjects with parafoveal, paramacular, and peripheral fixation, with a range of change per fixation across all subjects of 0.5 to 2.4 degrees. This increased variance in fixation locus in amblyopic eyes has recently been beautifully documented by Higgins et al. (1982) (Figure 5.3).

Avetisov (1968) studied fixation characteristics in a large sample of patients with amblyopia. Using a large table-mounted ophthalmoscope, the fixation area was estimated. He found 27.9% parafoveal fixation (< 2 degrees), 30.8% macular (3 to 4 degrees), 29.6% paramacular (5 to 8 degrees), and 11.7% peripheral fixation (> 8 degrees). With a photoscanning eye movement recording system, he recorded horizontal fixational movements in one amblyopic subject ranging from 4 to 28 degrees in amplitude. However, both lack of clinical data on the subjects and lack of calibration indicators in his records make interpretation of the results difficult.

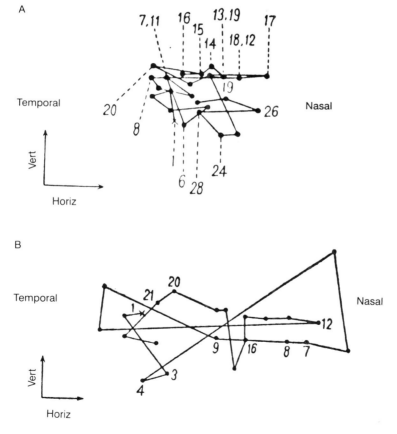

Figure 5.2 *Two-dimensional fixational eye movements in a normal (top) and amblyopic (bottom) eye during monocular fixation. (With permission of the publisher, from Hayashi 1961).*

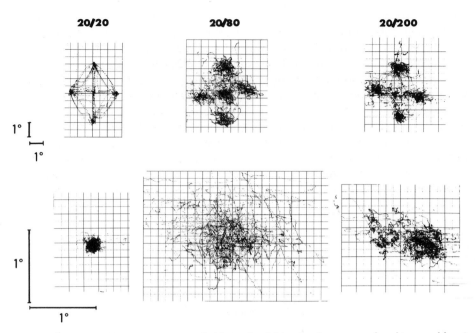

Figure 5.3   *Fixation patterns recorded from the right eyes of one normal and two amblyopic subjects. (Above) Data obtained by instructing subjects to "trace" out the pattern of the five fixation lights by shifting their fixation from one light to the next over a period of 1 minute. The spatial arrangement of the five fixation lights is readily evident from the eye movement pattern recorded from the normal eye, contrasting markedly with those of the two amblyopic eyes. (Below) Data obtained by instructing the subjects to attempt to maintain steady fixation of a single light in the array for a 1-minute period. Visual acuities of the three eyes are indicated at the top of each column. (With permission of the publisher, from Higgins et al. 1982.)*

Increased Drift

Increased drift refers to the abnormally large and/or rapid smooth drift amplitudes (up to about 3 degrees) and velocities (up to about 3 degrees per second), respectively, of the amblyopic eye during attempted maintained monocular fixation. It appears to be specific to amblyopia, once drugs, inattention, and visual fatigue are ruled out as possible contributory factors.

There have been several studies that have clearly documented the presence of increased drift in amblyopic eyes. Matteucci (1960) presented and compared electro-oculographic traces in one subject having amblyopia without strabismus with those of subjects with strabismic amblyopia. The amblyopic eyes of patients with strabismus appeared to exhibit more erratic fixation behavior than the amblyopic eye of the patient without strabismus; the subject having amblyopia showed much drift and a few large fixational saccades, while those with strabismic amblyopia showed much drift as well as many large fixational saccades. Lawwill (1968) observed the fundus of eight amblyopes with an infrared ophthalmoscope as they attempted to fixate letters on a visual acuity chart. Fading of the letters was related to the initiation of the ocular drift; reappearance of the target occurred when the drift terminated. Thus the subjective report of target fading was directly related to the observation of eye drift, which had amplitudes as great as 2 degrees; this has since been confirmed in one amblyopic subject with objective recording techniques using a reaction time paradigm (Ciuffreda et al. 1979e). Lawwill concluded that the poor fixation ability of the amblyopic eye was related, in part, to abnormally rapid local adaptation effects, leading to concurrent fading of the target.

Schor and Flom (1975) had five subjects with constant strabismic amblyopia (20/40 to 20/400), all with nasal eccentric fixation, fixate a very small spot of light and recorded eye movements photoelectrically (Figure 5.4). Several interesting phenomena were noted. First, contrary to normal subjects free from amblyopia and strabismus, who typically show randomness with respect to drift direction, *both* the normal eye of the subjects and the amblyopic eye, when tested separately, exhibited preferentially nasalward drift; other drift characteristics were within normal limits. However, saccadic movements during attempted steady fixation were larger in the amblyopic eye (40 to 200 minutes of arc, median amplitudes) than in the fellow normal eye (10 to 35 minutes of arc, median amplitudes). From an analysis of the drift direction, as well as saccadic direction and amplitude during fixation, these authors developed an asymmetric "dead zone" hypothesis to explain the eye position and eye movement abnormalities. Since the drift direction, as well as the saccadic direction in many instances, was directed nasally, they concluded that as a result of the hemiretinal suppression in the amblyopic eye during binocular viewing, this hemiretina had experienced a form of deprivation, thus resulting in reduced position sensitivity during monocular viewing. As a compensatory fixational strategy, error-producing saccades were executed in an attempt to move the eye nasally, along with the nasal drift, until a position error could be detected at the outer edge of the asymmetric (with respect to the fovea) zone of reduced sensitivity. They also regarded the abnormal eye position (i.e., the eccentric fixation), resulting from the preponderance of nasally directed drifts and saccades rather than the abnormal movements per se, to be partially responsible for the reduced visual acuity (i.e., the amblyopia) in these patients; thus motor factors were implicated in the visual acuity loss. However, interpretation of their data is seriously confounded by the abnormal eye movements (i.e., large nasally directed saccadic intrusions) found, in some of their subjects, in the *normal* eye (Schor 1972). Asymmetric fixational eye movement patterns consisting of small-amplitude (0.5 to 1.0 degrees) rapid movements have been previously observed but not objectively recorded by Pugh (1954) in 29% of her amblyopic test population. Later, Schor and Hallmark (1978) reported increased drift velocities (0.22 to 0.55 degrees per second) in amblyopic eyes.

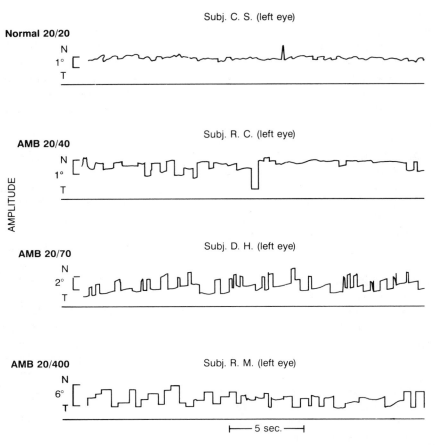

Figure 5.4   *Representative records of horizontal eye movements during attempted steady fixation from one normal eye (C.S.) and three amblyopic eyes (R.C., D.H., and R.M.) with acuities of 20/40, 20/70, and 20/400, respectively. (With permission of the publisher, from Schor and Flom 1975.)*

A comprehensive study of the drift in amblyopic eyes was conducted by Ciuffreda et al. (1980). The principal finding of their investigation was increased drift amplitude (> 12 minutes of arc) and velocity (> 20 minutes of arc per second) in all amblyopic eyes during monocular fixation. Increased drift occurred most frequently and with greatest magnitude in amblyopia without strabismus and in constant strabismic (exotropia) amblyopia, while it occurred least frequently and with smallest magnitude in intermittent strabismus. Increased drift was not present during either binocular fixation or monocular fixation with the dominant eye in any patient. Drift characteristics of each patient were similar for all five horizontal directions of gaze tested.

The presence of increased amblyopic drift is clearly seen in the eye movement records. In one representative patient (Figure 5.5) (amblyopia without strabismus), increased drift amplitude (up to 3.3 degrees) with a paucity of comparably sized saccades, as well as increased drift velocity (up to 1.7 degrees per second), was prominent throughout the record. Drifts rather than saccades appeared to be used to attempt to maintain eye position during fixation. Thus drifts functioned in both error-producing and error-correcting capacities. Comparison of monocular fixation in the amblyopic eye with monocular fixation in the fellow dominant eye is shown in Figure 5.6 (amblyopia without strabismus). The contrast between the extreme steadiness of the dominant eye (< 12 minutes of arc amplitude, < 20 minutes of arc per second velocity) and the increased drift in the amblyopic eye (1.8 degrees peak-to-peak amplitude and 1.7 degrees per second maximum velocity) is striking.

Further analysis of the drift was performed. The presence of abnormal drift (the number of 1-second intervals in which increased drift amplitude or velocity was found divided by the total number of seconds fixation was tested times 100) was calculated for each patient (Figure 5.7). Increased drift amplitude was found 50% of the time in constant strabismus amblyopia, occurring 35% of the time in the esotropes while increasing to 90% of the time in the exotropes. Increased drift velocity was found 55% of the time in constant strabismus amblyopia, occurring 45% of the time in the esotropes while increasing to 85% of the time in the exotropes. In amblyopia without strabismus, increased drift amplitude and velocity occurred 67% and 85% of the time, respectively. Increased drift amplitude was found 13% of the time in intermittent strabismus, occurring only 10% of the time in patients with 20/20 or better visual acuity while increasing to 20% of the time in patients with worse than 20/20 visual acuity. Increased drift velocity was found 30% of the time in intermittent strabismus, occurring only 25% of the time in patients with 20/20 or better visual acuity while increasing to 40% of the time in patients with worse than 20/20 visual acuity. In constant strabismic (esotropia) amblyopia, average maximum drift amplitude correlated well ($r = +0.975$, $p < 0.05$) with visual acuity of the amblyopic eye. Maximum peak-to-peak drift amplitude ($r = +0.90$, $p < 0.05$) and the presence of abnormal drift amplitude ($r = +0.90$, $p < 0.05$) also correlated well with visual acuity of the amblyopic eye in these five esotropic patients. In the four patients having amblyopia without strabismus, there was a strong trend ($r = +0.95$, $p > 0.05$) for average maximum drift amplitude and velocity to correlate well with visual acuity of the amblyopic eye. No other significant correlations or trends were found.

Increased drift was found in the amblyopic eyes of most of their patients. The increased drift amplitude and velocity were most pronounced in amblyopia without strabismus and constant strabismic (exotropia) amblyopia. It was evident to a lesser degree in constant strabismic (esotropia) amblyopia. Drift was either normal or nearly normal in the nondominant eyes of most patients having

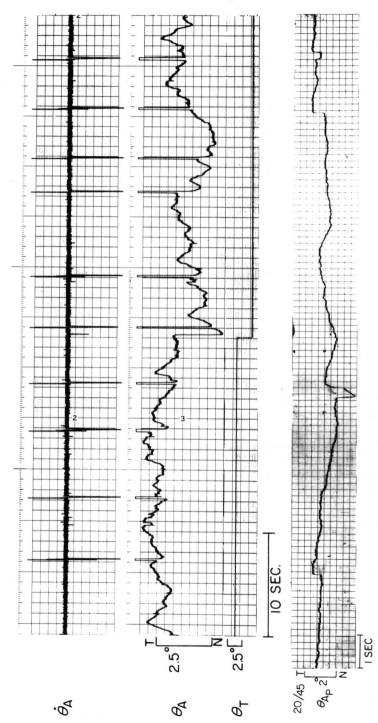

Figure 5.5   *(Above) Monocular fixation with the amblyopic eye. Amblyopia without strabismus (20/40). From top to bottom, eye velocity, eye position, and stimulus, respectively. Note increased drift amplitudes and velocities, and the paucity of saccades comparable in magnitude to the drifts. Deflections driving pens to the edge of the record are due to blinks. (N = nasalward eye movement; T = templeward eye movement; θ_T = target position; θ_A = eye position, amblyopic eye; and $\dot{\theta}_A$ = eye velocity, amblyopic eye.) (With permission of the publisher, from Ciuffreda et al. 1979e.) (Below) Monocular fixation with the amblyopic eye in a subject who had amblyopia without strabismus (20/110). Prominent features in the record are increased drift amplitudes and velocities. Same symbols as above. (With permission of the publisher, from Ciuffreda et al. 1980.)*

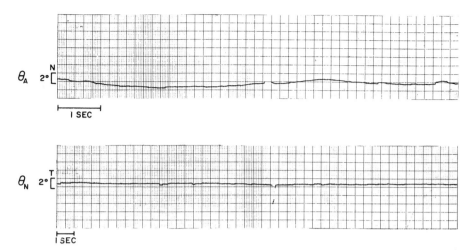

Figure 5.6 *Monocular fixation with the amblyopic (above) and dominant eye (below). Amblyopia without strabismus (20/40). Prominent drift in the amblyopic eye is in marked contrast to the steadiness evident in the dominant eye. (With permission of the publisher, from Ciuffreda et al. 1980).*

intermittent strabismus. Thus the results suggested that amblyopia and not strabismus was a necessary condition for the presence of significantly increased drift.

Increased drift amplitudes, without the occurrence of comparably sized corrective saccades (as was most dramatically found in patients having amblyopia without strabismus), suggest that drifts rather than saccades played a major role in the correction of fixation errors and in the maintenance of eye position in amblyopic eyes. Thus drift could be *either* error-producing *or* error-correcting in nature (Nachmias 1959, St. Cyr and Fender 1969, Stark 1971). It is interesting that Nachmias (1959), in analyzing his two-dimensional monocular fixation eye movement records in normal subjects, found correction of position error by drifts in those meridians in which microsaccadic corrections appeared to be ineffective. If this line of reasoning is applied to these patients, it suggests that the microsaccadic system, one of whose functions is to correct for drift-induced fixation errors, may be less effective in amblyopic eyes. Ineffectiveness of the microsaccadic system may involve failure to integrate eye velocity (drift velocity) into a position error for subsequent correction by the saccadic system and/or processing delays in initiation of appropriately sized microsaccades, similar to the processing delays found for larger tracking saccades in amblyopic eyes (Ciuffreda et al. 1978a and b). Increased drift amplitudes also might be found if processing delays in the smooth-pursuit velocity-correcting system (i.e., slow fixational control) were present. These hypotheses regarding possible mechanisms underlying increased amblyopic drift amplitude warrant further careful experimental testing.

Could part of the increased drift amplitudes observed in amblyopic eyes be due to normal drift characteristics of the oculomotor system for position errors

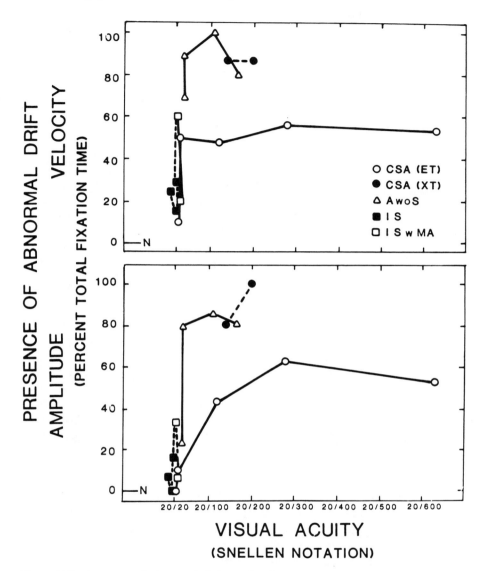

Figure 5.7 *Presence of abnormal drift amplitude and velocity as a function of visual acuity in the nondominant eye. CSA (ET) = constant strabismus amblyopia (esotropia); CSA (XT) = constant strabismus amblyopia (exotropia); AwoS = amblyopia without strabismus; IS = intermittent strabismus with visual acuity of 20/20 or better; ISwMA = intermittent strabismus with mild amblyopia (visual acuity worse than 20/20), and N = maximum normal drift level during either binocular fixation or monocular fixation with the dominant eye. (With permission of the publisher, from Ciuffreda et al. 1980.)*

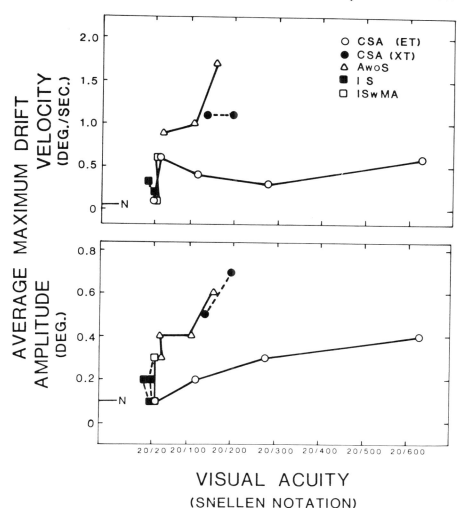

Figure 5.7 *(continued)*

generated in the retinal periphery? Results of Sanbury et al. (1973) support this idea. In their experienced normal subjects, as error signals were generated by more peripheral retinal regions, small increases (a few minutes of arc) in drift magnitude were found. Thus it seems reasonable to attribute a small part of the increased drift amplitudes observed in the untrained amblyopic patients to this factor, since they did fixate (on average) with nonfoveal regions; that is, eccentric fixation was present. The total extent over which the target image was displaced without execution of appropriate corrective movements may represent that region of the retina most adversely affected, in terms of eye position maintenance, by the amblyopia.

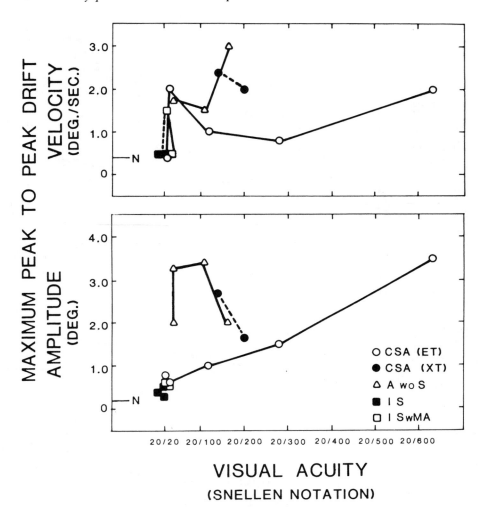

Figure 5.7   *(continued)*

Drift velocities as high as 3.0 degrees per second were found in amblyopic eyes. If drift rates were similar between the normal and amblyopic eyes, and only increased drift magnitudes were found in amblyopic eyes, this might point to a simple sensory basis for the abnormality in terms of defective sensing of position error over the affected (by amblyopia) retinal regions, thus allowing the eye to drift for a longer period of time, but with normal drift velocities, until the target image extended out of this relatively insensitive area. At that time, a position error would be sensed and a corrective movement initiated. That this might occur at times in amblyopic eyes has been discussed elsewhere (Ciuffreda 1977). More frequently, however, increased drift velocities were observed that may either be a consequence of delays resulting from amblyopia in the smooth-pursuit velocity-correcting system, thereby allowing long-duration drifts with high velocities to evolve, or may in part simply result from fixation with non-foveal retinal regions.

What effect would increased drift have on visual acuity and contrast sensitivity in amblyopic eyes? It has been clearly shown that retinal-image motion across the horizontal meridian of the fovea in normal persons must exceed 2.5 degrees per second before visual resolution is degraded (Westheimer and McKee 1975). If this result is applied to the amblyopic eyes, visual acuity should be little, if at all, affected by the increased drift velocities (generally < 1.0 degrees per second). However, increased drift amplitudes moving the retinal image onto more eccentric positions would reduce acuity, as shown by measures of the visual acuity gradient in the horizontal meridian in amblyopic eyes (Kirschen and Flom 1978), while increased drift amplitudes in any direction would contribute to increased variability in the acuity measure. Similarly, increased drift velocity would have little adverse effect on the contrast sensitivity function (CSF), since drift velocities were generally less than about 1 degree per second (Murphy 1978). Further, this is consistent with the experimental results in amblyopes (Hess 1977, Higgins et al. 1982).

The results of the study by Ciuffreda et al. (1980) can also provide insight into the clinical assessment of fixation in amblyopic eyes. During the visuscopic examination, the clinician estimates, with aid of a calibrated grid pattern projected onto the fundus, the magnitude (time-average position of the eye) and the range (maximum peak-to-peak drift amplitude with microsaccade amplitude superimposed) of eccentric fixation, as well as "steadiness" of fixation—a judgment based on some unknown combination of average and maximum drift amplitude and velocity with microsaccade amplitude superimposed. The presence of abnormal drift (in terms of percent total fixation time) is difficult to quantify accurately, and the absolute value of average or maximum drift velocity is impossible to ascertain. Recent findings obtained with an objective eye movement recording technique show, for example, that average maximum drift amplitude and velocity tend to become normal during orthoptic treatment (Ciuffreda et al. 1979c). These authors' results suggest that it is important to quantify accurately and completely measures of drift during treatment, and a visuscopic analysis alone is inadequate for such purposes. However, objective eye movement recording techniques also have a serious disadvantage. One generally does not know the location of the fovea with respect to the retinal image of the target. Thus, as advocated by Mackensen (1957a) and Ciuffreda et al. (1979c), use of both accurate eye movement recordings and visuscopic examination results (perhaps along with entoptically derived measures of the magnitude of eccentric fixation) are essential for a complete, quantitative description of fixation in amblyopic eyes.

More recent studies have confirmed and extended these earlier results. Higgins et al. (1982) found mean increased drift velocities in amblyopic eyes to range from 0.15 to 0.37 degrees per second; their normal subjects averaged 0.08

degrees per second with the SRI eye tracker. Srebro (1983) found increased drift (mean, maximum) amplitude (0.66 degree, 1 degree) and velocity (0.4 degree per second, 1.5 degrees per second) in amblyopic eyes; there was no evidence of a directional drift bias. Lastly, Westall and Aslin (1984) found drift variance to be four to five times greater in the amblyopic as compared with the fellow dominant eye during monocular fixation. They also found increased autokinesis when fixating with the amblyopic eye.

There is some evidence that orthoptic therapy can reduce the abnormal fixational drift in amblyopic eyes. In an adult anisometropic amblyope, Ciuffreda et al. (1979c) found drift amplitude and velocity to normalize, as did visual acuity and eccentric fixation, during a 8-month period of intensive therapy for remediation of the amblyopia (Figure 5.8). This suggests the presence of residual oculomotor/visual system plasticity in older amblyopes. Similar results have recently been reported in young amblyopes (Selenow and Ciuffreda 1983, 1986, Ciuffreda 1986). Flom et al. (1980) have demonstrated short-term reduction in abnormal drift amplitude and velocity in the amblyopic eye with oculomotor biofeedback therapy. However, additional study is needed to determine the long-term efficacy of such treatment.

Saccadic Intrusions

Saccadic intrusions refer to a pattern of movement in which there is a saccadic displacement of the visual axis away from the target, followed approximately 200 ms later by a return saccadic movement. However, variations of this pattern can occur; for example, there may only be an initial saccadic displacement followed by a return drift movement (Atkin and Bender 1964, Daroff 1977). Saccadic intrusions generally have amplitudes of 0.5 to 3.0 degrees and occur with a frequency of 1 to 4 per second (Troost et al. 1976). They have been recorded in patients with progressive supranuclear palsy (Troost et al. 1976), cerebellar atrophy (Baloh et al. 1975, Alpert et al. 1975), lesions of the cerebellum (Selhorst et al. 1976), and brainstem encephalitis (Jung and Kornhuber 1964). It has been hypothesized that saccadic intrusions represent a disorder of the microsaccadic system (Feldon and Langston 1977). These intrusive saccades also have been recorded in patients who were free of neurologic disease but who had strabismus (with or without amblyopia), as will be discussed in detail later in this chapter. To complicate matters even further, saccadic intrusions have recently been found to occur (generally intermittently, in about 10% of a neurooptometry clinic population) in individuals *free* of neurologic disease, strabismus, *and* amblyopia and who have normal or nearly normal visual acuities in each eye (Ciuffreda et al. 1983); these intrusive saccades were found in patients with reading disability, in anxious individuals, and as part of a predictive tracking strategy. Thus careful history and quantitative analysis of the eye movements (Sharpe et al. 1982) are required to pinpoint, if at all possible, the underlying etiologic factor for the presence of saccadic intrusions.

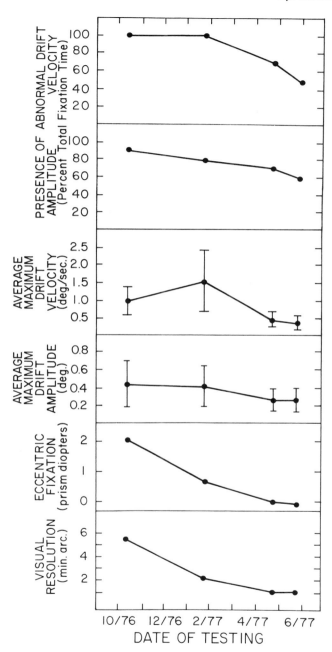

Figure 5.8 *Changes (for left eye) in presence of abnormal drift velocity and amplitude, average maximum drift velocity and amplitude (with standard deviations), eccentric fixation, and visual resolution during the last 8 months of orthoptic therapy. All show clear normalizing trends. (With permission of the publisher, from Ciuffreda et al. 1979c.)*

There have been several investigations over the past three decades or so dealing with saccadic intrusions in patients with amblyopia (and strabismus). Intrusions are evident in the fixation records of Mackensen (1957a) and of von Noorden and Mackensen (1962a). Saccadic intrusions and single large fixational saccades also were found by von Noorden and Burian (1958) and more recently by Hess (1977) during monocular fixation with the amblyopic eye. Schor and Flom (1975) found the median fixational saccadic amplitude (in minutes of arc) to be approximately equal to the Snellen fraction denominator describing visual

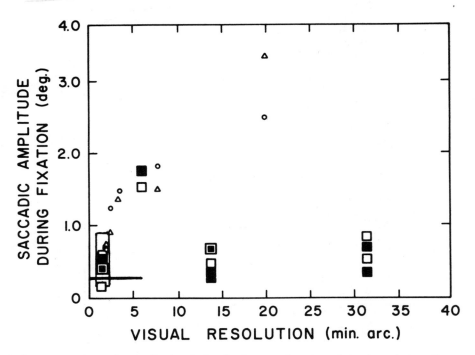

Figure 5.9 *Saccadic amplitudes during fixation as a function of visual resolution. Open squares represent mean saccadic amplitudes, and filled squares represent median saccadic amplitudes in amblyopic eyes for the subjects with constant strabismus; triangles represent mean amplitudes for templeward-directed saccades, and open circles represent mean amplitudes for nasalward-directed saccades of Schor's (1972) subjects with constant strabismic amblyopia. Range of mean and median saccadic amplitudes for intermittent strabismic subjects is represented by the vertical rectangle (in lower left corner). Saccadic amplitudes for the subjects having amblyopia without strabismus are represented by the horizontal line (in lower left corner); these are within normal limits. Note lack of any direct relationship between mean or median saccadic amplitude and visual resolution in the amblyopic (or nondominant) eye for subjects (excluding Schor's). Central tendencies are generally less than 1 degree. (With permission of the publisher, from Ciuffreda et al. 1979e.)*

acuity in the amblyopic eye (Figures 5.4 and 5.9); they also believed that the saccadic intrusions would have little adverse affect on visual acuity in the amblyopic eye.

Later, Ciuffreda et al. (1979e) confirmed and expanded on these most intriguing results. The principal finding of their investigation was the presence of saccadic intrusions during fixation in subjects with strabismus (Figure 5.10). Saccadic intrusions were found during most fixation conditions in three of four subjects with intermittent strabismus. They also were prominent during monocular fixation with the amblyopic eye in four of five subjects with constant strabismus and amblyopia. Saccadic intrusions were rarely found in the three subjects having amblyopia without strabismus. The initiation of saccadic intrusions did not depend on the presence of considerable preceding drift (i.e., drift amplitudes comparable in magnitude to saccadic amplitudes). In the vast majority of cases, the initial saccade of the intrusion was *not* corrective in nature.

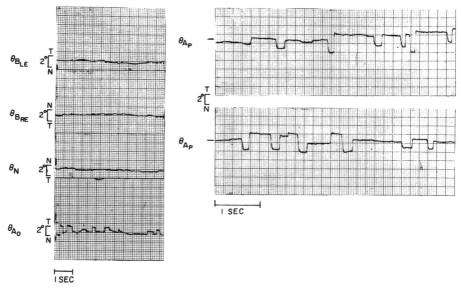

Figure 5.10   (Left) *Eye position as a function of time for a subject with constant strabismic amblyopia (20/277). From top to bottom, tracings are left and right eye during binocular fixation, monocular fixation with the normal eye, and monocular fixation with the amblyopic eye. Note the presence of saccadic intrusions only during monocular fixation with the amblyopic eye. (Right) Monocular fixation with the amblyopic eye for a subject with constant strabismic amblyopia (20/122). Trajectories and baseline of saccadic intrusions are clearly seen here with the faster chart speed. (With permission of the publisher, from Ciuffreda et al. 1979e).*

The group data are presented in Figure 5.9. Saccadic amplitude during fixation is plotted as a function of visual resolution. For subjects with either intermittent or constant strabismus, the central tendencies were typically 1 degree or less in amplitude. Thus there was no relationship between saccadic amplitude during fixation and visual resolution. Subjects having amblyopia without strabismus exhibited fixational saccades that were within normal amplitude limits (generally less than 20 minutes).

The preceding data illustrate rather clearly that the presence of saccadic intrusions was related to strabismus and not amblyopia. These findings confirm those of others regarding the presence of saccadic intrusions in constant strabismic amblyopia, but more important, they extend the data to include subjects with intermittent strabismus and exclude those with amblyopia alone. Thus, for the first time, a relationship between saccadic intrusions and strabismus was clearly demonstrated.

That intrusions do not adversely affect visual acuity was supported by the finding that they occurred in subjects with intermittent strabismus having normal visual acuity in each eye (20/20). Furthermore, the authors have recorded saccadic intrusions during fixation in subjects with normal visual acuity free from strabismus, amblyopia, or neurologic disease (unpublished data). This lack of interference by saccadic intrusions on visual acuity appears reasonable, since the intersaccadic interval for an intrusion was rarely shorter than 100 ms or longer than 400 ms, thereby allowing adequate visual processing time during these periods. Furthermore, since intrusions generally averaged less than 1 degree in amplitude, the change in visual resolution for those retinal areas used during the intrusion relative to the preferred fixation locus would not seriously impair resolving ability. It appears to go unnoticed in strabismic subjects during everyday binocular viewing conditions. Moreover, since saccadic intrusion frequency ranged from 0.3 to 2.0 per second, the interval during which a target and preferred fixation locus would be coincident also provided an adequate processing period. This lack of affect of saccadic intrusions on visual acuity in strabismics agrees with recent findings by Hess (1977), who, in a tangentially related study, found similar contrast thresholds in amblyopic eyes during both stabilized and normal viewing conditions. The fact that intrusion direction in the amblyopic eye frequently (more than 70% of the time) occurred in the same direction as the squint suggests a fixation bias induced by the strabismus. Subjects with constant exotropia, however, must be carefully studied and consistent results obtained before this hypothesis can gain support.

Can the amplitude of saccadic movements during fixation in an amblyopia eye be predicted based only on its visual resolution? Ciuffreda et al. (1979e) found no relationship between mean or median saccadic amplitude and visual resolution in the amblyopic eye for either group of subjects with strabismus (Figure 5.9). This result is in striking contrast to the findings of Schor and Flom (1975), who found a high correlation between these two variables in five constant strabismic amblyopes in whom median saccadic amplitude increased as visual acuity in the amblyopic eye decreased. They also developed a mathematical expression to predict median saccadic amplitude in the amblyopic eye based simply on its visual resolution. The lack of agreement between the data of Ciuffreda et al. (1979e) with constant strabismus and high amblyopia and theirs demonstrates the necessity of testing a large group of subjects before attempting to develop a general mathematical expression with high predictive power.

Several other facts regarding saccadic intrusions should be noted (Ciuffreda et al. 1979e). First, they appear to be unrelated to abnormal eye position error detection in the amblyopic eye resulting from an asymmetric "dead zone" caused by strabismic hemiretinal suppression, as was speculated by Schor and Flom (1975). Second, the intrusions do not appear to function to correct drift-induced position errors. Third, these intrusive saccades may be adaptive in nature and help to prevent fading of the retinal image owing to abnormally rapid visual adaptation, as was speculated by Lawwill (1968). Fourth, the presence of saccadic intrusions in the dominant eye of some strabismic amblyopes and intermittent strabismics without amblyopia suggests that the presence of strabismus may simply degrade fixation ability in both eyes. Fifth, the presence of these intrusions has recently been confirmed in strabismic amblyopes (Higgins et al. 1982) and alternating strabismics (Prakash et al. 1982). Sixth, these intrusions may convert to a jerk nystagmus in total darkness (Ciuffreda et al. 1979b). Lastly, they appear to be the "unnecessary" eye movement described by some (Flom 1958, Mehdorn and Kommerell 1978) during the cover test in certain strabismics.

The ability to reduce or "suppress" these saccadic intrusions, as has been well documented in normal individuals (Steinman et al. 1967, 1973), also has been objectively documented in amblyopes. Ciuffreda (1977) was the first to demonstrate this phenomenon. This was later confirmed and expanded by Ciuffreda et al. (1979a, b, e); they found that the frequency of these intrusive saccades could be reduced by as much as 10 times without influencing the amplitude of either the saccadic or the interspersed amblyopic drift component (Figure 5.11). Schor and Hallmark (1978) reported similar results, but their suppression could only be accomplished in the light and not in total darkness, suggesting that visual feedback was essential for successful completion of this higher-level, learned maneuver. They also found that the amblyopes could use oculomotor auditory biofeedback to suppress their fixational saccades (Figure 5.12).

There are two reports that provide objective documentation that orthoptic therapy can reduce these abnormal saccadic intrusions. Flom et al. (1980) demonstrated that eye movement auditory biofeedback could produce short-term improvement in fixational ability, including the saccadic intrusions, during monocular fixation with the amblyopic eye (Figure 5.13). However, the long-term effectiveness has yet to be established. Selenow and Ciuffreda (1983) provided before and after infrared recordings of fixational movements in the amblyopic eye of a 6-year-old with exotropia and high unilateral myopia (Figure 5.14). Marked improvement in all vision functions, including significant reduction in saccadic intrusions, was found following the termination of amblyopia therapy.

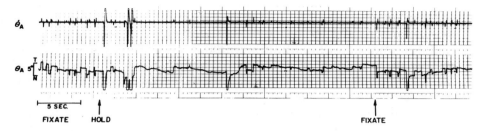

Figure 5.11 *Eye position (bottom trace) and eye velocity (top trace) as a function of time for a patient having constant strabismic (exotropia) amblyopia (20/122). Monocular fixation with the amblyopic eye. Patient was instructed either to "fixate carefully" or to "hold the eye steadily" in the light with the target present. During the "fixate" command, saccadic intrusions occurred frequently (~1 per second). Note the markedly reduced intrusion frequency during the "hold" command (~0.1 per second) and prominence of slow drift. Deflections driving pens to the edge of records are due to blinks. (T = templeward eye movement; N = nasalward eye movement; $\dot{\theta}_A$ = amblyopic eye velocity; θ_A = amblyopic eye position.) (With permission of the publisher, from Ciuffreda et al. 1979b.)*

Latent Nystagmus

Latent nystagmus is a disorder of the oculomotor system in which nystagmus is generally not present (or at least obvious) during binocular viewing, but upon occlusion of an eye, a conjugate jerk nystagmus with the fast phase directed toward the viewing eye ensues (Anderson 1954). It was first described by Faucon (1872) and named by Fromaget and Fromaget (1912). Besides occlusion as a means of inducing latent nystagmus, it can be induced by such procedures as shining a bright light into one eye (Clarke 1896, Simon and Slatt 1971) or introducing a high convex lens before an eye (Fromaget and Fromaget 1912). Latent nystagmus was reported to be improved by administration of a parasympathomimetic ocular drug, such as Cyclogyl, and this proved useful prior to and during occlusion therapy for treatment of unilateral amblyopia in these patients (Windsor 1968, Windsor et al. 1968, Alejo 1971, Walton 1972, Calcutt and Crook 1972). Fatigue may convert latent nystagmus into a manifest nystagmus (Anderson 1954). Sorsby (1931) stressed the variability of responses in patients with latent nystagmus, and he did not consider latent nystagmus to be a separate clinical entity, but rather a form of incomplete nystagmus. Abramson (1973) concluded from his identical-twin study that latent nystagmus probably resulted from postnatal trauma, such as convulsions, and not hereditary factors. Through a series of elegant experiments employing pseudoscopic viewing, van Vliet (1973) convincingly demonstrated that latent nystagmus was independent of retinal stimuli and instead resulted from the subject's intention of looking with one eye; thus the direction of the latent nystagmus was dependent on which eye the subject *thought* he or she was using rather than which eye actually received the visual stimulus.

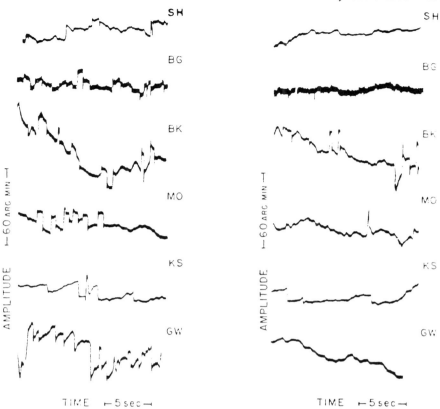

Figure 5.12 (Left) *Eye position during attempted steady fixation of a stationary target. Records are ranked according to the depth of amblyopia. The first subject had 20/15 acuity; the next two subjects had central fixation; and the latter three had eccentric fixation.* (Right) *Attempted steady fixation in the presence of auditory feedback for saccades. (With permission of the publisher, from Schor and Hallmark 1978.)*

The association between latent nystagmus and strabismus is well documented. Anderson (1954), and later Jung and Kornhuber (1964), found that 15% of patients with concomitant strabismus had latent nystagmus; conversely, 95% of patients with latent nystagmus had strabismus. Crone (1954) and Lang (1968) found that patients with latent nystagmus usually also had an alternating hyperphoria, strabismus of early onset that was convergent in nature, intorsion of the viewing eye and extorsion of the occluded eye, and abnormal head posture. Recently, it has been objectively documented that strabismus is a necessary condition for the presence of either latent or manifest-latent nystagmus (Dell'Osso et al. 1979, 1983).

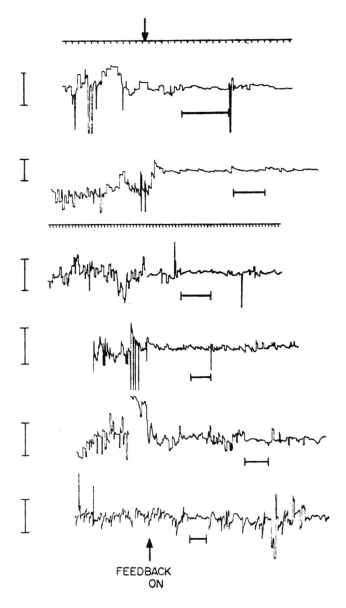

Figure 5.13 *Records of horizontal eye position show the fixation behavior of six amblyopic eyes without (left of arrows) and with (right of arrows) auditory feedback of eye position. Periods of steady foveal fixation (within ± 20 minutes of arc) are evident in each record when feedback is provided. One such period is shown for each subject by a horizontal line under the trace. Vertical calibration bars to the left of each trace are 3 degrees. Associated time scales (1-second divisions) are shown above the top two records and above the bottom four. Upward deflections denote eye movements to the left. (With permission of the publisher, from Flom et al. 1980.)*

BEFORE

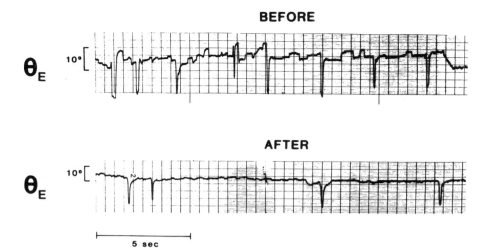

AFTER

├────────┤
   5 sec

Figure 5.14 *Fixational eye movements before and after orthoptic therapy. Amblyopic eye. Monocular viewing. Posttraining improvement is evident. Large, downward deflections represent blinks (θ_E = eye position). (With permission of the publisher, from Selenow and Ciuffreda 1983.)*

Although there have been numerous papers providing qualitative descriptions of latent nystagmus, only two reports with careful objective eye movement recordings exist. Ciuffreda and colleagues (Ciuffreda 1977, Ciuffreda et al. 1979a) recorded eye movements in two patients with documented "pure" latent nystagmus; that is, there was *no* nystagmus under binocular viewing conditions but appropriate jerk nystagmus under monocular viewing conditions. Examples of the fixational eye movements under monocular and binocular viewing conditions are presented and summarized in Figure 5.15. Evident is the low frequency and small amplitude of the jerk nystagmus under monocular conditions, making a diagnosis of latent nystagmus quite difficult in the absence of objective eye movement recordings. Similar results were found in the other patient. Latent nystagmus during monocular fixation with the dominant eye had a mean frequency of 1.7 Hz, a mean amplitude of about 1.0 degrees, and mean slow-phase peak velocity of 2.0 degrees per second. Latent nystagmus was found in 2 of 18 patients tested with strabismus; it was not found in any patient having amblyopia only, as correctly predicted by Dell'Osso et al. (1983). The nystagmus saccades had a normal peak velocity/amplitude relationship, suggesting normal neural control for saccade generation. More recently, Dell'Osso et al. (1983) presented binocular eye movement recordings of fixation, with and without monocular occlusion, in three patients with well-documented latent nystagmus. Records in one patient are presented in Figure 5.16, showing absence of nystagmus during binocular fixation but jerk nystagmus with the fast phase in the direction of the viewing eye once occlusion occurred, and the ocular deviation became manifest. Thus strabismus *is* a necessary condition for the latent nystagmus to be present.

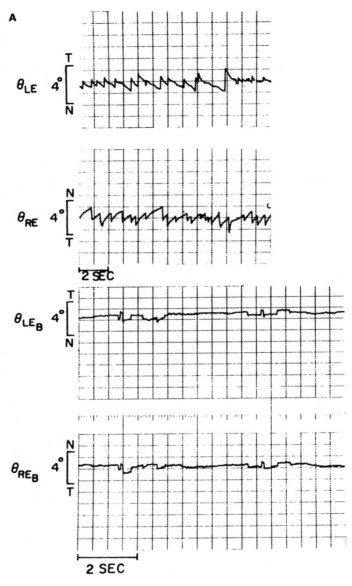

Figure 5.15 (A) *Eye position as a function of time for a subject with pure latent nystagmus. From top to bottom, monocular left eye position (θ_{LE}), monocular right eye position (θ_{RE}), and left (θ_{LE_B}) and right (θ_{RE_B}) eye positions during binocular viewing, respectively. Records show latent nystagmus during monocular viewing, but only intermittent saccadic intrusions during binocular viewing. Midline fixation. (B) Mean latent nystagmus frequency and amplitude as a function of gaze and fixating eye for this subject. Vertical bars represent ±1 standard deviation. (From Ciuffreda 1977.)*

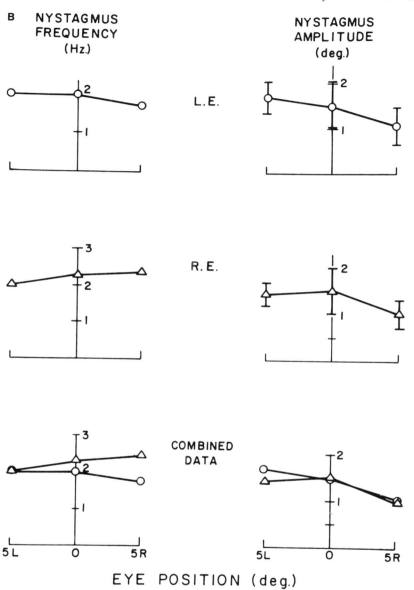

Figure 5.15 *(continued)*

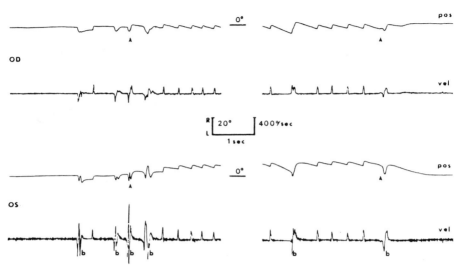

Figure 5.16   *Position (pos) and velocity (vel) tracings of the right (OD) and left (OS) eyes during covering (left arrows) and uncovering (right arrows) of the left eye while viewing a target in primary position. Primary position is indicated by the horizontal line labeled 0 degrees. Eye movement directions right (R) and left (L) are indicated, as are the blinks (b). (With permission of the publisher, from Dell'Osso et al. 1983.)*

Manifest Nystagmus

Manifest nystagmus is a disorder of the oculomotor system wherein the nystagmus (typically of the jerk variety, although pendular also could be included) is present (and obvious) during both monocular *and* binocular viewing conditions; this is in contrast to *latent nystagmus*, which is typically provoked by occlusion of an eye and is generally absent or much smaller when both eyes are unoccluded. Estimated incidence of manifest nystagmus in various populations include 0.005% by Norn (1964), 0.015% by Hemmes (1927), and 0.4% by Anderson (1954). Corrected visual acuity averaged 20/50 in a group of patients with nystagmus (Gamble 1934); 97% had visual acuities equal to or better than 20/200 (Norn 1964). Visual acuity and nystagmus intensity have been reported to be improved by orthoptics in some patients (Smith 1950, Healy 1952, 1962, Stegall 1973, Stohler 1973, Pearlman 1976).

The relationship between nystagmus and strabismus has received considerable attention. Gillies (1968) observed nystagmus in 17% of his clinical population; he found nystagmus in 10% of the patients having horizontal strabismus, in 30% of the patients having horizontal and vertical components to their strabismus, and in none of the patients having amblyopia alone or with a very small angular deviation. Wybar (1968) reported esotropia in 33% of the children with idiopathic nystagmus; he believed that nystagmus at an early age hindered the development of normal binocular vision, thus producing strabismus. Norn (1964) reported that approximately 50% of his patients with congenital idiopathic nystagmus had strabismus, while Gamble (1934) found that 40% of his patients with congenital nystagmus had strabismus. West (1939) presented a family pedigree showing that four of five individuals in the third generation with nystagmus also had strabismus. Coherty and Lee (1975) described two cases in which a unilateral vertical nystagmus appeared in the amblyopic eye during the course of treatment for amblyopia and strabismus. The high prevalence of strabismus in the various nystagmus populations is in marked contrast to the incidence of strabismus (4.8%) in a general population of school-aged children (M. C. Flom, personal communication, 1977).

Ciuffreda and colleagues (Ciuffreda 1977, Ciuffreda et al. 1979a) performed a quantitative analysis of fixation in four patients with manifest nystagmus and strabismus. Fixational eye movement responses are presented and summarized in a typical patient in Figure 5.17. The low frequency and amplitude of the jerk nystagmus once again make a simple clinical diagnosis difficult (Figure 5.17*A*); in many cases, use of high-resolution eye movement recordings is the only way to be certain of the diagnosis. Mean manifest nystagmus frequency ranged from 1.2 to 2.2, 0.9 to 2.3, and 0.7 to 1.9 Hz during midline fixation with the dominant eye, amblyopic eye, and both eyes, respectively. Mean nystagmus amplitude ranged from 0.24 to 1.4, 0.32 to 5.6, and 0.25 to 2.1 degrees during midline fixation with the dominant eye, amblyopic eye, and both eyes, respectively. Mean slow-phase nystagmus velocity ranged from 0.9 to 3.5, 1.0 to 8.0, and 1.0 to 3.5 degrees per second during midline fixation with the dominant eye, amblyopic eye, and both eyes, respectively. Mean nystagmus amplitude increased from 0.25 to 1.25 degrees and mean nystagmus slow phase velocity increased from 0.4 to 2.0 degrees per second when one patient changed from fixation in the light to "fixation" in total darkness (no other patients were tested in the dark) (Figure 17*B*). Nystagmus frequency remained unchanged at 1.75 Hz. This suggests that in the light a velocity-correcting system (probably smooth-pursuit slow-control) requiring visual feedback was operating to counteract the true nystagmus as revealed in the dark. Manifest nystagmus was found in 4 of 18 patients with strabismus, and in agreement with Gillies (1968) was not found in patients having amblyopia only. Suppression of nystagmus saccades was possible during the "hold" versus "fixate" command (Ciuffreda et al. 1979b, Ciuffreda 1979). Influence of changes in instruction (and apparently criteria for accurate fixation) is demonstrated during the "fixate" and "hold" trials in a later patient tested with manifest nystagmus and strabismus (Ciuffreda 1979) (Figure 5.18). Mean nystagmus fast-phase (saccadic) amplitude was 1.9 degrees during the "fixate" command, but only 1.4 degrees during the "hold" command (t test, $p < 0.001$). This result demonstrates the ability of a naive subject to reduce significantly the nystagmus amplitude simply by change of instruction. Reduction of nystagmus frequency during the "hold" command was not as consistent a finding, although as shown in the last portion of this trace, it could be decreased from an average of 3.7 to 3.1 Hz.

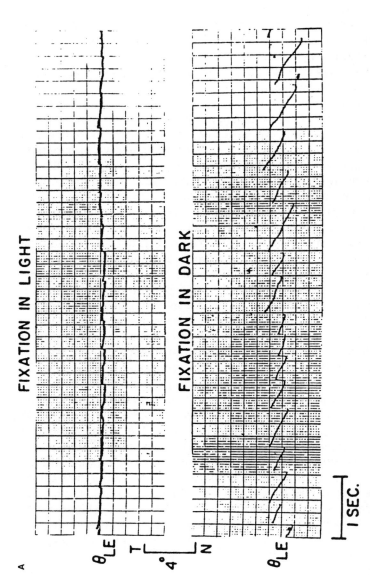

Figure 5.17 (A) Eye position as a function of time for midline fixation in a subject with manifest nystagmus. The top trace is eye position for fixation under normal test illumination conditions; bottom trace is fixation in total darkness immediately following extinguishing of the lights and target. Note increase in nystagmus amplitude and velocity in the dark but without much change in frequency. As fixation was continued in the dark, slow rightward drift of the eyes was superimposed on the large nystagmus movements. Ramp slow-phase waveform is prominent during the in-dark fixation. (B) Mean manifest nystagmus frequency and amplitude as a function of gaze and fixating eye for this subject. Vertical bars represent ±1 standard deviation. (From Ciuffreda 1977.)

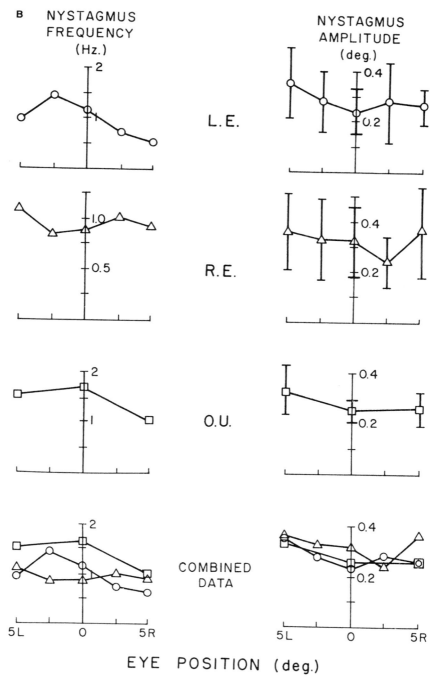

Figure 5.17   *(continued)*

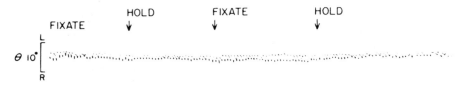

Figure 5.18 *Monocular fixation with the dominant eye. "Fixate" versus "hold" commands. (With permission of the publisher, from Ciuffreda 1979.)*

Use of the "hold" command during funduscopy may prove helpful in examination of patients exhibiting jerk nystagmus (or saccadic intrusions). Rather than being instructed "to fixate," the patient would be told "to hold the eye steady" as the posterior pole evaluation began. If the patient were capable of reducing jerk nystagmus frequency and/or amplitude, decreased "jerkiness" of the eye would result. This procedure, used in conjunction with the patient fixating in the "null" position (i.e., the gaze position of minimal nystagmus), would allow for a more careful funduscopic inspection by the examiner in such individuals.

The importance of precise, objective eye movement recordings to aid in clinical diagnosis is borne out in the case histories of two of the patients. They were now diagnosed as having manifest nystagmus of low amplitude, frequency, and slow-phase velocity. One patient had never been told she had nystagmus, although she had been examined on numerous occasions over the years. The other patient was referred to a neuro-optometry oculomotor clinic, not with a diagnosis of manifest nystagmus, but rather of "bilateral unsteady fixation."

With respect to treatment, two recent methods have been employed. Dell'Osso et al. (1979) reported improvement in both the overall nystagmus "intensity" and visual acuity in two patients with congenital manifest jerk nystagmus and strabismus following extraocular muscle surgery with these specific purposes in mind (Figure 5.19). Ciuffreda et al. (1982, 1983) have had much initial success using oculomotor biofeedback therapy in a patient with manifest nystagmus and strabismus, as well as other patients with either manifest, presumed latent, or pendular nystagmus; improvement was in both eye movements and visual acuity [See Ciuffreda and Goldrich (1983) for an extensive review of this area.] However, long-term effectiveness was not investigated.

SACCADIC EYE MOVEMENTS

Saccades are the very rapid (generally 20 to 45 ms duration), high velocity (up to 1000 degrees per second) movements of the eyes (Bahill et al. 1975a, b, Bahill and Stark 1978) used to foveate objects of interest. They are the predominant eye movement during such tasks as reading and scanning visual scenes. In amblyopic eyes, three abnormalities of the saccadic system have been reported: (1) increased latency, (2) reduced peak velocity, and (3) dysmetria.

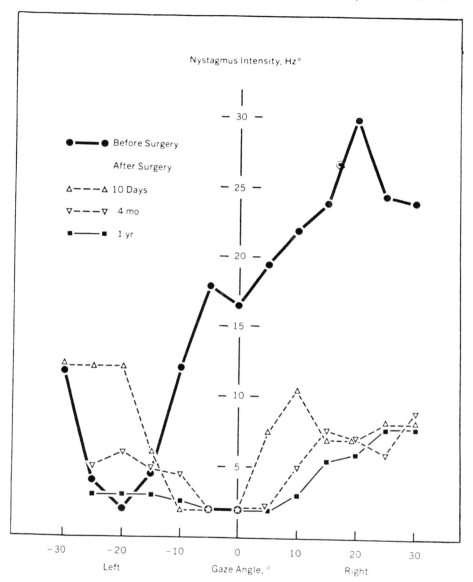

Figure 5.19 *Preoperative and postoperative plots of nystagmus intensity versus gaze angle for one patient showing the time course of improvement. (With permission of the publisher, from Dell'Osso and Flynn 1979.)*

Increased Saccadic Latency

Saccadic latency refers to the elapsed time between the change in stimulus, usually a rapid step displacement of the target, and the initiation of a saccadic eye movement to refixate the target. In visually normal individuals, saccadic latency averages about 200 ± 30 ms for objects located in the central visual field (Ciuffreda et al. 1978a, Leigh and Zee 1983).

There is a considerable body of evidence demonstrating the presence of increased saccadic latencies in most amblyopic eyes. One of the earliest investigations was that of Mackensen (1958). For targets randomly displaced ±15 degrees from the midline, he found saccadic latency to average about 250 ms in the amblyopic eyes and 225 ms in the fellow dominant eyes. This demonstrated some increased response delay to targets presented in the near periphery in the amblyopic eye. To determine if the central field was more severely affected by the amblyopia, as one might surmise, he then used an eye-hand reaction time paradigm with stimuli presented at the habitual fixation locus in the amblyopic eye and thus tested for central field delays. Now, however, the interocular difference increased to about 100 ms, with the amblyopic eye having the longer reaction time. This important result suggests that the effect of the amblyopia on reaction time is not uniformly distributed throughout the visual field, but rather has a more deleterious effect within the central few degrees. That eye-hand reaction time is indeed increased in the amblyopic eye in the central visual field has been confirmed and extended by von Noorden (1961) and by Hamasaki and Flynn (1981), with evidence to suggest that the increased reaction time was of a sensory rather than motor nature. Hamasaki and Flynn (1981) also demonstrated that the increased eye-hand reaction time (~ 45 ms) (Figure 5.20) (1) was related to the presence of amblyopia and not strabismus, (2) was not due to the presence of eccentric fixation, unsteady fixation, or retinal defocus in the amblyopic eye, and (3) was highly positively correlated with visual acuity in the amblyopic eye. However, the deeper the amblyopia, the greater was the difference in interocular reaction time (Figure 5.21).

There have been several other investigations of saccadic latency in amblyopic eyes that have extended the pioneering work of Mackensen (1958). Gerin et al. (1973) measured saccadic latencies and visual-evoked response (VER) implicit times in a group of 60 children with functional amblyopia. They (1) confirmed the presence of increased saccadic latencies in most amblyopic eyes, (2) found the increase in saccadic latency to be directly related to the severity of the amblyopia, and (3) found that the 100-ms average increase in saccadic latency in amblyopic eyes far exceeded the VER delay, suggesting that the neural pathway involved in the saccadic abnormality was beyond the site of generation of the VER in the primary visual cortex. More recently, Ciuffreda and colleagues (1978a and b) investigated saccadic latencies under monocular and binocular test conditions over the central visual field in normal individuals, amblyopes without strabismus, amblyopes with constant strabismus, and strabismics with little or no amblyopia. The primary finding of their investigation was that saccadic latency was increased in most amblyopic eyes (by up to 100 ms); a necessary condition for the occurrence of this increase was amblyopia and not strabismus, just as had been found by Hamasaki and Flynn (1981) for eye-hand reaction time in amblyopes. Thus amblyopes without strabismus always exhibited the delay, whereas strabismics without amblyopia did not (Figure 5.22).

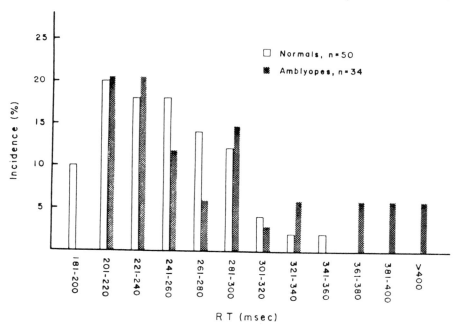

Figure 5.20 *Comparison of the distribution of mean reaction time of the normal subjects with that of the amblyopic patients. (Reprinted by permission of the publisher, from Hamasaki and Flynn 1981.)*

The finding of increased saccadic latencies in amblyopic eyes suggests a slowing in the sensory pathways that process visual information subsequently used by the oculomotor system in generating saccadic eye movements. These increased sensory processing times in amblyopic eyes, for both eye movements and eye-hand reaction times, are also consistent with results in amblyopes for visual masking (von Noorden and Burian 1960) and higher-level cognitive tasks (Burian et al. 1962).

In contrast to the sensory abnormalities found in amblyopic eyes, three findings provide evidence for normal motor control of their eye movements in amblyopic subjects. First, the saccades appear to be generated by normal pulse-step motoneuronal controller signals, as determined by the "main sequence" results, where saccadic amplitude is plotted against saccadic duration for the group (Figure 5.23) and peak velocity/peak acceleration/duration is plotted (Figure 5.24) for the normal and the amblyopic eyes of one subject; the data are in agreement with saccadic durations for normal subjects (Bahill et al. 1975a). Second, the precise synchronous movements of the two eyes under all test conditions further support the idea of normal neurologic control of saccadic eye movements, guided by two basic laws of oculomotor physiology—Descartes's law of reciprocal innervation (Ciuffreda and Stark 1975) and Hering's law of equal innervation (Bahill et al. 1976)—in these amblyopic subjects. Third,

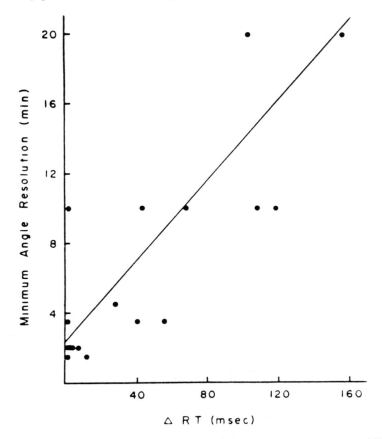

Figure 5.21 *Relationship between interocular difference in reaction time (ΔRT) and minimum angle of resolution in the amblyopic eye. The correlation coefficient is +0.82. (Reprinted by permission of the publisher, from Hamasaki and Flynn 1981.)*

saccadic latencies for binocular tracking, as well as for monocular tracking with the nonamblyopic eye, were within normal limits.

It is interesting to speculate on a possible neurophysiologic mechanism for producing increased saccadic latencies in amblyopic eyes. It has been advanced that the superior colliculus may be intimately involved in coding information regarding the location of objects in space relative to the fovea, the "foveation hypothesis" (Schiller and Stryker 1972), and in the initiation of saccadic eye movements. Cells have been found in the superior colliculus that appear to be related to the readiness to make an eye movement (Mohler and Wurtz 1976); it was suggested that these cells may be involved in early information processing for saccadic initiation. Increased saccadic latencies, approximately 150 to 300 ms greater than normal, have been measured in monkeys following focal lesions in the superior colliculus; accuracy of movement was not affected, and speed of

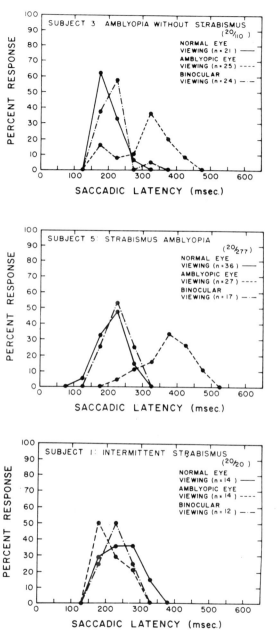

Figure 5.22 *Saccadic latency distributions for a subject from each of the three diagnostic groups. Note the pronounced distribution shift toward longer saccadic latencies in amblyopic eyes. Latency distributions are similar for all conditions in the subject having intermittent strabismus without amblyopia; in this subject, the "amblyopic eye" refers to the nondominant eye. (Reprinted by permission of the publisher, from Ciuffreda et al. 1978a.)*

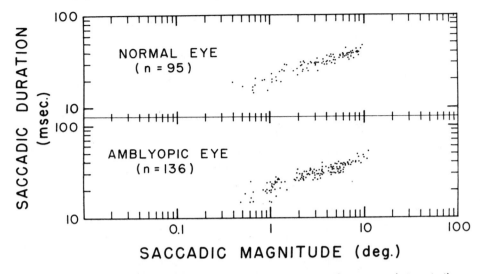

Figure 5.23   *Saccadic duration was found to be related to saccadic magnitude in a similar way in the 13 normal (fellow dominant) eyes and in the 13 amblyopic (or nondominant) eyes. (Reprinted by permission of the publisher, from Ciuffreda et al. 1978a.)*

movement was only minimally affected (Wurtz and Goldberg 1972). In kittens reared with unilateral strabismus (and presumably amblyopia), the ability of the strabismic eye to drive collicular cells was decreased (Gordon and Presson 1977). From these findings, it seems reasonable to suggest that in humans, as a result of abnormal visual experience (constant suppression and/or form deprivation producing amblyopia), certain cells in the sensory pathways leading either from the amblyopic eye directly to the superior colliculus or by means of the visual cortex, as well as cells and internal pathways within the superior colliculus itself, may be adversely affected, thus producing delays in information processing that result in abnormally long saccadic latencies.

Later, Ciuffreda et al. (1979c) reported a detailed account of changes in eye movements during the course of successful orthoptic therapy in an 18-year-old patient. Although several aspects of eye movement control improved with therapy, as did visual acuity, other aspects, such as saccadic latency, did not; it remained increased by about 100 ms (Figure 5.25). This result suggests that "transient" neural channels involved in saccadic initiation may either be more resistant to and/or are no longer amenable to recovery of vision function. However, more detailed investigations using a large clinical population undergoing therapy for remediation of their amblyopia must be studied in a double-blind controlled fashion before generalizations can be made.

Other studies have been conducted by the Japanese, who have a major commitment to understanding the mechanisms underlying amblyopia. Kato et al. (1980) found saccadic latencies to be greater for the nasal than temporal

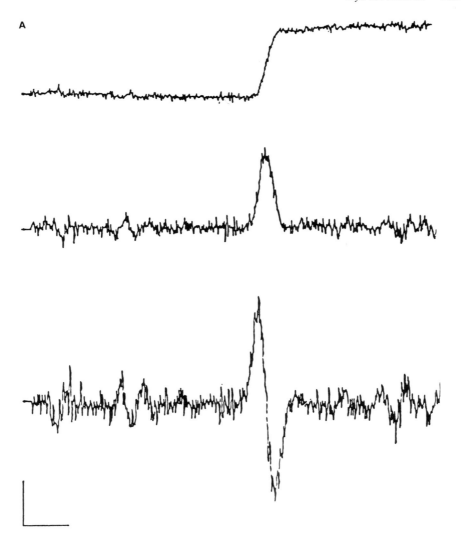

Figure 5.24 (A) *Eye position, velocity, and acceleration profiles (top to bottom) in an anisometropic amblyope (20/40) without strabismus. Calibration bar represents 1.3 degrees, 66 degrees per second, 3300 degrees per second squared, and 50 ms. Electronic tape noise in records is evident. (B) Main sequence plot of saccades in the dominant (closed circles) and amblyopic (triangles) eye. (From Ciuffreda KJ, Kenyon RV, and Stark L, unpublished findings.)*

hemiretina and for the superior than inferior hemiretina, suggesting differential retinal quadrant effects on saccadic processing time. Using an infrared TV fundus camera system, Mimura et al. (1981) have found saccadic latency to be increased in 16 of 18 patients tested for both horizontal *and* vertical saccadic

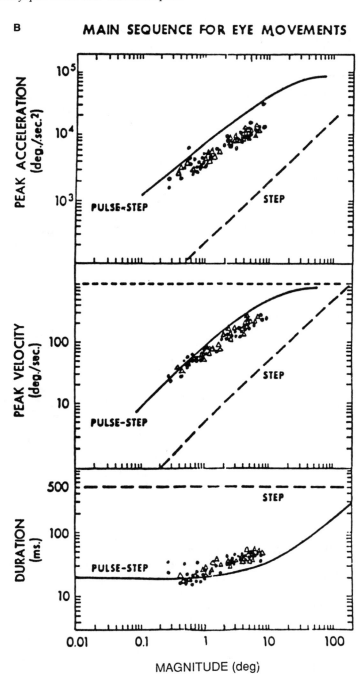

Figure 5.24   *(continued)*

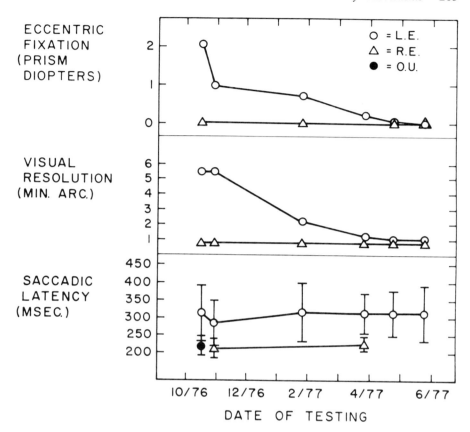

ECCENTRIC FIXATION (PRISM DIOPTERS)

VISUAL RESOLUTION (MIN. ARC.)

SACCADIC LATENCY (MSEC.)

O = L.E.
△ = R.E.
● = O.U.

DATE OF TESTING

Figure 5.25 *Changes in eccentric fixation, visual resolution, and saccadic latency for both eyes during the last 8 months of orthoptic therapy in an adult amblyope. Note centralization of fixation and normalization of visual resolution, but maintenance of increased saccadic latencies, in the left amblyopic eye. Plotted are the mean (and standard deviations for saccadic latency) of measures for each test session. (Reprinted by permission of the publisher, from Ciuffreda et al. 1979c.)*

tracking over the central field (± 5 degrees); the average reaction time was greater in strabismic (~300 ms) than anisometropic (~230 ms) amblyopes. This suggests that amblyopia adversely affects both the horizontal *and* vertical neural pathways subserving saccadic eye movements. Sensory rather than motor factors were again implicated. This notion was further reinforced by the recent work of Yamagata et al. (1983), who found normalization of saccadic latency in some amblyopic eyes when target energy (e.g., brightness) was increased. They, like Ciuffreda et al. (1979c), implicated the superior colliculus as the primary eye movement control center involved in such delays. Lastly, Fukushima and Tsutsui

(1984) performed a clever experiment which clearly demonstrated that increased saccadic latencies in amblyopic eyes were attributable to sensory rather than motor factors. They measured saccadic latency for both visual- and auditory-evoked saccades in amblyopic eyes. Saccadic latencies were increased for visual- but not auditory-evoked saccades in the amblyopic eye, with this increase being greater for strabismic than anisometropic amblyopes. Since there was no latency increase for visual-evoked saccades in strabismics without amblyopia, the results suggest that amblyopia and not strabismus was a necessary condition, as had been suggested earlier by Ciuffreda et al. (1978a and b). From this, Fukushima and Tsutsui (1984) suggested that the increased saccadic latencies found in amblyopic eyes were the result of visual processing delays in sensory pathways and, more specifically, that the dysfunction was localized in the occipital visual sensory areas. Lastly, they remarked that recovery of visual function in the amblyopic eye was greater the smaller the difference in interocular reaction time between the amblyopic and fellow dominant eye.

Normal Peak Saccadic Velocity and Duration

Although there are no direct comprehensive studies of saccadic velocities in amblyopic eyes, some preliminary work has been done that provides insight into this issue. In the unpublished findings of one adult anisometropic amblyope (20/40) without strabismus, Ciuffreda, Kenyon, and Stark found saccadic duration, peak velocity, and peak acceleration to be similar in each eye and without any obvious directional asymmetries (see Figure 5.24). These results suggest that the presence of the amblyopia did not differentially affect motor control; however, some values were very slightly depressed in each eye. Ciuffreda et al. (1978a), in a study primarily devoted to saccadic latency in amblyopia, found that saccadic durations in both the amblyopic and fellow dominant eye were normal and appropriate for their amplitude (see Figure 5.23). Thus, although the presence of increased saccadic latencies in amblyopic eyes suggested slowed sensory processing of visual information, the normal saccadic amplitude/duration/peak velocity relationship (i.e., "main sequence"; Bahill et al. 1975a) suggests normal motor control of saccadic eye movements. Thus the saccades were generated by normal pulse-step motoneuronal controller signals. However, a comprehensive investigation of saccadic duration, velocity, and acceleration in amblyopic eyes is yet needed to confirm and expand on these results to gain a more complete understanding in this area.

There have been two formal investigations of peak saccadic velocity and acceleration in strabismics having little or no amblyopia. Ishikawa and Terakado (1973) used electro-oculography to study refixation saccadic amplitude and peak velocity during the alternate cover test in esotropes and exotropes as well as normal patients. They found the peak saccadic velocities to be higher in exotropes than in esotropes; further, within each diagnostic group, the peak velocity was greater for movements in the same rather than opposing direction of the horizontal strabismic deviation. Normal subject data fell between these two groups. Unfortunately, the data are difficult to interpret in the absence of detailed clinic information regarding treatment history, especially with respect to extraocular muscle surgical manipulations, which may result in scar tissue formation that can act as a subtle mechanical hindrance to normal muscle dynamics. However, their saccadic velocity directional asymmetries are greater than those reported by Fricker (1976) in either normal individuals or postoperative strabismics. Lastly, the "supernormal" peak saccadic velocities of their exotropes leads one to suspect possible calibration artifacts. Again, more comprehensive studies with full clinical information and high-bandwidth eye movement recording will be necessary to resolve this important issue. Fricker (1976) used the dynamic parameters of saccadic velocity and acceleration to evaluate possible subtle changes in ocular movements following strabismus surgery. In three clinic patients with strabismus who were extensively tested, peak saccadic velocity and acceleration were within normal limits, thus suggesting that neither the presence of strabismus nor the extraocular muscle surgery adversely affected these two dynamic saccadic parameters.

Dysmetria

There has only been one detailed study of saccadic tracking in amblyopic eyes (Mackensen 1957b). Unfortunately, eye movements were recorded using electro-oculography and AC amplification; thus resolution was low, noise and drift were high, and postsaccadic fixation was contaminated by the short time constant (rapid decay) of the amplifiers. Further, many of the records presented are difficult to interpret owing to obvious contamination by prediction effects. The presence of marked hypometria (i.e., static undershooting), suggesting low gain of the saccadic system for large-amplitude (~ 30 degrees) movements, was the only clearly defined abnormality. Movements appeared to be conjugate. Mackensen interpreted his abnormal findings in terms of a sensory disturbance leading to inaccurate eye movements.

Other less comprehensive studies have provided additional important information regarding saccadic metrics. Schor (1975) noted marked and variable hypometria for predictable step target displacements into the nasal retina of the amblyopic eye (Figure 5.26); this was attributed to abnormal direction sense resulting from hemiretinal suppression in the habitually deviating amblyopic eye. However, the results are confounded by probable prediction effects. Two studies by Ciuffreda et al. (1979d and e) present some interesting but preliminary data related to this topic. In one adult amblyope monitored during the course of successful orthoptic therapy, marked static overshooting was evident during small-amplitude (0.6 degree) saccadic tracking, which did not diminish during the course of treatment (Ciuffreda et al. 1979d). Further, once steady-state fixation was attained, the movement amplitude was still much greater than the target step displacement (Figure 5.27). These results suggest grossly abnormal

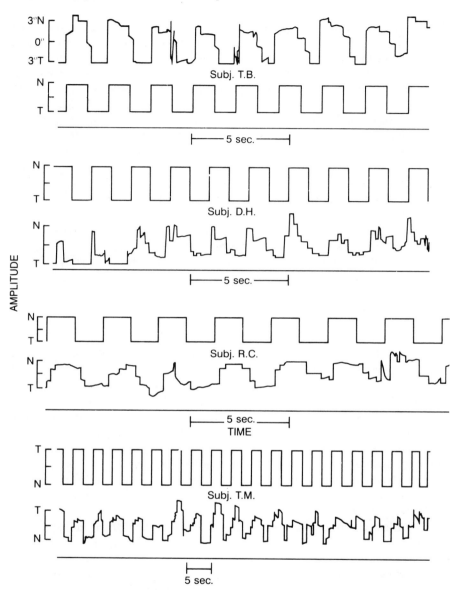

Figure 5.26 *Tracking responses of four amblyopic eyes to 0.5-Hz (first and second record) and 0.25-Hz (third and fourth record) square-wave stimuli contained a series of small saccades that were executed in the direction of each target displacement. The multiple saccades occurred most frequently in response to temporalward displacement of the test target (T) that corresponds to nasalward displacement of the retinal image. (Reprinted by permission of the publisher, from Schor 1975.)*

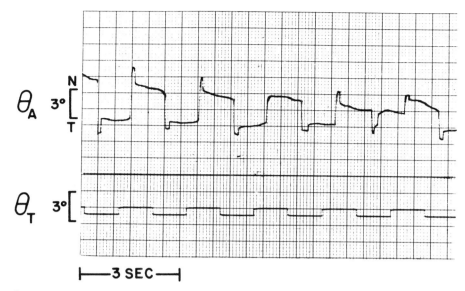

θ_A 3° [

N

T

θ_T 3° [

$\longmapsto$3 SEC$\longmapsto$

Figure 5.27 *Predictable, small-amplitude step tracking responses in the formerly ambly-opic eye (similar to that found in the same patient when visual acuity was 20/100). Upper trace is eye position, and lower trace is stimulus (0.5 Hz, 0.6-degree amplitude). Note static overshoots present in the majority of responses, suggesting increased gain of the saccadic eye movement system for small-amplitude displacements. (Reprinted by permission of the publisher, from Ciuffreda et al. 1979d.)*

spatial directional values in the central retina (Ciuffreda et al. 1979d), as has been reported by Schor (1972) and Bedell and Flom (1981, 1983). Later, Ciuffreda et al. (1979e) found evidence of marked hypometria and hypermetria in one patient with deep amblyopia (20/630) in response to nonpredictable 5-degree step target displacements. A series of large and small saccades was frequently required to refixate the target. Once again, saccadic inaccuracy was a common finding apparently related to abnormal sensory rather than motor factors.

PURSUIT EYE MOVEMENTS

The ability to follow a smoothly moving target, such as a speeding car or pitched baseball (McHugh and Bahill 1985), requires an intact pursuit system with enhancement by presence of a predictor operator (Stark 1968). Pursuit allows one to stabilize the target image on the retina, with addition of saccades for foveation to render its details more visible. Pursuit also may help in maintaining stability of gaze by counteracting drift of the eye during fixation. The stimulus for a pursuit eye movement is target or retinal-image velocity (Rashbass 1961, Robinson 1965), with target velocities up to 30 degrees per second or so accurately tracked, although some have reported olympic-quality tracking of up to 100 degrees per second (Lisberger et al. 1981). When target velocity exceeds this upper threshold, tracking is accomplished by some combination of pursuit and saccadic movements. In amblyopic eyes, abnormalities of pursuit include (1) reduced gain, (2) directional asymmetries, and (3) abnormal saccadic substitution.

Reduced Pursuit Gain

One of the earliest studies on pursuit eye movements in amblyopic eyes was conducted by von Noorden and Mackensen (1962). They used electro-oculography to measure pursuit movements to sinusoidally moving stimuli of various temporal frequencies over the central field (± 15 degrees) in a group of 30 strabismic amblyopes aged 7 to 21 years whose vision in the amblyopic eye ranged from 0.03 to 0.6. They found the "critical frequency," i.e., the target frequency for which pursuit tracking became saccadic (which indirectly reflects system gain), to be reduced in the amblyopic eye as compared with the fellow dominant eye (0.33 versus 0.53 Hz). Of interest was the finding that the critical frequency was slightly reduced in the fellow dominant eye as compared with either eye of visually normal subjects (0.53 versus 0.65 Hz), suggesting that the dominant eyes of amblyopes also may be slightly abnormal. This has recently been reported by Fukai and colleagues (Fukai 1974, Fukai et al. 1976) along with the presence of an increased frequency of saccadic and asymmetric pursuit in the dominant eyes of amblyopes; they speculated that such patients, generally strabismic amblyopes, had a reduced number of binocular cortical units that ultimately were used to drive the pursuit system. However, this asymmetric saccadic pursuit could, in part, also be due to the presence of small-amplitude jerk nystagmus, a common finding in *each* eye of such patients (Ciuffreda 1977). Low-resolution electro-oculography, as used by Fukai and colleagues (1974, 1976), would not be sensitive enough to discern such abnormal movements. While there was no clear relationship between pursuit ability and depth of amblyopia, von Noorden and Mackensen (1962) did find that those with the most severe amblyopia had the lowest critical frequencies. However, they also found that the critical pursuit frequency decreased as magnitude of eccentric fixation increased in the amblyopic eye. They believed that the presence of eccentric fixation was the key to the pursuit abnormality. If central fixation were preserved and the fovea remained as the sensory-motor zero reference point, then little if any pursuit disturbance should be observed. However, if eccentric fixation were present and the spatial properties of the eccentric fixation locus were indistinct, then pursuit should be disturbed, since they believed that the spatial "indistinctness" increased as eccentric fixation increased. This finding of reduced pursuit gain has been documented in several subsequent investigations (Figures 5.28 to 5.31). (Fukai and Tsutsui 1973, Schor 1975, Fukai et al. 1976,

Ciuffreda 1977, Tsutsui and Fukai 1978, Ciuffreda et al. 1979c and d, Quere 1980, Barard et al. 1980, Stark et al. 1982, 1984, Schor 1983, Tsutsui et al. 1984, Tychsen et al. 1985).

Asymmetric Pursuit

Asymmetric and saccadic pursuit, i.e., pursuit gain being grossly different for opposing directions of movement, has been reported by many investigators. Fukai and Tsutsui and colleagues (Fukai and Tsutsui 1973, Tsutsui and Fukai 1978, Tsutsui et al. 1984) have been the major proponents of this finding and its theoretical implications. Asymmetric pursuit was generally observed in strabismic amblyopes with eccentric fixation, wherein pursuit was relatively smooth and accurate (i.e., exhibiting normal gain) in one direction but saccadic in the opposing direction, suggesting low pursuit gain. However, the presence of jerk nystagmus with an otherwise intact and normal pursuit system can give the same

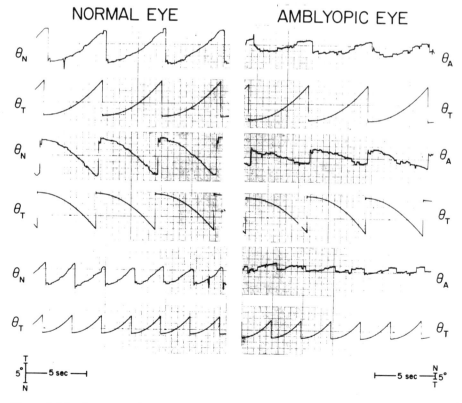

Figure 5.28 *Pursuit tracking in an anisometropic amblyope (20/180) for parabolic (i.e., constant acceleration) stimuli of 0.8 degrees per second squared. Reduced gain in the amblyopic eye is evident. (From K.J. Ciuffreda unpublished findings.)*

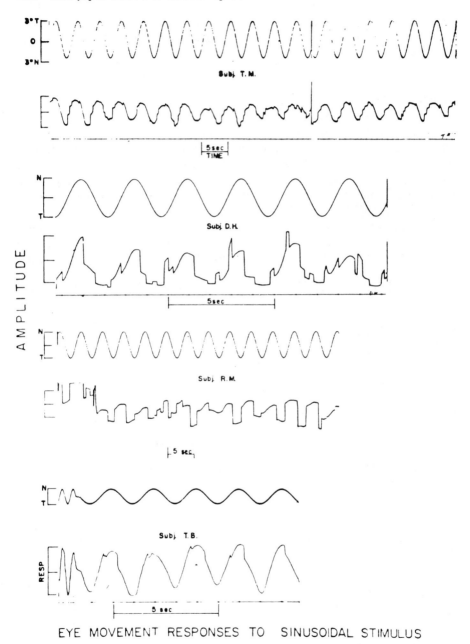

EYE MOVEMENT RESPONSES TO SINUSOIDAL STIMULUS

Figure 5.29   *The pursuit responses of amblyopic eyes to sinusoidal stimuli were composed of brief acceleration segments and uniform velocity segments interrupted by saccades. The abnormal acceleration control of the amblyopic eye appears to result from reduced sensitivity for velocity that disrupts prediction of future target motion. (Reprinted by permission of the publisher, from Schor 1975.)*

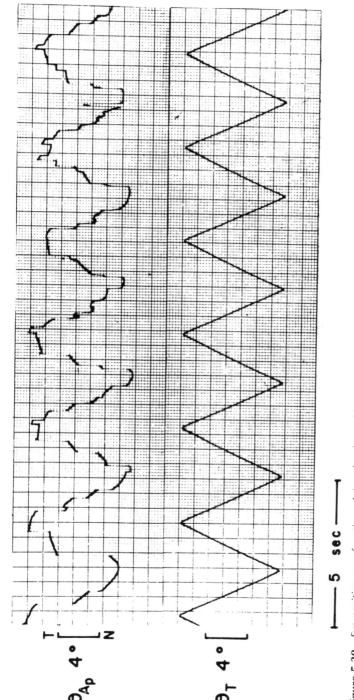

Figure 5.30 *Eye position as a function of time for the amblyopic eye. Strabismus amblyopia (20/277). Top trace is eye position, and bottom trace is stimulus (10 degree amplitude and 6.25 degrees per second velocity). Marked variability of pursuit performance is clearly indicated. (From Ciuffreda 1977.)*

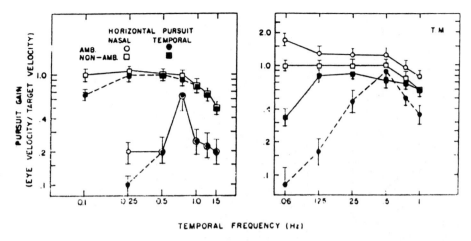

Figure 5.31   *Frequency response curves are compared for the normal and amblyopic eyes of two subjects for horizontal pursuit stimulated by a 6-degree peak-to-peak triangular stimulus at temporal frequencies ranging from 0.1 to 1.5 Hz. (Reprinted by permission of the publisher, from Schor 1983.)*

result when the nystagmus slow phases and target movement are in opposing directions as a result of (partial) velocity summation or cancelation at the retina (Ciuffreda 1977). In fact, this has been confirmed by the recent work of Bedell et al. (1990), who demonstrated that the pursuit asymmetry is markedly reduced following compensation for the fixational drift biases. In some cases, they speculated that this was due to a "disorganized, nondecussated visual pathway." However, a recent study by Tsychsen et al. (1985) suggests that a true pursuit asymmetry does indeed exist, with temporally directed pursuit being impaired, at least in patients with documented infantile (versus noninfantile) strabismus. This has been attributed in part to defective motion processing (Tsychen et al. 1986). In a recent retrospective study, Tsutsui et al. (1984) reported that patients with asymmetric pursuit (and asymmetric OKN) had the poorest prognosis for recovery of binocular vision function. However, it was in two studies by Schor (1975, 1983) that such asymmetric pursuit was most convincingly demonstrated in some amblyopic eyes (Figures 5.29 and 5.31). There was a marked directional impairment, with the gain being grossly reduced for nasalward versus temporalward target movement on the retina. Schor (1975) speculated that this was the result of hemiretinal suppression effects reducing velocity sensitivity over the nasal retina. Presence of monocular spatial distortion, being most pronounced in the nasal retina, also could be a major contributing factor (Ciuffreda et al. 1979d, Bedell and Flom 1981, 1983). Ciuffreda (1977) also found evidence of asymmetric pursuit in amblyopic eyes, but it was not a consistent finding and was quite variable in nature, even within the same subject tested over a period of only a few seconds (Figure 5.32). Asymmetric vertical pursuit also has been documented in some amblyopic eyes (Schor 1983) (Figure 5.33). Thus asymmetric and saccadic

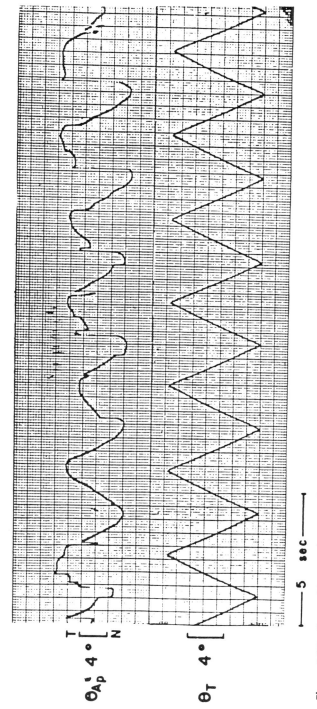

Figure 5.32 *Eye position as a function of time for the amblyopic eye. Strabismus amblyopia (20/630). Top trace is the eye position record, and bottom trace is the stimulus (10 degree amplitude and 6.35 degrees per second velocity). Last four cycles show the most marked directional asymmetry observed in any subject during pursuit. Note preceding one cycle of accurate pursuit. (From Ciuffreda 1977.)*

pursuit are clearly present in some amblyopic eyes, even when tested at the clinic level (Sherman 1974, George 1976), although its extent, consistency, and clinical impact remain debatable.

Abnormal Saccadic Substitution

A most unusual finding in amblyopic eyes was uncovered by Ciuffreda et al. (1979c, d). In normal individuals, when target velocity begins to approach the upper tracking threshold, saccades are added to the pursuit movements to reduce the accumulating position error, with saccade amplitude always being *less* than the full target excursion. However, when many amblyopes attempted to track a target moving over a relatively small spatial extent (no greater than 2

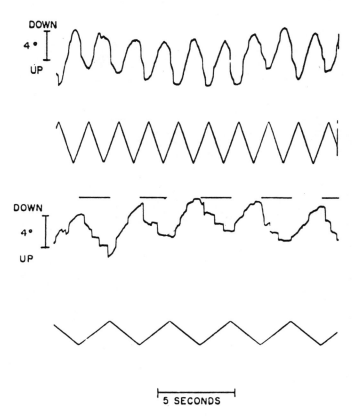

Figure 5.33 *Vertical pursuit response of an amblyopic eye to an 8-degree peak-to-peak triangular stimulus of 0.5 Hz (top) and 0.25 Hz (bottom). (Reprinted by permission of the publisher, from Schor 1983.)*

degrees), Ciuffreda et al. (1979d) found that they primarily used saccades whose amplitudes were two to four times *greater* than the target amplitude (Figures 5.34 and 5.35). This response pattern was referred to as *abnormal saccadic substitution*. It was related to the presence of amblyopia and not strabismus or eccentric fixation and did not improve with therapy (Ciuffreda et al. 1979c).

Although there is no single clear mechanism to explain the phenomenon of abnormal saccadic substitution, there are at least three possibilities (Ciuffreda et al. 1979d). The first is abnormal direction sense in amblyopic eyes. As a result of amblyopia, a depression of the directional-sensitivity gradient over the central retina may occur. This could result in impaired and/or marked variability of

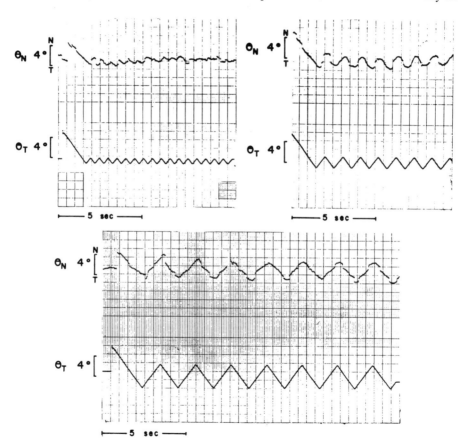

Figure 5.34   *Eye position as a function of time for the dominant eye (20/15) of a patient having amblyopia without strabismus. In each pair of records, the upper trace is eye position, and the lower trace is the stimulus. Target amplitudes are 1 degree (upper left), 2 degrees (upper right), and 4 degrees (below). T and N near calibration bars indicate templeward and nasalward movement of the eye, respectively. No evidence of abnormal saccadic substitution was present. Pursuit gain was within normal limits. (Reprinted by permission of the publisher, from Ciuffreda et al. 1979d.)*

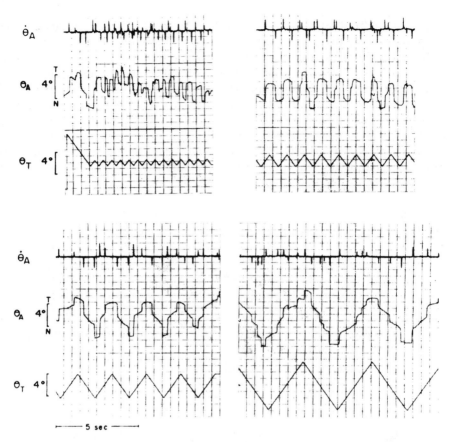

Figure 5.35   *Eye position as a function of time for the amblyopic eye of a patient having amblyopia without strabismus (20/110). Each set of traces shows eye velocity, eye position, and stimulus, respectively, from top to bottom. Target amplitudes are 1 degree (upper left), 2 degrees (upper right), 4 degrees (lower left), and 8 degrees (lower right). T and N near the calibration bars indicate templeward and nasalward movement of the eye, respectively. Abnormal saccadic substitution is clearly seen for the 1- and 2-degree stimuli, as well as some smooth movements at the turnaround points; for the 4-degree stimulus, saccadic pursuit is evident, with the overall tracking response amplitude still being somewhat larger than the stimulus amplitude; for the 8-degree stimulus, saccadic pursuit is evident, but the overall tracking response amplitude is now approximately equal to the stimulus amplitude. Thus, as the target amplitude increased (but with constant velocity maintained), pursuit became more normal. (Reprinted by permission of the publisher, from Ciuffreda et al. 1979d.)*

direction sense, including errors or biases in estimation of angular distance of targets relative to the preferred fixation locus. In the present situation, overestimation of small target movements on the retina would result in the inappropriately large eye movement exhibited by patients. If this abnormal direction sense hypothesis is correct and is generalized for all types of tracking, one would predict that hypermetria [i.e., static overshooting (Bahill et al. 1975b) and single large saccades] would be commonly found during small-amplitude step tracking. Although hypermetria was found in amblyopes, it was not as consistent a finding as was abnormal saccadic substitution. However, it appears reasonable to assume that a constantly moving target providing repeated information regarding target direction by stimulating retinal regions in an orderly sequence would elicit this response in a more consistent manner than would a target that moves in relatively infrequent, discrete, random steps and only stimulates small, isolated retinal regions. This idea of abnormal direction sense in amblyopic eyes is in agreement with that of other investigators. Mackensen (1957a, b) believed that the physiologic superiority of the fovea and the graded sensory function of the macula region had been transformed, due to the amblyopia, into a region of equivalent sensory characteristics. Mackensen (1966) also believed that eccentric fixation represented a transposition of the principal visual direction; von Noorden (1967) believed that amblyopes possessed a vagueness of directional sense; and Griffin (1976) believed that direction sense in an amblyopic eye with eccentric fixation is impaired and results in pastpointing. Bedell and Flom (1981, 1983) found increased spatial distortion and uncertainty in amblyopic eyes. These factors related to direction could contribute to the anomalous tracking responses found in amblyopic eyes. It is interesting to speculate that our notion of abnormal direction sense in amblyopic eyes, based on *dynamic* test results, may be related to eccentric fixation, which is based on *static* test results. Eccentric fixation is found in the majority of amblyopic eyes (Brock and Givner 1952, Girard et al. 1962), and its presence suggests a shift in the zero sensorimotor directional reference point under "steady state" monocular test conditions. A second mechanism, possibly related to the first, is suppression. It is a well-established fact that suppression is commonly found in amblyopic eyes under binocular test conditions (Travers 1938, Nawratzki and Jampolsky 1958). Suppression may result in an overall reduction in sensitivity over the central retinal region of the amblyopic eye. This sensorially depressed central zone would correspond to all or part of the area undergoing suppression in the amblyopic eye during binocular viewing. If this is true, a strategy of placing the target just outside this depressed region might be adopted during monocular tracking with the amblyopic eye. Impaired or vague direction sense would prevent the phenomenon of eccentric viewing from being reported. Thus the average size of these large tracking saccades (~ 2.5 degrees) may represent the horizontal angular dimension of this abnormal region. Direction, amplitude, and velocity of target movement could be processed for a longer period of time as target amplitude increased (and target movement on the retina increased). This could provide a possible explanation for the abnormal tracking response (large tracking saccades and absence of smooth movements) found for small-target excursions and the more normal tracking response (lack of large tracking saccades and presence of smooth movements) for larger-target excursions. This would be consistent with the notion of increased information-processing delays in amblyopic eyes (Ciuffreda et al. 1978a and b, Mackensen 1958, von Noorden and Burian 1960, von Noorden 1961, Burian et al. 1962, Goldstein and Greenstein 1971). A third explanation might simply be that abnormal saccadic substitution represents a normal phenomenon for small-amplitude pursuit tracking with the peripheral retina. However, the persistence of this abnormal response in one subject whose fixation centralized during orthoptic therapy does not lend support to this idea (Ciuffreda et al. 1979b). Moreover, recent findings by Fukai and Tsutsui (1973) suggest that nonfoveal tracking would result in asymmetric pursuit rather than the symmetric abnormal saccadic substitution found in our patients. That tracking small-amplitude stimuli binocularly or monocularly with the dominant eye never resulted in abnormal saccadic substitution further points to a sensory rather than motor basis for this pursuit defect.

VESTIBULAR-OPTOKINETIC MOVEMENTS

The vestibular-optokinetic system functions to maintain stability of images on the retina during movement of the head; thus it stabilizes one's gaze and ensures clear vision during self-movement, such as when one looks about while walking. The dual-component nature of the system is related to its dynamic characteristics. During sustained rotation, there is habituation of the vestibular system. The optokinetic system is then called on to maintain compensatory slow-phase eye movements to sustain retinal-image stability (Leigh and Zee 1983). In amblyopes, abnormalities in these joint systems include asymmetric and reduced optokinetic and vestibular responses.

Asymmetric/Reduced Optokinetic Responses

There have been numerous reports of asymmetric optokinetic responses in amblyopic eyes. The first was in a clinic investigation by Nicolai (1959). He found such responses in about half of the 99 strabismic amblyopes tested. The optokinetic responses were greater for temporal-to-nasal than for nasal-to-temporal movement. In 50 patients with strabismic amblyopia and eccentric fixation, asymmetric optokinetic nystagmus was found in 39 of the amblyopic eyes and in 25 of the fellow dominant eyes (Loewer-Sieger 1962). Schor and Levi (1980) found reduced and asymmetric optokinetic slow-phase gain under (normal) closed-loop test target conditions in the amblyopic eye (Figure 5.36). This abnormal response also was found in the fellow dominant eye of some of the amblyopes; such a finding is consistent with a report showing reduced and asymmetric optokinetic responses in each eye of cats reared throughout the critical period with surgically induced exotropia (Cynader and Harris 1980), suggesting that it was more related to the presence of strabismus than to any presumed amblyopia. While there was a reduction in pattern and motion sensitivity in the amblyopic eye, this deficit was not direction-dependent; thus such a symmetric sensory disturbance of perceived motion could not account for the optokinetic

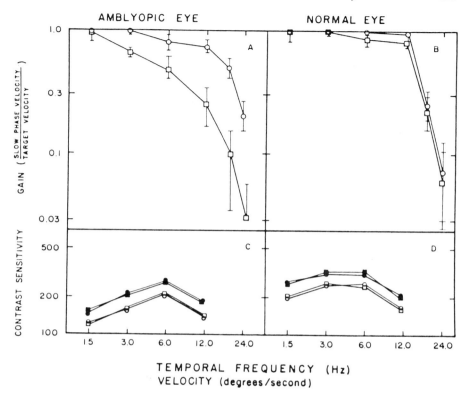

Figure 5.36 (A, B) *Gain (eye velocity/target) of the slow-phase of OKN for the moderately amblyopic eye (20/70) and nonamblyopic eye is plotted as a function of velocity of a 1 cycle per degree vertical sine wave grating drifting either nasalward (circles) or temporalward (squares) at velocities ranging from 1.5 to 25 degrees per second. Gain of the temporal slow phase of the amblyopic eye is abnormally reduced at velocities above 6 degrees per second. Gain for the nasalward slow phase of the amblyopic eye and both directions of slow phase for the nonamblyopic eye is the same as observed for the normal control subjects. (C, D) Contrast sensitivity to a 1 cycle per degree sinusoidal grating for the amblyopic and normal eye, respectively. Pattern sensitivity (open symbols) and movement sensitivity (closed symbols) are plotted in response to velocities ranging from 1.5 to 12 degrees per second in either the nasal (circles) or temporal (squares) direction. Sensitivity to nasalward and temporalward drifting gratings is symmetrical for both the amblyopic and nonamblyopic eye. (Reprinted by permission of the publisher, from Schor and Levi 1980.)*

motor system asymmetry. Similar results were found in four adults whose amblyopia was fully corrected in childhood. Further, there was not a direct relationship between the degree of optokinetic abnormality and visual acuity in the amblyopic eye, although the most severe amblyopes showed a greater deficit than those with moderate degrees of amblyopia. The authors presented arguments to suggest that the asymmetry was greater than could be accounted for by the presence of either latent nystagmus or fixational drift biases. Lastly, Schor and Levi speculated that the asymmetric optokinetic nystagmus was due to incomplete development of binocular vision, more specifically to cortical mechanisms mediating temporally driven optokinetic responses, prior to the age of 4 years. These basic ideas were summarized and expanded upon later by Schor (1983), who now also implicated subcortical pretectal mechanisms underlying these abnormal responses. Mein (1983) only found asymmetric optokinetic responses in patients having strabismus, nystagmus, *and* dissociated vertical divergence, and not in other patients with either early or late onset of strabismus. Only when nystagmus was *absent* did the optokinetic asymmetry no longer prevail. Asymmetry of optokinetic nystagmus also was reported in strabismics (generally with amblyopia) by Flynn et al. (1984). Schor and Westall (1984) believed the optokinetic directional asymmetry in amblyopic eyes was a result of extraretinal drift bias, as well as abnormal visually based nasal drift bias and reduced position sensitivity. However, their results may be confounded by unwarranted assumptions (such as linear summation of motor responses) and the presence of jerk nystagmus in some patients. Most recently, Westall and Schor (1985) studied optokinetic asymmetries as related to size and location of the retinal stimulating area under open-loop test target conditions. All amblyopic eyes exhibited greater responses for nasal than for temporal target movement for the large central, small central, and peripheral concentric stimulating fields. The responses were reduced for temporal versus nasal hemiretinal stimulation. These authors speculated that the asymmetric optokinetic responses were due to reduced cortical input to subcortical structures, as well as to binocular cortical suppression effects in the amblyopic eye. Such reasoning would account for the presence of optokinetic asymmetry in *each* eye of the amblyopes, as found in some of the patients in this and an earlier study (Schor and Levi 1980) under closed-loop conditions, assuming absence of any jerk nystagmus. In two other studies it was reported that optokinetic nystagmus gain was either very low (Urist 1961) or normal (Enokkson and Mortensen 1968) in the amblyopic eye.

Asymmetric/Reduced Vestibular Responses

There have been only a handful of studies involving vestibular function in the amblyopic eye. Salman and von Noorden (1970) found caloric-induced nystagmus in strabismics (many presumably with amblyopia due to the early onset of the strabismus) to have a more variable amplitude and frequency, as compared with normal children, and to be similar to what may be found in a variety of neurologic disorders. Thus they emphasized the need for clinicians to be aware of such "abnormal" responses in an otherwise apparently healthy population, especially as related to differential diagnosis in patients suspected of having organic or neurologic disease. It should be noted that many of their patients probably had latent nystagmus, which could confound both the eye movement record and the diagnosis. Similar results were reported earlier by Doden and

Adams (1957). Ciuffreda (1977), however, found normal vestibulo-ocular responses during sinusoidal head rotation with gaze fixed on a midline target in a strabismic amblyope with latent nystagmus (Figure 5.37). The frequency of saccades, as evidenced in the velocity trace, was similar to that found during normal midline fixation with the amblyopic eye. This suggested that the resultant motor output was due to summation (not necessarily linear) between the vestibular signals and those neural signals responsible for nystagmus generation. Hoyt (1982) reported reduced vestibulo-ocular responses in 14 of 24 congenital esotropes (without apparent nystagmus) during clinic testing. Flynn and colleagues (Flynn 1982, Flynn et al. 1984) reported gaze-dependent failure to suppress the vestibulo-ocular response in some patients with congenital esotropia. Schor and Westall (1984) found vestibular imbalance in the dark in amblyopes; that is, the saccade-free slow-phase component of the response to sinusoidal head rotation in darkness exhibited a directional preference. This directional preference was the same as found during dark fixation in these same subjects. These authors speculated that the vestibular imbalance could account for one-half the variance in dark drift, although the logic (other than from their correlational analysis) for such a relationship is not obvious. More recently, Westall and Schor (1985) found asymmetric vestibulo-ocular adaptation in strabismic amblyopes; the vestibulo-ocular gain increased more following adaptation to nasal versus temporal field motion. There was no difference in adaptive capability between the amblyopic and fellow dominant eye, suggesting that this abnormality was related to the presence of strabismus and not the amblyopia. However, recent work by Tyschen et al. (1985) shows normal vestibular responses when contamination from the (defective) pursuit system is absent in infantile strabismus.

VERGENCE EYE MOVEMENTS

Disparity Vergence with and without the Accommodative Contribution

Until recently, vergence eye movements recorded from amblyopic and/or strabismic patients either have been confined to static measures of eye position or were inferred from subjective responses. Bielschowsky (1900), Schlodtmann (1900), and Burian (1941) all reported fusional abilities in strabismic patients. Burian (1941), using an elaborate system of projectors and polarizers, presented identical images haploscopically into the periphery of each eye. When these images were made disparate, the strabismic subject was instructed to report the position of two fiduciary marks in the (blanked out) center of his visual field. Realignment of these marks, which did occur, was interpreted to be the result of peripheral fusional eye movements. Hallden (1952) found similar results when measuring the static vergence angle. His measurements were taken at 1-minute

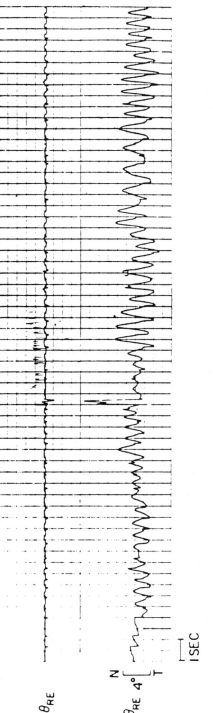

Figure 5.37 *Eye position as a function of time during vestibular testing in a strabismic amblyope with latent nystagmus. Top trace is right eye velocity, and bottom trace is right eye position. Head of subject was rotated at several frequencies by the examiner as the subject was instructed to fixate a midline target. Note the nystagmus prominent throughout; see especially the velocity trace. (From Ciuffreda 1977.)*

intervals, and he reported that strabismic patients took several minutes (up to 40 minutes) to realign their eyes following a change in target disparity. Results similar to Hallden's were recently reported by Bagolini and his group (Bagolini 1974, 1976; Campos and Catellani 1978; Campos et al. 1988, 1989). An alternative interpretation of Burian's result was proposed by Kretschmar (1955) and later by Mariani and Pasino (1964). They demonstrated how sensory changes related to the angle of anomaly could account for some or all of the preceding results. Kertesz (1983) reported improvement in fusional ability following wide-angle (57-degree) fusional stimulation training in exotropes, with maintenance of the effects 3½ years later. Eye position was not measured in any of these studies, however. Furthermore, in most of these studies, the time course of the presumed disparity vergence (several seconds to several minutes) was much greater than for typical vergence movements in normal individuals (about 1 second) (Westheimer and Mitchell 1956, Riggs and Neihl 1960, Rashbass and Westheimer 1961, Zuber and Stark 1968). This suggests involvement of slow tonic vergence rather than the very rapid disparity vergence system. Further studies are needed to lend support to this speculation.

Only recently have objective dynamic vergence eye movements been measured in strabismic and/or amblyopic patients (Kenyon 1978, Quere 1979, Kenyon et al. 1980a and b, 1981, Schoessler 1980, Boman and Kertesz 1985). Schoessler (1980) presented normal and strabismic subjects having anomalous retinal correspondence (ARC) with an asymmetric disparity stimulus using a modified haploscope. With the dominant eye's target held stationary at the fovea, target position and thus disparity was changed in the strabismic eye. Vergence responses were recorded in all subjects. The direction of the disparity or fusional vergence response changed appropriately when the stimulus was displaced through the subject's ARC point in the nondominant eye rather than the fovea as found in normal subjects. This is consistent with the idea of a foveal-to-nonfoveal binocular zero sensorimotor coordinate correspondence system in ARC rather than a foveal-to-foveal system as found in normal retinal correspondence (NRC).

Unlike the previous studies that presented targets haploscopically and introduced changes in target disparity only, Kenyon and colleagues (1978, 1980a and b, 1981) introduced vergence stimuli by having subjects fixate targets at different physical distances; thus these targets stimulated both the disparity and accommodative vergence systems and provided congruent stimuli similar to that found in everyday viewing. Peripheral retinal contribution to vergence was reduced by using small targets of 2 degrees that moved approximately 3 degrees into the periphery. Thus disparity and defocus changes were confined to the foveal and near-parafoveal regions. Under conditions in which both target disparity and target distance were randomly changed, strabismic patients used accommodative vergence instead of disparity vergence to shift their eyes to the new target position. In comparing normal symmetric vergence movements with those of the strabismic patients (Figures 5.38 to 5.40), dramatic differences were evident. Instead of a smooth and equal disjunctive movement, patients made a saccade to place the fovea of the dominant eye on the target, followed by an unequal vergence movement, i.e., accommodative vergence (Kenyon et al. 1978, 1980a, b). Patients with intermittent strabismus, constant strabismus with or without amblyopia, and some amblyopes without strabismus showed these abnormal responses. Presence of amblyopia alone appeared to have a less dramatic effect than strabismus alone, since amblyopes without strabismus did not always produce these abnormal responses, whereas strabismics (with or without amblyopia) *always* did. Neither the amount of strabismus nor the degree of amblyopia in patients with constant strabismic amblyopia had any effect on the response to symmetric vergence stimuli. Patients with small-angle strabismus and deep amblyopia produced abnormal symmetric vergence responses similar to those of patients who had small-angle strabismus and mild amblyopia. These abnormal vergence responses were made independent of the presence of ARC. Quere (1979) reported similar results, as well as marked inequality of interocular disparity vergence amplitude, in response to symmetric disparity stimuli in many amblyopes and strabismics. Pickwell and Hampshire (1981) have provided clinical confirmation. Recently, Boonstra et al. (1988) have presented results using objective eye movement recordings in microstrabismus that confirm the findings of Kenyon and colleagues, as well as those of Boman and Kertesz (1985).

Targets aligned along the dominant eye (i.e., to elicit asymmetric vergence) revealed responses with a similar lack of normal disparity vergence (Kenyon 1978, Kenyon et al. 1980b, 1981). Thus differences between patient and control responses to symmetric and asymmetric vergence stimuli demonstrated a general lack of disparity vergence in these patients and the consequent frequent use of accommodative vergence under these test conditions with small central targets.

The striking absence of disparity vergence in these patients may be related to stimulus form. At the time, it was speculated that with use of either large-field stimuli or stimuli having equal perceptual efficacy in each eye (e.g., created by placing neutral-density filters in front of the dominant eye until target "sensations" are equal in the two eyes), true disparity vergence responses might have been elicited. This possibility is consistent with their notion of suppression as a common factor in strabismics and amblyopes.

Work by Boman and Kertesz (1985) has helped to resolve in part a current controversy regarding vergence responses in strabismics. While many clinicians claim to have observed normal fusional vergence responses in strabismics, the laboratory investigations of Kenyon et al. (1980a and b, 1981) do not support such observations. The key to this dilemma, as originally speculated by Stark et al. (1982, 1984), is the size of the target used to stimulate the fusional vergence system. Boman and Kertesz (1985) objectively recorded binocular horizontal eye movements in older strabismics (with and without amblyopia) (Figure 5.41). First, they replicated the test conditions used by Kenyon et al. (1980a) and confirmed their original findings. When small central test stimuli were used, strabismics did not execute normal vergence responses; they responded with a (dominant eye) foveating saccade and an accommodative vergence movement. Then, in these same subjects (as well as in several others tested), use of a large

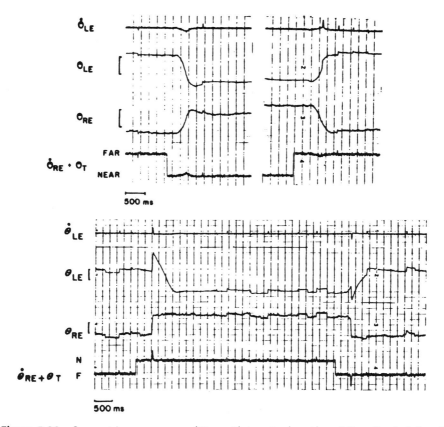

Figure 5.38 *Symmetric vergence condition with targets along the midline. Symbols for all figures unless otherwise noted are θ_{LE} = left eye position; θ_{RE} = right eye position; $\dot{\theta}_{LE}$ = left eye velocity; $\dot{\theta}_{RE} + \theta_T$ = right eye velocity summed with target position. Downward deflections represent rightward movements. Calibration bars for position represent 2 degrees, and time markers represent 500 ms. (Above) Normal control subject shows normal responses to symmetric vergence stimuli. (Below) Patient having intermittent strabismus without amblyopia exhibits abnormal responses. Saccade occurring early in the response is used to foveate the new target with the dominant right eye. Accommodative vergence occurs primarily in the strabismic left eye. (Reprinted by permission of publisher, from Kenyon et al. 1980a.)*

($\sim$ 40- by 50- degree) disparity-only stimulus (presented in 0.5-degree steps) *was* indeed sufficient to produce more normal-appearing disparity vergence responses, although the average group response amplitude was reduced by about 33% when compared with that of control subjects. Thus these results support the speculation of Kenyon et al. (1980a) that central suppression acted to block the disparity input to the oculomotor system; however, once the disparity stimulus extended outside this presumed region of binocular suppression, the disparity input could be processed, resulting in disparity vergence responses.

Further, the new findings of Boman and Kertesz (1985) support the preliminary results of Noordenbos and Crone (1976), who used an objective photographic technique to provide evidence for a motor vergence component when large-field disparity-only stimuli were used in patients with small-angle esotropia. However, once again, response amplitudes were generally reduced.

Based on these experiments, one can begin to consider possible causes for the abnormal vergence movements. A purely peripheral and/or motor dysfunction encompassing the extraocular muscles, oculomotor neurons, and/or brainstem

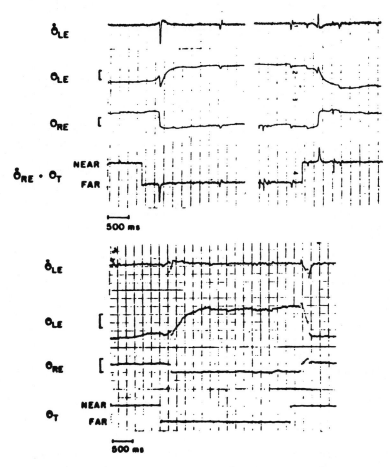

Figure 5.39 *Symmetric vergence condition. (Above) Patient with constant strabismic amblyopia (20/122) showing similar abnormal responses consisting of predominant accommodative vergence in the amblyopic left eye and an early foveating saccade driven by the dominant right eye. Note unequal non-Hering's law saccades during the responses, especially for convergence. (Below) Patient having amblyopia without strabismus (20/38). Similar abnormal responses were found in this patient, but they only occurred intermittently. (Reprinted by permission of the publisher, from Kenyon et al. 1980a.)*

nuclei is unlikely in these patients, since accommodative vergence had normal dynamics and latencies (Kenyon 1978, Kenyon et al. 1980a and b, 1981). Also, the intermittent nature of these abnormal responses in some patients demonstrated that the basic vergence motor nuclei and controller were capable of generating motoneuronal signals to which the extraocular muscles could respond to produce appropriate and normal disparity vergence movements (Kenyon 1978, Kenyon et al. 1980b). Higher-level defects are much harder to specify precisely. Suppression is a likely mechanism to block disparity, especially in patients with strabismus having deviations greater than 10 prism diopters (Travers 1938, Jampolsky 1955, Pratt-Johnson et al. 1967, Pratt-Johnson and Wee 1969). Such a suppression mechanism also may block information to disparity-processing centers, effectively leaving only information from the dominant eye. Interestingly, Blake and Lehmkuhle (1976) have demonstrated normal grating aftereffects in the presence of suppression associated with strabismus. This suggests that the site for suppression is beyond the site of the grating aftereffect (probably area 17 of the visual cortex). A similar higher-level central site may be responsible for suppression of disparity information used in the control of disparity vergence eye movements. Markedly reduced visual acuity in some of the amblyopic eyes also may explain their poor responses; however, the intermittent nature of the abnormal vergence in some patients having only amblyopia suggests that strabismus had a much stronger effect on disparity vergence than did the presence of amblyopia and its related sensory abnormalities (Kenyon et al. 1980a and b, 1981). Finally, it is possible, although highly speculative, that lack of disparity vergence may be a result of reduced binocular stimulation to corresponding retinal points during childhood. Animal

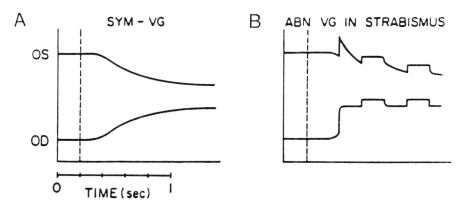

Figure 5.40 *Vergence eye movements. Schematized responses. (A) Symmetrical vergence. Vertical dashed line indicates instant of target distance change; upward displacement on ordinate is leftward for left eye (OS) and the right eye (OD); time in seconds is on the abscissa. (B) Abnormal vergence in a patient with strabismus showing an asymmetrical response to a symmetrical stimulus, as well as multiple saccadic intrusions. (Adapted and reprinted by permission of the publisher, from Stark 1983.)*

Figure 5.41
Responses by four strabismics to 5-degree convergent or divergent disparity presentations contained in the full-field stimulus. The overall motor compensation and the change in each eye's line of sight are given in degrees of arc. (A) Patient 9, a microtrope. (B) Patient 6, an intermittent exotrope. (C) Patient 8, an accommodative esotrope. (D) Patient 1, a small-angle esotrope with amblyopia. (Reprinted by permission of the publisher, from Boman and Kertesz 1985.)

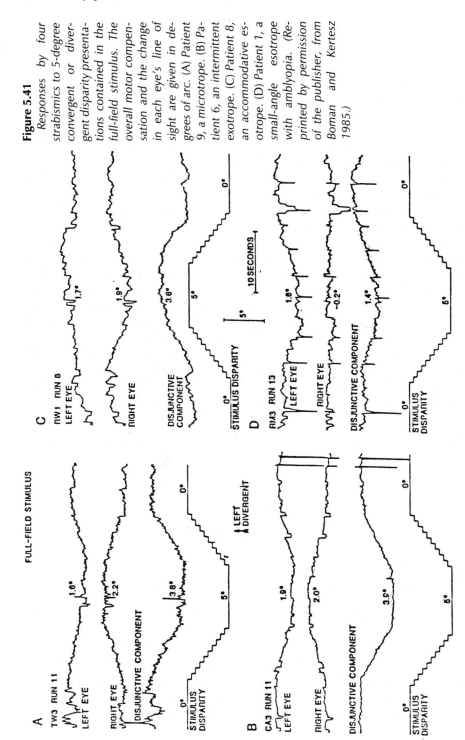

studies in which strabismus (and amblyopia) were artificially produced showed a reduction in the number of binocular cortical cells (Hubel and Wiesel 1965, Ikeda and Tremain 1977, Baker et al. 1974, Ikeda and Wright 1974). If cells that process and code disparity information used in the control of vergence eye movements are similarly affected, the lack or decreased number of these cells might reduce vergence response capability and/or amplitude. Further experiments that simultaneously monitor eye movements and single-unit responses from the visual cortex and oculomotor nuclei in both natural and artificially rendered strabismic and amblyopic animals should help to clarify these points.

Orthoptic Effects

Within the group of patients studied by Kenyon et al. (1980a and b, 1981), three adults were successfully treated for either amblyopia or strabismus. One patient received orthoptic therapy for amblyopia and eccentric fixation in the left eye. After training, his visual acuity improved from 20/110 to 20/20, and the eccentric fixation reduced from 2 prism diopters to zero in the amblyopic eye. His vergence movements, recorded shortly after termination of the orthoptic treatment, contained the same characteristic abnormal vergence response pattern as recorded in all the other strabismic patients. Thus, even after normalization of visual acuity and centralization of fixation, disparity vergence responses were still abnormal in this former amblyope. Interestingly, some other oculomotor findings such as saccadic latency and smooth pursuit also remained abnormal during and subsequent to successful amblyopia therapy (Ciuffreda et al. 1979c). Another adult patient who had an exophoria at the time of testing was operated on at age 8 years to correct an esotropia. His abnormal symmetric vergence responses were similar to those of the other patients having strabismus but who were not surgically corrected. However, yet another patient who had an esotropia surgically corrected at age 3 years and had an esophoria at the time of testing exhibited intermittent episodes of normal convergence interspersed with more frequent abnormal responses.

Accommodative Vergence

Given the reduced visual acuity and contrast sensitivity, as well as the presence of eccentric fixation, in amblyopes, one would predict reduced accommodation and therefore reduced accommodative vergence (Ciuffreda and Kenyon 1983). Kenyon and colleagues (1978, 1980b, 1981) have shown reduced accommodative vergence amplitudes in some patients when the amblyopic eye, as compared with the fellow dominant eye, viewed the accommodative stimulus. Small to moderate reductions in visual acuity (20/40 to 20/120) had little if any effect on the accommodative vergence response in the few patients examined (Figure 5.42). A noticeable drop in accommodative vergence amplitude, however, was found when the visual acuity was less than 20/400. However, their preliminary study was not broad enough to analyze either a wide range or a large sample of

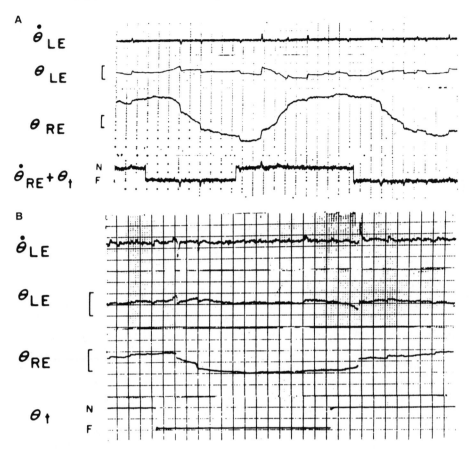

Figure 5.42 *Accommodative vergence responses with targets aligned along the line of sight of the nondominant eye, with the fellow eye covered. The effect of deep amblyopia on accommodative vergence is evident. (A) Left intermittent strabismus (exotropia); normal visual acuity (20/20) in each eye. Normal accommodative vergence amplitudes and dynamics in the nondominant left eye shown here, similar to that found in the dominant right eye. (B) Amblyope (20/38) without strabismus. Normal accommodative vergence amplitude and dynamics similar to dominant right eye responses. (C) Amblyope (20/400) without strabismus. No discernible normal accommodative vergence response was evident when the nondominant right eye fixated and focused on the target. (Reprinted by permission of the publisher, from Kenyon et al. 1981.)*

amblyopes. Nevertheless, a pronounced reduction in accommodative vergence does seem to occur in deep amblyopia. Further experiments will be necessary to determine the relationship between degree of amblyopia and/or eccentric fixation and static and dynamic characteristics of accommodative vergence.

c

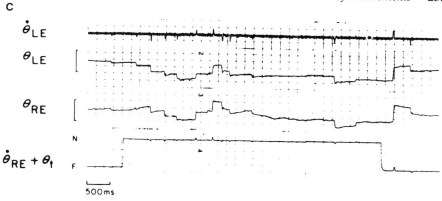

$\dot{\theta}_{LE}$

θ_{LE}

θ_{RE}

N

$\dot{\theta}_{RE} + \theta_t$ F

500ms

Figure 5.42   *(continued)*

REFERENCES

Abramson DH. (1973) Latent nystagmus in identical twins. *Arch. Ophthalmol.* 89:256–7.

Adler FH, Fliegelman M. (1934) Influence of fixation on the visual acuity. *Arch. Ophthalmol.* 12:475–83.

Alejo R. (1971) Latent nystagmus: A case report. *Philippine J. Ophthalmol.* 3:115–7.

Alpert JN, Coats AC, Perusquia E. (1975) Saccadic nystagmus in cerebellar atrophy. *Neurology* 25:676–80.

Anderson JR. (1954) Latent nystagmus and alternating hyperphoria. *Br. J. Ophthalmol.* 1:2–12.

Atkin A, Bender MB. (1964) Lightening eye movements in ocular myoclonus. *J. Neurol. Sci.* 1:2–12.

Avetisov ES. (1968) Methods and Results in Examination of Fixation in Amblyopia. In *Strabismus*, pp. 14–19. New York: Karger.

Bagolini B. (1974) Sensory and sensorio-motorial anomalies in strabismus. *Br. J. Ophthalmol.* 58:313–19.

Bagolini B. (1976) Sensory anomalies in strabismus. *Doc. Ophthalmol.* 41:1–22.

Bahill AT, Stark L. (1978) The trajectories of saccadic eye movements. *Sci. Am.* 240:108–17.

Bahill AT, Clark MR, Stark L. (1975a) The main sequence: A tool for studying human eye movements. *Math. Biosci.* 24:191–204.

Bahill AT, Clark MR, Stark L. (1975b) Dynamic overshoot in saccadic movements is caused by neurological control signal reversals. *Exp. Neurol.* 48:107–22.

Bahill AT, Ciuffreda KJ, Kenyon RV, Stark L. (1976) Dynamic and static violations of Hering's law of equal innervation. *Am. J. Optom. Physiol. Opt.* 53:786–96.

Baker FH, Grigg P, von Noorden GK. (1974) Effects of visual deprivation and strabismus on the response of neurons in the visual cortex of monkeys including studies on the striate and prestriate cortex in the normal animal. *Brian Res.* 66:185–208.

Baloh RW, Konrad HR, Konrubia V. (1975) Vestibulo-ocular function in patients with cerebellar atrophy. *Neurology* 25:160–8.

Bedell H, Flom MC. (1981) Monocular spatial distortion in strabismic amblyopia. *Invest. Ophthalmol. Vis. Sci.* 20:263–8.

Bedell H, Flom MC. (1983) Normal and abnormal space perception. *Am. J. Optom. Physiol. Opt.* 60:426–35.

Bedell HE, Yap YL, Flom MC. (1990) Fixational drift and nasotemporal pursuit asymmetries in strabismic amblyopes. *Invest. Ophthalmol. Vis. Sci.* 31:968–76.

Berard PV, Tassy A, Deransart-Ferrero JC, Mouillac-Gambarelli N. (1980) Valeur semeiologique de l'electro-oculographie motrice de poursuite dans les esotropies de l'amblyopie strabique. *J. Fr. Ophthalmol.* 3:719–30.

Bielschowsky A. (1900) Untersuchungen ubert das Sehen der Schielender. *Arch. Klin. Exp. Ophthalmol.* 50:406.

Blake R, Lehmkule SW. (1976) On the site of strabismic suppression. *Invest. Ophthalmol. Vis. Sci.* 15:660–3.

Boman DR, Kertesz AE. (1985) Fusional responses of strabismics to foveal and extrafoveal stimulation. *Invest. Ophthalmol. Vis. Sci.* 26:1731–9.

Boonstra FM, Koopmans SA, Houtman WA. (1988) Fusional vergence in microstrabismus. *Doc. Ophthalmol.* 70:221–6.

Brock FW, Givner I. (1952) Fixation anomalies in amblyopia. *Arch. Ophthalmol.* 47:775–86.

Burian HM. (1941) Fusional movements in permanent strabismus: A study of the role of central and peripheral retinal regions in the act of binocular vision in squint. *Arch. Ophthalmol.* 20:626–52.

Burian HM, Benton AE, Lipsius AR. (1962) Visual cognitive functions in patients with strabismic amblyopia. *Arch. Ophthalmol.* 68:785–91.

Calcutt C, Crook W. (1972) The treatment of amblyopia in patients with latent nystagmus. *Br. Orthopt. J.* 29:70–2.

Campos EC, Bolzani R, Cipolli C. (1988) Role of the central field in disparity-induced vergence movements in strabismus. *Graefes Arch. Clin. Exp. Ophthalmol.* 226:119–121.

Campos EC, Bolzani R, Gualdi G, Cipolli C. (1989) Recording of disparity vergence in comitant esotropia. *Doc. Ophthalmol.* 71:69–76.

Campos EC, Catellani T. (1978) Further evidence for the fusional nature of the compensation (or "eating up") of prisms in concomitant strabismus. *Int. Ophthalmol.* 1:57–62.

Ciuffreda KJ. (1977) Eye Movements in Amblyopia and Strabismus. Ph.D. dissertation, School of Optometry, University of California, Berkeley.

Ciuffreda KJ. (1979) Jerk nystagmus: Some new findings. *Am. J. Optom. Physiol. Opt.* 56:521–30.

Ciuffreda KJ. (1986) Visual System Plasticity in Human Amblyopia. In Sheffield J, Hilfer R (Eds.), *Development of Order in the Visual System*, pp. 211–44. New York: Springer-Verlag.

Ciuffreda KJ, Goldrich SG. (1983) Oculomotor biofeedback therapy. *Int. Rehabil. Med.* 5:111–17.

Ciuffreda KJ, Goldrich SG, Neary C. (1982) Use of eye movement auditory biofeedback in the control of nystagmus. *Am. J. Optom. Physiol. Opt.* 59:396–409.

Ciuffreda KJ, Kenyon RV, Stark L. (1978a) Processing delays in amblyopic eyes: Evidence from saccadic latencies. *Am. J. Optom. Physiol. Opt.* 55:187–96.

Ciuffreda KJ, Kenyon RV, Stark L. (1978b) Increased saccadic latencies in amblyopic eyes. *Invest. Ophthalmol. Vis. Sci.* 17:697–702.

Ciuffreda KJ, Kenyon RV, Stark L. (1979a) Fixational eye movements in amblyopia and strabismus. *J. Am. Optom. Assoc.* 50:1251–8.

Ciuffreda KJ, Kenyon RV, Stark L. (1979b) Suppression of fixational saccades in strabismic and anisometropic amblyopia. *Ophthalmic Res.* 11:31–9.

Ciuffreda KJ, Kenyon RV, Stark L. (1979c) Different rates of functional recovery of eye movements during orthoptic treatment in an adult amblyope. *Invest. Ophthalmol. Vis. Sci.* 18:213–19.

Ciuffreda KJ, Kenyon RV, Stark L. (1979d) Abnormal saccadic substitution during small-amplitude pursuit tracking in amblyopic eyes. *Invest. Ophthalmol. Vis. Sci.* 18:506–16.

Ciuffreda KJ, Kenyon RV, Stark L. (1979e) Saccadic intrusions in strabismus. *Arch. Ophthalmol.* 97:1673–79.

Ciuffreda KJ, Kenyon RV, Stark L. (1980) Increased drift in amblyopic eyes. *Br. J. Ophthalmol.* 64:7–14.

Ciuffreda KJ, Kenyon RV, Stark L. (1983) Saccadic intrusions contributing to reading disability: A case report. *Am. J. Optom. Physiol. Opt.* 60:242–9.

Ciuffreda KJ, Stark L. (1975) Descartes' law of reciprocal innervation. *Am. J. Optom. Physiol. Opt.* 52:663–73.

Clarke E. (1896) A rare form of nystagmus. *Trans. Ophthalmol Soc. U.K.* 17:327–8.

Cogan DG. (1956) *Neurology of the Ocular Muscles*, 2d Ed. Springfield, Ill.: Thomas.

Coherty PT, Lee C. (1975) Two cases of unilateral vertical nystagmus. *Br. Orthopt. J.* 32:122–3.

Cornsweet TN. (1957) Determination of the stimuli for involuntary drifts and saccadic eye movements. *J. Opt. Soc. Am.* 46:987–93.

Crone RA. (1954) Alternating hyperphoria. *Br. J. Ophthalmol.* 38:591–2.

Crone RA. (1977) Amblyopia: The pathology of motor disorders in amblyopic eyes. *Doc. Ophthalmol.* 11:9–17.

Cynader M, Harris L. (1980) Eye movement in strabismic cats. *Nature* 286:64–5.

Daroff RB. (1977) Ocular oscillations. *Ann. Otol. Rhinol. Laryngol.* 86:102–7.

Dell'Osso LF, Flynn JT. (1979) Congenital nystagmus surgery: A quantitative evaluation of the effects. *Arch. Ophthalmol.* 97:462–9.

Dell'Osso LF, Schmidt D, Daroff RB. (1979) Latent, manifest latent and congenital nystagmus. *Arch. Ophthalmol.* 97:1877–87.

Dell'Osso LF, Traccis S, Abel LA. (1983) Strabismus: A necessary condition for latent and manifest latent nystagmus. *Neuro-ophthalmol.* 3:247–57.

Doden W, Adams A. (1957) Elektronystagmographische Ergelvisse der Prufung des optisch vestibularen Systems bei Schielender. *Ber. Deutsch. Ophthalmol. Ges.* 60:316–17.

Enoksson P, Mortensen K. (1968) Optokinetic ocular dominance and unilateral amblyopia. *Acta Ophthalmol.* 46:915–19.

Faucon A. (1872) Nystagmus par insuffisance des droits externes. *J. Ophthalmol. (Paris)* 1:233.

Feldon SE, Landston JW. (1977) Square-wave jerks: A disorder of microsaccades? *Neurology* 27:278–81.

Flom MC. (1958) Some interesting eye movements obtained during the cover test. *Am. J. Optom. Arch. Am. Acad. Optom.* 35:69–71.

Flom MC, Kirschen DG, Bedell HE. (1980) Control of unsteady, eccentric fixation in amblyopic eyes by auditory feedback of eye position. *Invest. Ophthalmol. Vis. Sci.* 19:1371–81.

Flynn JT. (1982) Vestibulo-optokinetic interactions in strabismus. *Am. Orthoptic. J.* 32:36–47.

Flynn JT, Pritchard C, Lasley D. (1984) Binocular Vision and OKN Asymmetry in Strabismic Patients. In Reinecke R (Ed.), *Strabismus II*, pp. 35–43. New York: Grune & Stratton.

Fricker SJ. (1976) Use of Velocity and Acceleration Measurements in the Evaluation of Strabismus Patients. In Moore S, Mein J, Stockbridge L (Eds.), *Orthoptics: Past, Present, Future*, pp. 113-21. New York: Stratton.

Fromaget C, Fromaget H. (1912) Nystagmus latent. *Ann. Ocul.* 147:344-50.

Fukai S. (1974) Studies on the sensory motor anomalies in amblyopia and strabismus: IV. Abnormal pursuit movement of the fellow eye in amblyopia with strabismus. *Acta Soc. Ophthalmol. Jpn.* 78:475-81.

Fukai S, Tsutsui J. (1973) Asymmetric version in pursuit eye movement under extrafoveal fixation. *Jpn. J. Ophthalmol.* 17:30-9.

Fukai S, Tsutsui J, Nakamura Y. (1976) Abnormal Pursuit Movements of the Fellow Eye in Amblyopia with Strabismus. In Moore S, Mein J, Stockbridge L (Eds.), *Orthoptics: Past, Present, Future*, pp. 75-91. New York: Stratton.

Fukushima M, Tsutsui J. (1984) Visually and Auditory Evoked Saccadic Reaction Time in Amblyopia. In Reinecke R (Ed.), *Strabismus II*, pp. 443-49. New York: Grune & Stratton.

Gamble RC. (1934) The visual prognosis for children with congenital nystagmus. *Trans. Am. Ophthalmol. Soc.* 32:485-96.

George ML. (1976) Training with a post-surgical exotrope. *J. Am. Optom. Assoc.* 47:692.

Gerin P, Peronnet F, Maynard P. (1973) Relation entre temps de reaction et alteration de la perception visuelle dans l'amblyopie fonctionnelle. *Electroencephalogr. Clin. Neurophysiol.* 35:49-57.

Gillies WE. (1968) The Significance of Nystagmoid Movement in Amblyopia. In Arruga A (Ed.), *International Strabismus Symposium*. New York: Karger.

Girard LJ, Fletcher MC, Tomlinson E, Smith B. (1962) Results of pleoptic treatment of suppression amblyopia. *Am. Orthoptic. J.* 12:12.

Goldstein JH, Greenstein F. (1971) Eye-Hand Coordination in Strabismus. In Fells P (Ed.), *The First Congress of the International Strabismological Association* St. Louis: Mosby.

Gordon B, Presson J. (1977) Effects of alternating occlusion on receptive fields in cat superior colliculus. *J. Neurophysiol.* 40:1406-14.

Griffin JR. (1976) *Binocular Anomalies: Procedures for Vision Therapy*, pp. 74-75, 95-96. Chicago: Professional Press.

Hallden U. (1952) Fusional phenomena in anomalous correspondence. *Acta. Ophthalmol.* 37(Suppl. 1):1-93.

Hamasaki DI, Flynn JT. (1981) Amblyopic eyes have longer reaction times. *Invest. Ophthalmol. Vis. Sci.* 21:846-53.

Hayashi S. (1961) Studies on the fixation movement of the eyeball. *Jpn. J. Ophthalmol.* 4:235-44.

Healy E. (1952) Nystagmus treated by orthoptics. *Am. Orthopt. J.* 2:53-5.

Healy E. (1962) Nystagmus treated by orthoptics: A second report. *Am. Orthopt. J.* 12:89-91.

Hemmes GD. (1927) Hereditary nystagmus (abstract). *Am. J. Ophthalmol.* 10:149-50.

Hess RF. (1977) Eye movements and grating acuity in strabismic amblyopia. *Ophthalmic Res.* 9:225-37.

Higgins KE, Daugman JG, Mansfield RFW. (1982) Amblyopic contrast sensitivity: Insensitivity to unsteady fixation. *Invest. Ophthalmol. Vis. Sci.* 23:113-20.

Hokoda SC, Ciuffreda KJ. (1986) Different rates and amounts of vision function recovery during orthoptic therapy in an older strabismic amblyope. *Ophthalmic. Physiol. Opt.* 6:213–20.

Hoyt CS. (1982) Abnormalities of the vestibulo-ocular response in congenital esotropia. *Am. J. Ophthalmol.* 93:704–8.

Hubel D, Wiesel TN. (1965) Binocular interactions in striate cortex of kittens reared with artificial squint. *J. Neurophysiol.* 28:1041–59.

Ikeda H, Tremain KE. (1977) Different causes for amblyopia and loss of binocularity in squinting kittens. *J. Physiol.* 299:26–7.

Ikeda H, Wright MJ. (1974) Is amblyopia due to inappropriate stimulation of the sustained pathways during development? *Br. J. Ophthalmol.* 58:165–75.

Ishikawa S, Terakado R. (1973) Maximum velocity of saccadic eye movements in normal and strabismic subjects. *Jpn. J. Ophthalmol.* 17:11–21.

Jampolsky A. (1955) Characteristics of suppression in strabismus. *Arch. Ophthalmol.* 54:683–96.

Jung R, Kornhuber HH. (1964) Results of Electronystagmograpy in Man: The Value of Optokinetic, Vestibular and Spontaneous Nystagmus for Neurologic Diagnosis and Research. In Bender M (Ed.), *The Oculomotor System*, New York: Harper & Rowe.

Kato H, Mimura O, Shimo-oku M. (1980) Saccadic latencies in amblyopia using two-dimensional stimulus. *Folia Ophthalmol. Jpn.* 31:1818–22.

Kenyon RV. (1978) Vergence Eye Movements in Strabismus and Amblyopia. PhD. dissertation, School of Optometry, University of California, Berkeley.

Kenyon RV, Ciuffreda KJ, Stark L. (1978) Binocular eye movements during accommodative vergence. *Vision Res.* 18:545–55.

Kenyon RV, Ciuffreda KJ, Stark L. (1980a) Dynamic vergence eye movements in strabismus and amblyopia: Symmetric vergence. *Invest. Ophthalmol. Vis. Sci.* 19:60–74.

Kenyon RV, Ciuffreda KJ, Stark L. (1980b) Unexpected role for normal accommodative vergence in strabismus and amblyopia. *Am. J. Optom. Physiol. Opt.* 57:566–77.

Kenyon RV, Ciuffreda KJ, Stark L. (1981) Dynamic vergence eye movements in strabismus and amblyopia: Asymmetric vergence. *Br. J. Ophthalmol.* 65:167–76.

Kertesz AE. (1983) The effectiveness of wide-angle fusional stimulation in strabismus. *Am. Orthopt. J.* 33:83–90.

Kirchen DK, Flom MC. (1978) Visual acuity at different retinal loci of eccentrically fixating functional amblyopes. *Am. J. Optom. Physiol. Opt.* 55:144–50.

Krauskopf J, Cornsweet TN, Riggs LA. (1960) Analysis of eye movements during monocular and binocular fixation. *J. Opt. Soc. Am.* 50:572–8.

Kretschmar S. (1955) Lafausse correspondence retnienne. *Doc. Ophthalmol.* 9:46.

Lang J. (1968) Squint Dating from Birth or with Early Onset. In Kimpton H (Ed.), *The First International Congress of Orthoptists*, pp. 231–7. London: Kimpton.

Lawwill T. (1966) The fixation pattern of the light-adapted and dark-adapted amblyopic eye. *Am. J. Ophthalmol.* 61:1416–19.

Lawwill T. (1968) Local adaptation in functional amblyopia. *Am. J. Ophthalmol.* 65:903–6.

Leigh J, Zee DS. (1983) *The Neurology of Eye Movements.* Philadelphia: Davis.

Lisberger SG, Evinger C, Johanson GW, Fuchs AF. (1981) Relation between eye acceleration and retinal-image velocity during foveal smooth pursuit in man and monkey. *J. Neurophysiol.* 46:229–41.

Loewer-Spieger DH. (1962) Amblyopie een studie over de kenmerken en de behandeling. *J. Ruysendaal Amsterdam.* 52:107–19.

Mackensen G. (1957a) Das fixationsverhalten amblyopischer augen. *Arch. Ophthalmol.* 159:200–11.

Mackensen G. (1957b) Blickbewegungen amblyopischer augen. *Arch. Ophthalmol.* 159:212–32.

Mackensen G. (1958) Resktionszeitmessungen bei Amblyopie. *Arch. Ophthalmol.* 159:636–42.

Mackensen G. (1966) Diagnosis and phenomenology of eccentric fixation. *Int. Ophthalmol. Clin.* 6:397–409.

Mariani G, Pasino L. (1964) Variations in the angle of anomaly and fusional movements in cases of small angle convergent strabismus with harmonious anomalous correspondence. *Br. J. Ophthalmol.* 48:439–43.

Matteucci P. (1960) Strabismic amblyopia. *Br. J. Ophthalmol.* 44:577–82.

McHugh DE, Bahill AT. (1985) Learning to track predictable target waveforms without a time delay. *Invest. Ophthalmol. Vis. Sci.* 26:932–37.

Mehdorn E, Kommerell G. (1978) Rebound-saccade in the prism cover test. *Int. Ophthalmol.* 1:63–6.

Mein J. (1983) The OKN response and binocular vision in early onset strabismus. *Aust. Orthopt. J.* 20:13–17.

Mimura O, Kato H, Kani K, Shimo-oku M. (1981) Saccadic latencies in amblyopia using infrared television fundus camera with two-dimensional stimuli. *Jpn. J. Ophthalmol.* 25:248–57.

Mohler CW, Wurtz RH. (1976) Organization of monkey superior colliculus: Intermediate layer cells discharging before eye movements. *J. Neurophysiol.* 39:722–65.

Murphy BJ. (1978) Pattern thresholds for moving and stationary gratings during smooth eye movements. *Vision Res.* 18:521–30.

Nachimias J. (1959) Two-dimensional motion of the retinal image during monocular fixation. *J. Opt. Soc. Am.* 49:901–8.

Nawratski I, Jampolsky A. (1958) A regional hemiretinal difference in amblyopia. *Am. J. Ophthalmol.* 46:339–44.

Nicolai H. (1959) Differenzen zwischen optokinetischem Recht-und Links-nystagmus bei einseitiger Schiel Amblyopie. *Klin. Mbl. Augenheilk.* 134:245–50.

Noordenbos AM, Crone RA. (1976) Motor Fusion in Small-Angle Esotropia. In Moore S, Mein J, Stockbridge L (Eds.), *Orthoptics: Past, Present, Future.* New York: Stratton.

Norn MS. (1964) Congenital idiopathic nystagmus. *Acta Ophthalmol.* 42:889–96.

Pearlman CA. (1976) A case study. *J. Am. Optom. Assoc.* 47:396–8.

Pickwell LD, Hampshire R. (1981) Jump-convergence test in strabismus. *Ophthalmic. Physiol. Opt.* 1:23–4.

Prakash P, Grover AK, Khosia PK, Gahlot DK. (1982) Ocular motility in alternating squints: An electro-oculographic study. *Br. J. Ophthalmol.* 66:258–63.

Pratt-Johnson J, Wee HS. (1969) Suppression associated with exotropia. *Can. J. Ophthalmol.* 2:136–44.

Pratt-Johnson J, Wee HS, Ellis S. (1967) Suppression associated with exotropia. *Can. J. Ophthalmol.* 4:284–91.

Pugh M. (1954) Foveal vision in amblyopia. *Br. J. Ophthalmol.* 38:321–31.

Quere MA. (1980) Abnormal ocular movements in amblyopia. *Trans. Ophthalmol. Soc. U.K.* 99:401–6.

Rashbass C. (1961) The relationship between saccadic and smooth tracking eye movements. *J. Physiol.* 159:326-38.

Rashbass C, Westheimer G. (1961) Disjunctive eye movements. *J. Physiol.* 159:339-60.

Ratliff F, Riggs LA. (1950) Involuntary motions of the eye during monocular fixation. *J. Exp. Psychol.* 40:687-701.

Riggs LA, Niehl EW. (1960) Eye movements recorded during convergence and divergence. *J. Opt. Soc. Am.* 50:913-20.

Riggs LA, Ratliff F. (1951) Visual acuity and the normal tremor of the eyes. *Science* 114:17-18.

Riggs LA, Armington JC, Ratliff F. (1954) Motions of the retinal image during fixation. *J. Opt. Soc. Am.* 44:315-21.

Robinson DA. (1965) The mechanics of human smooth pursuit eye movement. *J. Physiol.* 180:569-91.

Salman SD, von Noorden GK. (1970) Induced vestibular nystagmus in strabismic patients. *Ann. Otol. Rhinol. Laryngol.* 79:352-7.

Sansbury RV, Skavenski AA, Hadded GM, Steinman RN. (1973) Normal fixation of eccentric targets. *J. Opt. Soc. Am.* 63:612-14.

Schiller PH, Stryker M. (1972) Single-unit recording and stimulation in superior colliculus of the alert rhesus monkey. *J. Neurophysiol.* 35:915-24.

Schoessler JP. (1980) Accommodative and fusional vergence in anomalous correspondence. *Am. J. Optom. Physiol. Opt.* 57:676-80.

Schor CM. (1972) Oculomotor and Neurosensory Analysis of Amblyopia. PhD dissertation, University of California School of Optometry, Berkeley.

Schor CM. (1975) A directional impairment of eye movement control is strabismus amblyopia. *Invest. Ophthalmol. Vis. Sci.* 14:692-7.

Schor CM. (1983) Subcortical binocular suppression affects the development of latent and optokinetic nystagmus. *Am. J. Optom. Physiol. Opt.* 60:481-501.

Schor CM, Flom MC. (1975) Eye Position Control and Visual Acuity in Strabismus Amblyopia. In Lennerstrand G, Bach-y-rita P (Eds.), *Basic Mechanisms of Ocular Motility and Their Clinical Implications*, pp. 555-9. New York: Pergamon Press.

Schor CM, Hallmark W. (1978) Slow control of eye position in strabismic amblyopia. *Invest. Ophthalmol. Vis. Sci.* 17:577-81.

Schor CM, Levi DM. (1980) Disturbances of small-field horizontal and vertical optokinetic nystagmus in amblyopia. *Invest. Ophthalmol. Vis. Sci.* 19:668-83.

Schor CM, Westall C. (1984) Visual and vestibular sources of fixation instability in amblyopia. *Invest. Ophthalmol. Vis. Sci.* 25:729-38.

Schlodtmann W. (1900) Studien uber anomale Sehrich-tungsgemunschaft bei Schielenden. *Arch. Ophthalmol.* 51:526-34.

Selenow A, Ciuffreda KJ. (1983) Vision function recovery during orthoptic therapy in an exotropic amblyope with high unilateral myopia. *Am. J. Optom. Physiol. Opt.* 60:659-66.

Selenow A, Ciuffreda KJ. (1986) Vision function recovery during orthoptic therapy in an adult strabismic amblyope. *J. Am. Optom. Assoc.* 57:132-40.

Selhorst JB, Stark L, Ochs AL, Hoyt WF. (1976) Disorders in cerebellar ocular motor control: II. Macrosaccadic oscillation; an oculographic control system and clinico-anatomical analysis. *Brain.* 99:522-90.

Sharpe JA, Herishanu YO, White OB. (1982) Cerebral square wave jerks. *Neurology* 32:57–62.

Sherman A. (1974) Case report of an anisometropic amblyopic patient. *J. Optom. Vis. Ther.* 5:46–9.

Simon F, Slatt BJ. (1971) Light induced nystagmus. *Can. J. Ophthalmol.* 6:128–32.

Skavenski AA, Steinman RM. (1970) Control of eye position in the dark. *Vision Res.* 10:193–203.

Smith W. (1950) *Clinical Orthoptic Procedures*, pp. 336–38. St. Louis: Mosby.

Sorsby A. (1931) Latent nystagmus. *Br. J. Ophthalmol.* 15:1–18.

Srebro R. (1983) Fixation of normal and amblyopic eyes. *Arch. Ophthalmol.* 101:214–17.

Stark L. (1968) *Neurological Control Systems*. New York: Plenum Press.

Stark L. (1971) The Control System for Versional Eye Movements. In Bach-y-rita P, Collins CC (Eds.), *The Control of Eye Movements*. New York: Academic Press.

Stark L, Ciuffreda KJ, Kenyon RV. (1982) Abnormal Eye Movements in Strabismus and Amblyopia. In Lennerstrand G, Zee DS, Keller EL (Eds.), *Functional Basis of Ocular Motility Disorders*, pp. 71–82. New York: Pergamon Press.

Stark L, Ciuffreda KJ, Kenyon RV. (1984) Similarities and Differences between Strabismus and Amblyopia: An Eye Movement Study. In Reinecke RD (Ed.), *Strabismus II*, pp. 401–27. New York: Grune & Stratton.

St. Cyr G, Fender DH. (1969) The interplay of drifts and flicks in binocular fixation. *Vision Res.* 9:245–65.

St. Cyr GJ. (1973) Signal and noise in the human oculomotor system. *Vision Res.* 13:1979–91.

Stegall FW. (1973) Orthoptic aspects of nystagmus. *Am. Orthopt. J.* 23:30–4.

Steinman RM, Cunitz RJ, Timerlake GT, Herman M. (1967) Voluntary control of microsaccades during maintained monocular fixation. *Science* 155:1577–9.

Steinman RM, Hadded GM, Skavenski AA, Wyman D. (1973) Miniature eye movement. *Science* 181:810–19.

Stohler T. (1973) After-image treatment in nystagmus. *Am. Orthopt. J.* 23:65–7.

Travers TB. (1938) Suppression of vision in squint and its association with retinal correspondence and amblyopia. *Br. J. Ophthalmol.* 22:577.

Troost BT, Daroff RB, Dell'Osso LF. (1976) Quantitative analysis of the ocular motor deficit in progressive supranuclear palsy (PSP). *Trans. Am. Neurol. Assoc.* 101:1–4.

Tsutsui J, Fukai S. (1978) Human Strabismic Cases Suggestive of Asymmetric Projection of the Visual Pathway. In Reinecke R (Ed.), *Strabismus*, pp. 79–88. New York: Grune & Stratton.

Tsutsui J, Fukai A, Kimura H. (1984) Pursuit Movement Disorders and the Prognosis of Strabismus Treatment. In Reinecke R (Ed.), *Strabismus II*, pp. 459–65. New York: Grune & Stratton.

Tychsen L, Hurtig RR, Scott WE. (1985) Pursuit is impaired but the vestibulo-ocular reflex is normal in infantile strabismus. *Arch. Ophthalmol.* 103:536–9.

Tyschen L, Lisberger SG. (1986) Maldevelopment of visual motion processing in humans who had strabismus with onset in infancy. *J. Neurosci.* 6:2495–501.

Urist MJ. (1961) Fixation anomalies in amblyopia ex anopsia. *Am. J. Ophthalmol.* 52:19–28.

van Vliet AGM. (1973) On the central mechanism of latent nystagmus. *Acta Ophthalmol.* 66:772–81.

von Noorden GK. (1961) Reaction time in normal and amblyopic eyes. *Arch. Ophthalmol.* 66:695–701.

von Noorden GK. (1967) Pathogenesis of eccentric fixation. *Doc. Ophthalmol.* 23:263–317.

von Noorden GK, Burian HM. (1958) An electro-oculographic study of the behavior of the fixation of amblyopic eyes in light- and dark-adapted state: A preliminary report. *Am. J. Ophthalmol.* 46:68–77.

von Noorden GK, Burian HM. (1960) Perceptual blanking in normal and amblyopic eyes. *Arch. Ophthalmol.* 54:817–22.

von Noorden GK, Mackensen G. (1962a) Phenomenology of eccentric fixation. *Am. J. Ophthalmol.* 53:642–61.

von Noorden GK, Mackensen G. (1962b) Pursuit movements of normal and amblyopic eyes: II. Pursuit movements in amblyopic patients. *Am. J. Ophthalmol.* 53:477–87.

von Noorden GK, Allen L, Burian HM. (1959) A photographic method for the determination of the behavior of fixation. *Am. J. Ophthalmol.* 48:511–14.

Wald G, Burian HM. (1944) The dissociation of form vision and light perception in strabismic amblyopia. *Am. J. Ophthalmol.* 27:950–63.

Walton J. (1972) Occlusion in Latent Nystagmus. In Mein J, Bierlaagh JJM, Brummelkamp-Dons TEA (Eds.), *Orthoptics: Proceedings of the Second International Orthoptic Congress.* Amsterdam: Excerpta Medica.

West L. (1939) Coincident inheritance of strabismus and nystagmus. *J. Hered.* 30:496–8.

Westall CA, Aslin RA. (1984) Fixational eye movements and autokinesis in amblyopes. *Ophthalmic. Physiol. Opt.* 4:333–7.

Westall CA, Schor CM. (1985) Asymmetries of optokinetic nystagmus in amblyopia: The effect of selected retinal stimulation. *Vision Res.* 25:1431–1438.

Westall CA, Schor CM. (1985) Adaptation of the vestibulo-ocular reflex in amblyopia. *Invest. Ophthalmol. Vis. Sci.* 26:1724–30.

Westheimer G, McKee SP. (1975) Visual acuity in the presence of retinal image motion. *J. Opt. Soc. Am.* 65:847–50.

Westheimer G, Mitchell AM. (1956) Eye movement responses to convergent stimuli. *Arch. Ophthalmol.* 55:848–56.

Windsor CE. (1968) Modification of latent nystagmus, Part II. *Arch. Ophthalmol.* 80:352–3.

Windsor CE, Burian HM, Milojevic B. (1968) Modification of latent nystagmus, Part I. *Arch. Ophthalmol.* 80:657–63.

Wurtz RH, Goldberg ME. (1972) Activity of superior colliculus in behaving monkey: IV. Effects of lesions on eye movements. *J. Neurophysiol.* 35:587–96.

Wybar K. (1968) Nystagmus in Childhood. In Kimpton H (Ed.), *The First International Congress of Orthoptists.* London: Kimpton.

Yamagata Y, Haruta R, Mimura O, Shimo-oku M. (1983) Saccadic latency in amblyopia with special reference to the target energy. *Folia Ophthalmol. Jpn.* 34:47–53.

Zuber BL, Stark L. (1968) Dynamical characteristics of fusional vergence eye movement system. *IEEE Trans. Syst. Sci. Cybernet.* 4:72–9.

Zuber BL, Stark L, Cook G. (1965) Microsaccades and the velocity-amplitude relationship for saccadic eye movements. *Science* 150:1459–60.

Chapter 6

Accommodation

Accommodation refers to a change in the refractive state of the eye due to alteration in the curvature of the crystalline lens and is initiated to focus and maximize spatial contrast of the foveal retinal image (Fujii et al. 1970, Krishnan et al. 1973). Although a primary stimulus to accommodation is blur (Troelstra et al. 1964, Phillips and Stark 1977, Kruger and Pola 1986, Ciuffreda in press *a*), disparity (during binocular viewing) (Fincham and Walton 1957, Hung et al. 1983a), perceptual factors (Ittleson and Ames 1950, Hokoda and Ciuffreda 1983, Kruger and Pola 1985, McLin et al. 1988), the tonic innervation level (Owens and Leibowitz 1983), and voluntary effort (Ciuffreda and Kruger 1988) serve as additional drives to the accommodation system (Toates 1972, Semmlow and Jaeger 1972, Hung and Semmlow 1980, Hung et al. 1983b). Other factors that influence the accommodative response include the spatial frequency composition (Heath 1956, Phillips 1974, Charman and Tucker 1977, 1978, Charman and Heron 1979, Owens 1980, Bour 1981, Ciuffreda and Hokoda 1983, Ciuffreda et al. 1987, Tucker and Charman 1987, Dul et al. 1988, Ciuffreda in press *b*) contrast (Heath 1956, Phillips 1974, Bour 1981, Ciuffreda and Rumpf 1985, Ward 1987), and retinal eccentricity (Phillips 1974, Semmlow and Tinor 1978, Bullimore and Gilmartin 1987, Gu and Legge 1987) of the target. In this chapter we will review and discuss the static and dynamic aspects of accommodation and their related sensory aspects in amblyopic eyes. See Chapters 8 to 10 for clinical aspects of accommodation related specifically to the diagnosis and treatment of amblyopia.

ACCOMMODATIVE AMPLITUDE

One of the simplest and most frequently performed tests of accommodation in patients is determination of the age-dependent amplitude (Borish 1970). By doing so, one is measuring the maximum motor output in response to a blur (and sometimes size also) stimulus of increasingly greater optical vergence demand. The distance from the eye to the point of first slight sustained blur, converted dioptrically, is the *clinical amplitude*. It is typically measured monocularly, with slightly greater values obtained binocularly owing to the addition of vergence accommodation. In visually normal individuals, the accommodative amplitude is approximately the same in each eye (Turner 1958, Wold 1967, Hokoda and Ciuffreda 1982).

However, in amblyopia, one might expect unequal monocularly determined accommodative amplitudes owing to the early years of abnormal visual experience, especially from the monocular contrast deprivation that may occur in uncorrected anisometropia. Reduced amplitude is indeed a consistent finding in amblyopic eyes (even in amblyopic monkeys; Kiorpes and Boothe 1984). This was first documented in brief reports by clinicians (Urist 1950, Abraham 1961, Sherman 1970, Wick and Grisham 1980). More recently, in a comprehensive series of experimental and modeling studies investigating static aspects of accommodation in response to high contrast, square-wave-type stimuli (i.e., reduced Snellen chart letters) in amblyopic eyes, Ciuffreda and colleagues (Hokoda and Ciuffreda 1982, Ciuffreda et al. 1983, 1984, Hung et al. 1983b) found the minus lens accommodative amplitude to be the *best* discriminator between amblyopic and normal eyes when compared with several other measures of accommodative functions. *All* the amblyopes showed reduced accommodative amplitude in the amblyopic eye. The difference in accommodative amplitude between the amblyopic and fellow dominant eye ranged from ½ to 5 diopters (Figure 6.1), corresponding to an average interocular difference of about 25% (range 10% to 50%). Accommodative amplitude was normal in the fellow eye, as was its consensually driven accommodation.

Recently, the effects of orthoptic therapy on accommodative amplitude in amblyopic eyes have been studied. In a case report, Wick and Grisham (1980) found the amplitude to increase to a normal level in a young amblyope following orthoptic therapy. Three detailed studies investigating the recovery of accommodation and related vision functions following intensive orthoptic therapy have been conducted by Ciuffreda and his clinical colleagues (Ciuffreda 1986). In a 6-year-old exotropic amblyope, Selenow and Ciuffreda (1983) found the accommodative amplitude to increase dramatically with concomitant but even more rapid improvement in visual acuity and fixation (Figure 6.2). In an 11-year-old, small-angle esotropic amblyope, Hokoda and Ciuffreda (1986) found that the accommodative amplitude rapidly and markedly improved, while visual acuity and fixation showed a slower but consistent change toward normal levels following a long and intensive orthoptic program (Figure 6.3). In a 29-year-old, small-angle esotropic amblyope, Selenow and Ciuffreda (1986) found the amplitude to become normal after 6 months of rigorous orthoptic therapy, but only once the patient learned that his best (subjective) focus was obtained by using the fovea rather than the habitual eccentric fixation point (3 degrees nasal). Thus these findings clearly demonstrate the positive effects of conventional orthoptic therapy on accommodative amplitude function in amblyopic eyes.

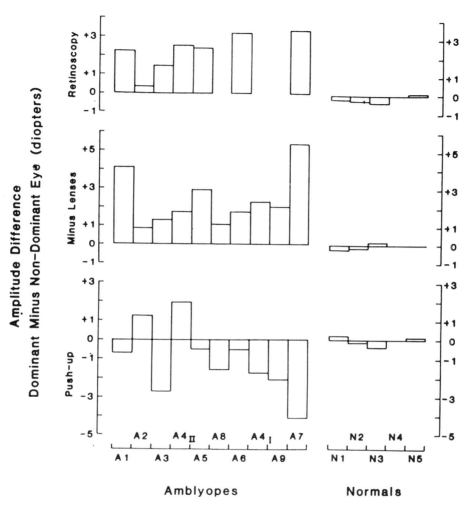

Figure 6.1 *Difference in accommodative amplitude between the dominant and non-dominant eye of each subject plotted in order of decreasing visual acuity in the amblyopic eye (left to right). Reduced accommodative amplitude in the amblyopic eye was consistently found using the minus lens and dynamic retinoscopy objective push-up techniques, but not with the subjective push-up technique, which resulted in inflated values. Normal subjects showed little difference in accommodative amplitude between the two eyes with any of the techniques. (Reprinted, with permission, from Hokoda and Ciuffreda 1982.)*

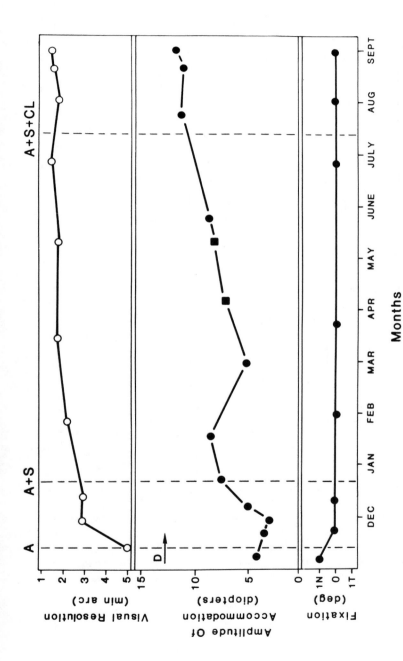

Figure 6.2 *Changes in visual resolution, accommodative amplitude, and fixation during the course of intensive orthoptic therapy in a 7-year-old patient with strabismus (exotropia), anisometropia (axial myopia), and partial ptosis. Improvements in all three vision functions were evident. (A = amblyopia therapy, S = strabismus therapy, CL = prescription of contact lens, and D = accommodative amplitude in the dominant eye determined with the minus lens technique.) (Reprinted, with permission, from Ciuffreda et al. 1983.)*

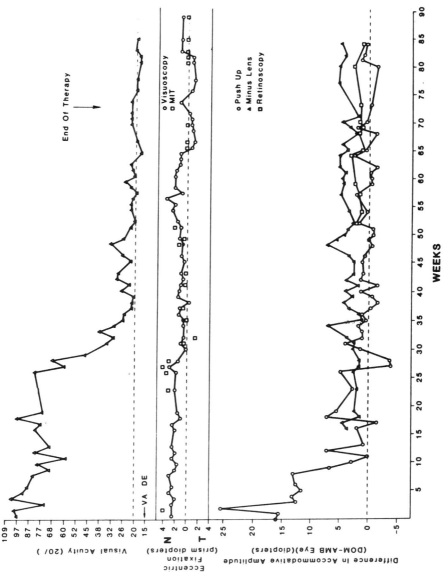

Figure 6.3 *Visual acuity, fixation, and difference in accommodative amplitude between the two eyes of an 11-year-old strabismic amblyope during the course of intensive orthoptic therapy. (Reprinted, with permission, Hokoda and Ciuffreda 1986.)*

ACCOMMODATIVE STIMULUS-RESPONSE FUNCTION AND THE MODEL

While the accommodative amplitude represents an important clinical and experimental measure reflecting maximum accommodative ability, its diagnostic
value in the prepresbyopic patient population lies primarily as a comparative
"maximum effort-type" indicator of accommodative dysfunction within or between patients having some underlying functional or organic disorder. Further,
until the onset of presbyopia, one rarely functions habitually or even for brief
periods of time at such close distances. In general, adults and children typically
focus on objects whose distances range from a few hundred feet to somewhat closer
than arm's reach. Thus, if we wish to assess steady-state accommodative function in
either patients or laboratory subjects under more naturalistic stimulus distances,
determination of the accommodative response and, in turn, the accommodative
error over the range of about 0 to 5 diopters or so would be most meaningful.

Stimulation of the accommodative system by introducing random dioptric
step changes in the target with concurrent measures of the average static or

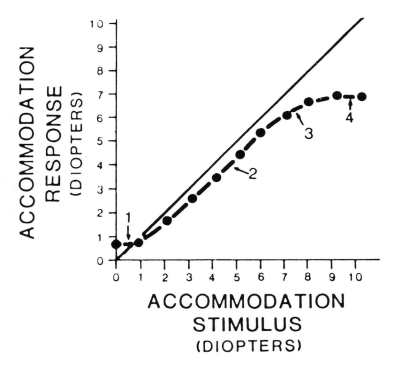

Figure 6.4 *Static accommodative stimulus-response curve for a young adult normal
subject. [1 = initial non-linear region, 2 = linear region, 3 = transitional soft saturation
(non linear) region, and 4 = hard saturation (nonlinear) presbyopic region.] (Reprinted,
with permission, from Ciuffreda and Kenyon 1983.)*

steady-state response results in a plot of the accommodative stimulus-response curve (Morgan 1944a and b, 1968, Ciuffreda and Kenyon 1983) (Figure 6.4). Stimuli may encompass the entire response range, which includes the following:

1. The initial nonlinear portion of the curve from 0 to about 1.5 diopters of accommodative stimulus over which the accommodative response is approximately constant or shows relatively little change, with mean population values ranging from 0.5 to 1.5 diopters. This response is strongly influenced by the tonic or accommodative bias level, as well as the depth of focus (Hung and Semmlow 1980, Hung et al. 1983b).
2. The linear manifest zone over which a change in accommodative stimulus produces a proportional change in accommodative response. This response is typically less than the stimulus, producing the so-called lazy lag of accommodation primarily as a result of the proportional control property of the steady-state accommodation system (Toates 1972) and depth of focus of the eye (approximately ± 0.35 diopter) (Campbell 1957, Green et al. 1980), which is influenced slightly by pupil diameter under normal conditions.
3. The nonlinear transition zone (region of soft saturation), over which further increases in the stimulus produce an increase in response, but progressively smaller than would be found for the same stimulus change over the manifest zone.
4. The nonlinear latent zone (region of hard saturation), which defines the amplitude of accommodation, over which still further increases in the stimulus fail to produce any additional increase in response. However, ciliary body force continues to increase in this zone, but presumed sclerosis of the crystalline lens and capsule impedes further rounding of the lens to increase lenticular dioptric power, and thus functional presbyopia is attained (Saladin and Stark 1975).

There have been four groups who investigated the accommodative stimulus-response function in amblyopes. Otto and colleagues (1967, 1974, 1976) used either a retinoscope or a Hartinger coincidence optometer to measure steady-state accommodative responses in amblyopic eyes at distance and near while fixating letters on a Snellen chart. They found accommodation to be imprecise and variable in the functionally amblyopic eyes, with all patients presumably having central scotomas (Figure 6.5). Similar results were found in their patients with organic disease involving either the macula region or optic nerve. They concluded that the effect of the central scotoma, resulting from abnormal visual experience in the functional amblyopes and disease processes in the organic amblyopes, was similar in both groups, disturbing signal processing in the central retinal cones used for initial control of accommodation (Campbell 1954). Further, Otto and colleagues believed that the immediately adjacent nonaffected retina was therefore used in the initiation and maintenance of the accommodative response and that this peripherally generated cone response was of necessity inaccurate (presumably due to the reduced cone population and

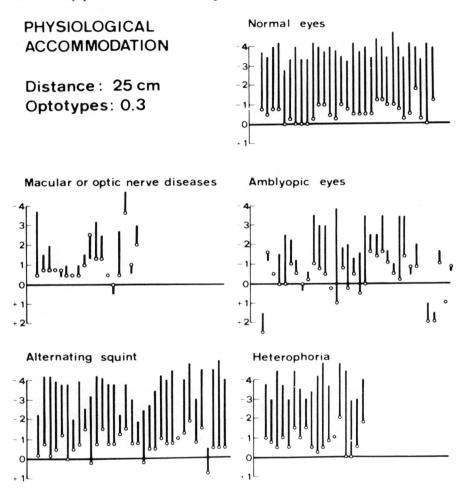

Figure 6.5   (Above) *Normal eyes. Accommodation is accurate for required distance. If smaller optotypes are used, accommodation becomes more precise (not shown here). (Center) Eyes with permanent central scotoma due to either organic lesions or functional amblyopia. Without the possibility of "steering" (i.e., accurate sensing of the defocused retinal image), accommodation is completely irregular. (Below) Eyes with either alternating or periodic central scotoma. Accommodation is similar to normal eyes but with less accuracy. In all cases, open circles indicate the initial state of accommodation and end of line segment indicates the final state of accommodation to the 4-diopter Snellen letter stimuli. (Reprinted, with permission, from Otto and Safra 1976.)*

increased retinal receptive field size in the near retinal periphery) (Phillips 1974). In patients exhibiting suppression (with or without strabismus but without amblyopia), the accommodative responses were not as precise and were slightly more variable than those found in their visually normal population. As before, the scotoma hypothesis was invoked to explain these results. Wood and Tomlinson (1974) used a laser optometer to measure the accommodative stimulus-response function in five functional amblyopes. The amblyopic eye exhibited more overaccommodation at low stimulus levels and more under-accommodation at high stimulus levels than found in the fellow normal eye in most cases, and thus there was reduced slope to the response profile as determined by linear regression analysis. Wood and Tomlinson believed the results suggested a loss of contrast sensitivity, especially at the higher spatial frequencies. Their results in amblyopes are similar to those found in normal individuals by Heath (1956) when the target was optically defocused and thus had an overall effective reduction in contrast and high spatial frequency content. Kirschen et al. (1981) used an eye movement auditory biofeedback procedure to train foveation in amblyopes (Kirschen and Flom 1978). They found slightly increased accommodative responses (~ 0.25 diopter) when eccentrically fixating amblyopes now fixated with their fovea during accommodation on Snellen letters at low and moderate dioptric levels (Figure 6.6). This result suggests that eccentricity of fixation contributes to a small part of the increased steady-state accommodative error commonly found in amblyopic eyes. We will now discuss the background and results of Ciuffreda and colleagues' recent detailed investigation in this area.

It is important to understand accommodative function in amblyopic eyes and in what regard it differs from accommodative performance in normal individuals. Such an understanding necessitates a standardized set of measures to assess accommodative ability. From a model of accommodation developed using systems analysis (Hung and Semmlow 1980), it was demonstrated that only three parameters were essential to describe static accommodative behavior in a comprehensive, quantitative manner: the slope of the stimulus-response curve, the depth of focus, and the tonic level. These three parameters can be obtained by either experimental or clinical measurement procedures. In addition to providing a quantitative description of static accommodative function, these three parameters can be related to the elements of a theoretical model of accommodative control (Hung and Semmlow 1980, Hung et al. 1983b), thus providing additional insight into the mechanisms and/or component contribution underlying the abnormal accommodative behavior typically found in amblyopic eyes (Figure 6.7).

Previous studies of accommodative stimulus-response function in amblyopia have had serious limitations with respect to sample size (Wood and Tomlinson 1974, Kirschen et al. 1981), stimulus range (Otto and Graemiger 1967, Otto and Safra 1974, 1976, Kirschen et al. 1981), and/or range and magnitude of visual acuity and eccentric fixation of subjects (Wood and Tomlinson 1974, Kirschen et al. 1981). Further, none of the preceding studies measured all three parameters *essential* to describing static accommodative behavior completely. Thus Ciuffreda and colleagues conducted a more comprehensive investigation of static accommodation in human amblyopia. Using wide-range stimulating and measuring optometers and the three essential parameters described earlier,

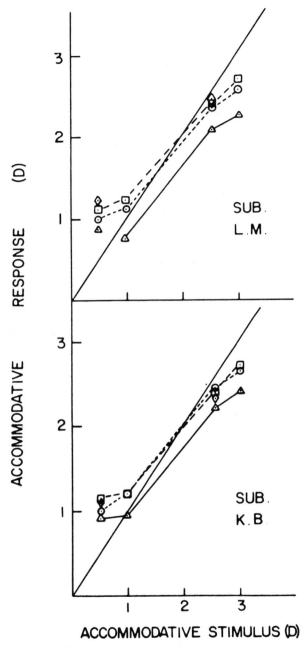

Figure 6.6 *Accommodative responses of normal subjects* (squares) *compared with the responses by the dominant eye of an amblyope* (circles) *and the amblyopic eye of an amblyope* (triangles) *viewing the target with unsteady and eccentric fixation. The diamonds at 0.50- and 2.50-diopter stimuli indicate the mean accommodative response of the amblyopic eye when it is fixating steadily and foveally with the aid of auditory feedback. (Reprinted, with permission, from Kirschen et al. 1981.)*

they quantified static accommodative function: (1) in a large group of amblyopes encompassing a representative range of visual acuity and eccentric fixation levels, (2) in strabismics without amblyopia to estimate the contribution of strabismus alone to the accommodative deficits found in strabismic amblyopes, and (3) in amblyopes during the course of orthoptic therapy, as well as several years after successful orthoptic therapy, to determine the magnitude of recovery of accommodation in the amblyopic eye.

Four measures of accommodation were taken. The first was the accommodative stimulus-response function, which provides a quantitative description of the relationship between the accommodative stimulus and response for a wide range of stimulus levels and is used to obtain the closed-loop gain of the accommodation system (e.g., ratio of accommodative response to accommodative stimulus). The second was tonic accommodation, which represents the accommodative response when accommodative feedback (i.e., blur) is rendered ineffective (as in total darkness, a ganzfeld, or with pinhole viewing conditions) (Phillips 1974) and vergence drive to the accommodative system (i.e., vergence accommodation) is absent (Hung and Semmlow 1980, Ciuffreda and Kenyon 1983); thus the accommodative system is open-looped. The third measure was depth of focus, which represents the total dioptric range over which a target can be displaced and yet be perceived as in focus without a change in mean accommodative level. With this information, the open-loop gain of the accommodation system can be calculated (Ciuffreda et al. 1984). [See Equation (6.3) below.] The

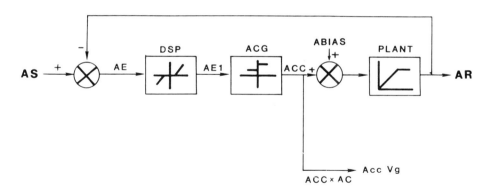

Figure 6.7 *Block diagram of the static model of the accommodative system from Hung and Semmlow. Accommodative error (AE) is the difference between accommodative stimulus (AS) and accommodative response (AR). Deadspace (±DSP) reflects depth of focus of the eye. Output (AE1) from the deadspace operator goes into the accommodative controller, which exhibits nonlinear accommodative controller gain (ACG). Output (ACC) from the accommodative controller is summed at the summing junction and also cross-linked to the vergence system (Acc Vg) by means of gain AC. Accommodative bias (ABIAS) or tonic accommodation under the "no stimulus" condition (i.e., open-looped vergence and accommodation) is also summed here. Output from the summing junction goes through a saturation element, which reflects plant saturation (i.e., amplitude) of the accommodative system. (Adapted, with permission, from Ciuffreda et al. 1983.)*

fourth measure was accommodative amplitude, which represents the maximum response of the accommodative system. For all testing, the target consisted of letters on a reduced Snellen chart presented in a Badal optical system.

Accommodative stimulus-response curves and related measures of accommodative function in normal subjects are presented in Tables 6.1 and 6.2 and Figures 6.8 and 6.9. Slopes of the accommodative stimulus-response curves were within normal limits (Wood and Tomlinson 1974, Ciuffreda and Kenyon 1983), statistically equivalent in the two eyes, and exhibited close correspondence between the accommodative stimulus and average accommodation response in all four subjects. Depth of focus (Campbell 1957) and tonic accommodative levels (Hung and Semmlow 1980) were similar in the two eyes and normal.

Table 6.1　Clinical and Experimental Findings of Representative Subjects in Each Diagnostic Group

Subject	Visual Acuity (S-Chart)	EF($\triangle$)	Minus Lens AMP(D)	Slope	ACG	DF(D)	ABIAS(D)
N2	20/15*	0	8.11	0.78	21	0.28	1.07
	20/13	0	7.72	0.89	21	0.28	1.12
A11	20/120	3.0	3.36	0.72	6.5	1.51	0.79
	20/15	0	9.90	0.91	21	0.63	1.52
FA3	20/13	0	11.05	1.17	21	0.78	1.76
	20/18†	0	9.26	0.98	21	0.56	0.76
S4	20/23*	1.0	9.39	0.92	13.2	0.65	0.56
	20/22	0.25	10.50	1.00	19	0.53	2.31

*Nondominant eye.
†Formerly amblyopic eye.
Source: Reprinted, with permission, from Ciuffreda et al. 1983.

Table 6.2　Summary of Accommodative Data for All Subjects in Each Diagnostic Group

	A	FA	S	N
ACG	AE < DE* 9/11	FAE < DE 1/5	NDE < DE 1/4	NDE = DE 4/4
Slope	AE < DE 9/11	FAE < DE 2/5	NDE < DE 2/4	NDE < DE 4/4
DF	AE > DE 9/11	FAE > DE 2/5	NDE > DE 3/4	NDE > DE 4/4
ABIAS	AE < DE 7/11	FAE < DE 4/5	NDE < DE 4/4	NDE < DE 2/4
AMP	AE < DE 11/11	FAE < DE 4/5	MDE < DE 4/4	NDE < DE 1/4

*Symbols: AE, amblyopic eye; FAE, former amblyopic eye; DE, dominant eye; NDE, nondominant eye; A, amblyopes; FA, former amblyopes; S, strabismics without amblyopia; and N, normal individuals.
Source: Reprinted, with permission, from Ciuffreda et al. 1983.

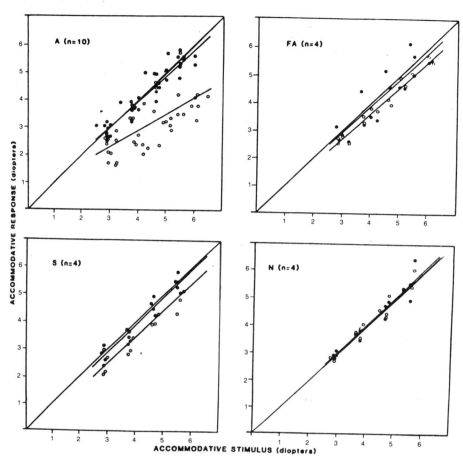

Figure 6.8 *Accommodative stimulus-response curves in a group of amblyopes* (A), *former amblyopes* (FA), *strabismics* (S), *and normal individuals* (N). *Closed circles represent the dominant eye responses, and open circles represent nondominant eye responses. Reduced accommodative responses are evident in the amblyopic eyes. There was a statistically significant difference in slope of the linear regression lines in the dominant and amblyopic eyes (t test, p < 0.05). No such interocular difference was found in the other three groups (t test, p > 0.05). (Reprinted, with permission, from Ciuffreda and Kenyon 1983.)*

Accommodative amplitude values were within normal limits (Borish 1970) (for their age) and were equal in the two eyes (Turner 1958, Wold 1967, Hokoda and Ciuffreda 1982).

Accommodative stimulus-response curves and related measures of accommodative function in amblyopic subjects are presented in Figures 6.8 and 6.9 and Tables 6.1 and 6.2. Slope of the accommodative stimulus-response curve was reduced in the amblyopic eye with respect to the fellow dominant eye in 9 of the 11 subjects; this slope difference was statistically significant in 8 subjects. These

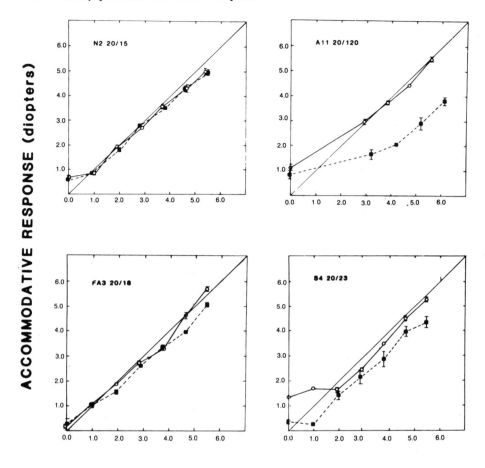

ACCOMMODATIVE STIMULUS (diopters)

Figure 6.9   *Representative accommodative stimulus-response curves in the four popula-*
tions tested. Each eye of the normal subject (N2) showed normal accommodative re-
sponses. In contrast, nondominant eyes (filled squares) of most amblyopes (A11), some
former amblyopes (FA3), and some strabismics without amblyopia (S4) showed reduced
accommodative responses as compared with their dominant eye responses (open circles).
$\bar{X} \pm 1$ SD is plotted. (Reprinted, with permission, from Ciuffreda et al. 1983.)

results were confirmed by dynamic retinoscopy (Figure 6.10) (Ciuffreda et al.
1983). In addition, there was increased variability of accommodative responses in many (7 of 11) of the amblyopic eyes. Depth of focus was greater
in the amblyopic eye when compared with the fellow dominant eye in 9 of the
11 subjects, with increases as great as fivefold over the fellow dominant eye
value. Tonic accommodative values were within normal limits in the two

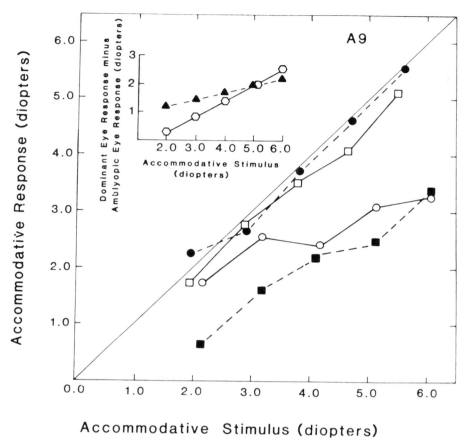

Figure 6.10 *Accommodative stimulus-response curves in an amblyopic subject measured with the Hartinger optometer (open symbols) and with dynamic retinoscopy (filled symbols). Both techniques clearly discriminated between accommodative responses in the amblyopic (open circles, filled squares) and fellow dominant eye (filled circles, open squares). Inset showing interocular differences in response in each eye as a function of stimulus level is derived from linear regression analysis of the raw data. (Reprinted, with permission, from Ciuffreda et al. 1983.)*

eyes, although differences between the two eyes could be large. Accommodative amplitude was reduced in the amblyopic eye as compared with the fellow dominant eye in *all* 11 subjects.

Accommodative stimulus-response curves and related measures of accommodative function in formerly amblyopic subjects are presented in Figures 6.8 and 6.9 and Tables 6.1 and 6.2. While the slope of the accommodative stimulus-response curve was generally similar in each eye, there was a larger range of values than found in the normal subjects. Slightly reduced accommodative responses were particularly evident at the higher stimulus levels in some subjects. Depth of focus values were within normal limits in each eye. Tonic accommodative level was reduced in four of the five formerly amblyopic eyes when compared with the fellow eyes, with this interocular difference being noteworthy in two subjects. Accommodative amplitude was reduced in the formerly amblyopic eye with respect to the fellow eye by 0.5 to 2.0 diopters in four of the five subjects.

Accommodative stimulus-response curves and related measures of accommodative function in strabismics without amblyopia are presented in Figures 6.8 and 6.9 and Tables 6.1 and 6.2. Slope of the accommodative stimulus-response curve was reduced in the nondominant (deviated, nonsighting, nonpreferred) eye with respect to the fellow dominant eye in two subjects, with this slope difference being statistically significant in one. This subject also exhibited markedly increased accommodative response variability in the nondominant eye. Consistent reduction of accommodative response in the nondominant eye with respect to the dominant eye was evident in three subjects over most of the stimulus range. In three of the four subjects, depth of focus was slightly increased, but still within normal limits, in the nondominant eye as compared with the fellow dominant eye. Tonic accommodative level was slightly reduced but generally within normal limits in the nondominant eye as compared with the fellow dominant eye in these subjects. Accommodative amplitude was reduced in the nondominant eye as compared with the fellow dominant eye in all four subjects by 1 to 2 diopters.

Additional analyses were performed on the group data (Figure 6.8 and Table 6.2) (Ciuffreda and Kenyon 1983). There was a statistically significant difference in the slope of the accommodative stimulus-response curve in the amblyopic as compared with the fellow dominant eyes, with the slope being reduced in the amblyopic eyes; there was no significant difference in slope between the dominant and nondominant eyes in the other three diagnostic groups. As the difference in interocular fixation increased, the difference in interocular accommodative amplitude showed a strong trend toward increasing in the amblyopic subjects (Figure 6.11). However, there was no correlation between visual acuity and slope of the accommodative stimulus-response curve in the amblyopic eye, nor between interocular difference in slope of the accommodative stimulus-response curve and difference in interocular fixation locus in the amblyopic subjects. Sample size in the other three diagnostic groups was too small for statistical consideration.

Orthoptic therapy had a positive effect on accommodative function in amblyopic eyes. It increased the slope of the accommodative stimulus-response curve in all four of the treated subjects. In two of the treated subjects, the slope was now statistically similar to that found in the dominant eye. This effect was most striking in the 11-year-old amblyope, whose pre- and postorthoptic accommodative stimulus-response curves were now virtually identical (Ciuffreda et al. 1983, Hokoda and Ciuffreda 1986) (Figure 6.12). Such improvements in accommodative function probably reflect changes in the neurosensory pathways involved in processing of the blur input, and such processing would include those computations that result in maximizing contrast of the foveal retinal image. There are orthoptic-related changes, also presumably of neural origin, in other systems that can influence effectiveness of the retinal stimulus on the accommodation system and thus enhance its response. For example, improvement in dynamic characteristics of fixational eye movements and decrease in magnitude of eccentric fixation could result in increased accommodative responses. The rather minor accommodative deficits found in the nondominant eye of many of the former amblyopes suggests that the orthoptic therapy was sufficient to provide relatively good long-term recovery and maintenance of accommodative function (Ciuffreda 1986).

Lastly, let us consider the results as related to a recently proposed model (Figure 6.7) of steady-state accommodation in normal (Hung and Semmlow 1980) and amblyopic (Hung et al. 1983b) eyes. As mentioned earlier, with this model, determination of three parameters is sufficient to describe the static accommodative behavior in amblyopic eyes during monocular viewing. This includes accommodative controller gain (*ACG*), which represents the open-loop gain of the accommodation system and is directly related to the slope of the

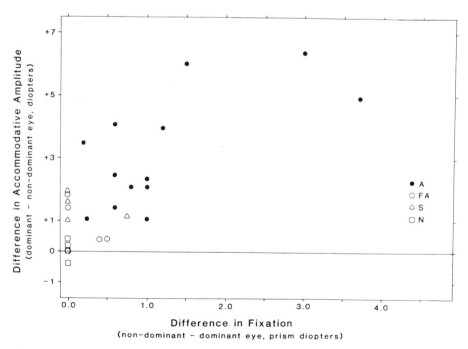

Figure 6.11 *Interocular difference in accommodative amplitude as a function of difference in fixation locus. There was a trend (ρ = +0.52, p < 0.10) for the difference in accommodative amplitude between the two eyes to increase as the difference in fixation locus between the two eyes increased in amblyopic subjects. (Adapted, with permission, from Ciuffreda et al. 1984.)*

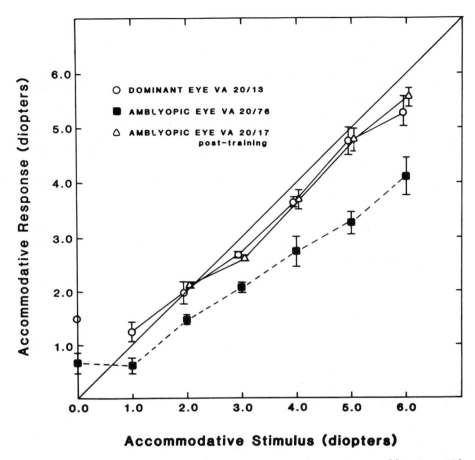

Figure 6.12 *Accommodative stimulus-response curves in an 11-year-old patient with strabismic amblyopia before and after intensive orthoptic therapy. After therapy, monocular accommodative responses were similar in each eye. In the dominant eye (open circles), visual acuity (VA) is 20/13; in the amblyopic eye before therapy (filled squares), VA is 20/76; in the amblyopic eye after therapy (open triangles), VA is 20/17. X̄ ± 1 SD is plotted. (Reprinted, with permission, from Ciuffreda et al. 1983.)*

accommodative stimulus-response curve (i.e., closed-loop gain), tonic accommodative response or bias (*ABIAS*), and the depth of focus (±*DSP*).

The following equation (of the general form $y = mx + b$) can be used to estimate the contribution made by each of the three model parameters (*ABIAS*, *DSP*, and *ACG*; see Figure 6.7) to the reduced accommodative responses found in amblyopic eyes:

$$AR = \frac{ACG}{1+ACG}(AS) + \left[(-DSP)\frac{ACG}{(1+ACG)} + (ABIAS)\frac{1}{(1+ACG)}\right] \quad (6.1)$$

ABIAS has a constant biasing or offsetting effect on the accommodative stimulus-response curve. Presence of a low *ABIAS* as found in a few amblyopic eyes would act in only a very minor way to reduce accommodative responses by some constant amount. *DSP* also produces a bias effect on the accommodative stimulus-response curve. If *DSP* is sufficiently increased, accommodative responses might be markedly reduced (theoretically by some constant amount at each stimulus level) yet *not* be inappropriate, provided the target remained within this extended subjective range of clear retinal imagery. Based on computations involving mean accommodative response level and the associated depth of focus in each subject, it appears that *DSP* has a moderate influence on reducing the accommodative responses in amblyopic eyes, especially at intermediate target vergence levels. Simulation studies (Hung et al. 1981, 1983b) show that the open-loop gain parameter *ACG* has the major independent influence on the slope of the accommodative stimulus-response curve (Figure 6.13). From the preceding equation, it is evident that this influence becomes pronounced at high stimulus levels, where

$$AR \cong \frac{ACG}{1+ACG}(AS) \qquad \begin{array}{l} \text{for } AS \gg DSP \\ AS \gg ABIAS \end{array} \qquad (6.2)$$

It is at these high stimulus levels that the difference in accommodative response between the dominant and amblyopic eye was most evident in the subjects. Thus *ACG* appears to be the primary parameter involved in producing the reduced accommodative responses found in amblyopic eyes, although the other two parameters also play a role. For example, if an amblyopic eye has reduced *ACG*, reduced *ABIAS*, and increased *DSP*, the accommodative stimulus-response profile would have reduced slope (attributed to *ACG*) and downward displacement (primarily due to increased *DSP*, but also to reduced *ABIAS*) with respect to either the 1:1 stimulus-response line or to the normal response profile in the fellow dominant eye.

CLINICAL PROCEDURES TO ASSESS STEADY-STATE ACCOMMODATIVE FUNCTION COMPREHENSIVELY IN AMBLYOPIC EYES USING THE MODEL

Uniform assessment of accommodative function during orthoptic therapy can be used to evaluate a patient's progress. Since the experimental apparatus and procedures Ciuffreda and colleagues used are too complicated, specialized, and time-consuming for all but the research laboratory, they have developed and tested clinical procedures centered around use of the retinoscope that will allow the clinician to obtain reasonable *estimates* of the various accommodative measures and/or model parameters (Ciuffreda et al. 1984). All measures are taken with the subjective refraction in place. The following measures were taken:

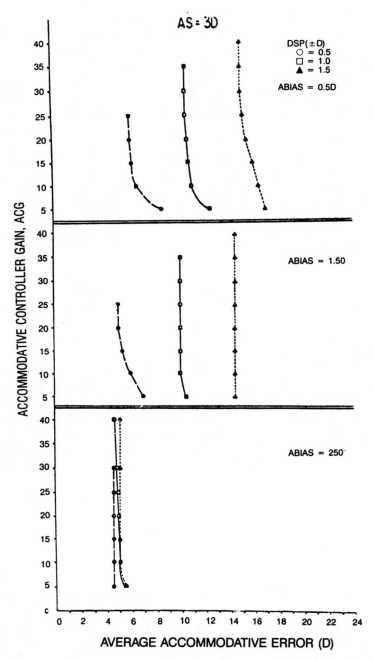

Figure 6.13   *Each computer-simulated plot shows the accommodative controller gain value as a function of accommodative error for the full range of experimentally derived values of DSP and ABIAS (see Figure 6.7 for model symbols). (Reprinted, with permission, from Hung et al. 1983b.)*

Tonic Accommodation (ABIAS)   The patient is placed in a totally darkened room with the nontested eye patched. The patient fixates, for 60 seconds or so, a small, dim, diffuse light source (such as an LED) mounted above the retinoscope. The experimenter then very briefly exposes the retinoscope beam, scans the pupil in quick sweeps, and rapidly changes the test distance until the neutral reflex is observed. This distance converted into diopters represents the tonic accommodation (resting state of accommodation, dark focus), which corresponds to the tonic accommodative bias (*ABIAS*) in the model.

The fixation target (Hennessy and Leibowitz 1971) and the retinoscope beam (Owens et al. 1980) are presumably poor stimuli to accommodation and thus allow the accommodation system to shift gradually to (or toward) its natural tonic level. Occlusion of the nontested eye "opens the loop" of the disparity vergence system and thus precludes introduction of stimulus-driven vergence accommodation into the measurement. The 60-second pretest period in the dark room generally provides sufficient time for completion of accommodation transients that occur in shifting from the initial accommodative level to the tonic level of accommodation (Phillips 1974), although longer times (2 to 3 minutes) may be better.

Slope of the Accommodative Stimulus-Response Function (Closed-loop Accommodative Gain)   The patient is placed in a darkened room, and the nontested eye is patched. A nearpoint card, consisting of a front-illuminated reduced Snellen chart, is presented at different distances representing several accommodative stimulus levels (generally 3 to 6 diopters). The patient is instructed to keep a row of threshold Snellen letters in sharp focus. The experimenter, viewing through a small aperture in the card, scans the pupil with quick sweeps and moves away from the patient (since the accommodative response is typically less than the accommodative stimulus over the range tested) until the "with" motion is neutralized. This distance converted into diopters represents the accommodative response. However, when "against" motion (indicating overaccommodation) is initially observed, the monocular estimate method (Borish 1970) together with the target-to-retinoscopic distance are used to calculate the accommodative response. The mean accommodative response at each stimulus level is plotted, and the slope is found by estimating by eye the straight line of best fit through the data points. The slope is directly related to the neural accommodative controller gain (*ACG*).

Accommodative Amplitude   The apparatus and procedures are similar to those used to determine the accommodative slope function. However, in this case, the experimenter moves the stimulus (a front-illuminated reduced Snellen card) as close as possible to the patient's eye until no further increase in accommodative response is observed with the retinoscope (i.e., consistent "with" motion is now present). This distance converted into diopters represents the response or objective (rather than stimulus or subjective) accommodative amplitude.

Depth of Focus (±DSP)   Two small pieces of clear lucite are mounted on a rod at near. On the fixed lucite plate, a small, just-above-threshold letter X is present. On the movable lucite plate, several small letters just above threshold are placed so that they appear to surround the fixated letter X closely. This stimulus arrangement is similar to that used by Campbell (1957). The patient is instructed to fixate carefully on the X. As the experimenter slowly moves the lucite plate having multiple letters, the patient is instructed to indicate when the multiple letters become slightly blurred. The accommodative response, which should remain relatively constant, is monitored periodically by scanning the patient's pupil through the lucite plates (or through an auxiliary half-silvered mirror) with the retinoscope. The proximal and distal range, converted into diopters, represents the total depth of focus; this value, divided by 2, will give the depth of focus model parameter ($\pm DSP$).

Accommodative Controller Gain (ACG) (Open-Loop Accommodative Gain)
With the preceding information, this model parameter can be either calculated or determined quickly in clinic patients using available computer-simulation results (Figure 6.13) (Hung et al. 1981, Hung et al. 1983b, Ciuffreda et al. 1983, 1984):

$$ACG = \frac{(AR - ABIAS)}{(AE - DSP)} \tag{6.3}$$

EFFECT OF SPATIAL FREQUENCY

In all the studies described so far, the stimulus (generally letters on a Snellen chart) contained high contrast (> 90%) contours with sharply defined borders. The individual components of such a target can be described as having a periodic broadband square-wave nature, since it is formed by zero-phase addition of the higher-frequency, odd-harmonic sinusoidal components to the fundamental sine wave according to the following equation:

$$L(x) = L_0 \{1 + \frac{4m}{\pi} [\sin (2\pi fx) + \frac{1}{3} \sin 3(2\pi fx) + \frac{1}{5} \sin 5(2\pi fx) +]\} \tag{6.4}$$

where $L(x)$ = the luminance profile of a square-wave grating, L_0 = the space-averaged luminance of the grating, f = the spatial frequency (cycles per degree) of the square-wave having unit amplitude, x = the spatial extent of the grating luminance profile in x space, and m = the modulation or contrast in percent. This conforms to Fourier's general theorem, which states that *any* periodic function can be expressed as the summation of a series of simple harmonic terms having frequencies that are multiples of that of the given function (Longhurst 1967). This concept is clearly demonstrated in Figure 6.14. As increasingly higher frequency (but with proportionally decreasing amplitude), odd-harmonic sine waves are added with zero phase to the fundamental sine wave (which has the same frequency as the intended square wave), a square wave is approximated. By applying minor variations to the preceding equation, with respect to the frequency, amplitude, and phase of the higher-order sinusoidal components related to the fundamental sine wave, one can, in addition, describe the luminance/contrast profiles of real-life objects having such basic configurations as a sawtooth or triangle, as well as more complex waveforms (Bateman 1980).

The opposite of Fourier synthesis is Fourier analysis. By this we mean that any complex periodic function or waveform can be decomposed into its basic simple sinusoidal harmonic components. This notion has direct and important bearing on understanding the process of accommodation. Various theories of accommodative control have been proposed that involve the spatial frequency component contribution to the steady-state accommodative response (see Ciuffreda and Kenyon 1983 for a review). For example, Charman and Tucker (1977) believe that the low spatial frequencies provide a "coarse" guide to the accommodation system, with the high spatial frequencies being used to "fine-tune" the accommodative response to make it more accurate (fine focus control hypothesis). In contrast, Owens (1980) believes that the intermediate spatial frequencies (~ 4 cycles per degree), where contrast sensitivity is maximum, are most important for accurate accommodation (contrast control hypothesis). Ciuffreda and Hokoda (1983) explored these ideas in a relatively large group of visually normal subjects and found evidence that could support either or neither hypothesis (Figure 6.15). Thus the relationship between target spatial frequency and accommodation is not a simple one, with addition of voluntary and perceptual aspects of accommodation playing a role to varying (and perhaps unpredictably and

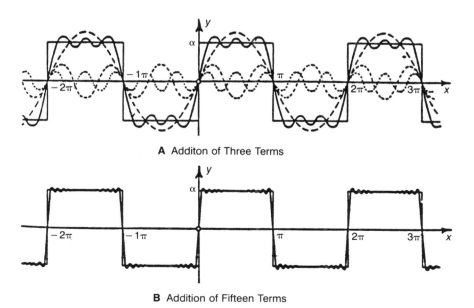

A Additon of Three Terms

B Addition of Fifteen Terms

Figure 6.14 *The addition of sine waves to synthesize a square wave. (Reprinted, with permission, from Longhurst 1967.)*

somewhat uncontrollably) extents in different individuals, leading to the mixed results Ciuffreda and Hokoda found when a sufficiently large number of subjects *were* carefully tested. Recently, Dul et al. (1988) provided evidence suggesting a luminance/contrast gradient hypothesis underlying accommodation to complex gratings in normal observers.

But what about amblyopes? Do they also exhibit spatial frequency dependence of the accommodative response, as found earlier in most normal individuals? Do they favor either hypothesis? Are responses to simple sine-wave stimuli reduced, as was the case for square-wave targets? Are portions of the accommodative-related spatial frequency spectrum no longer functioning and

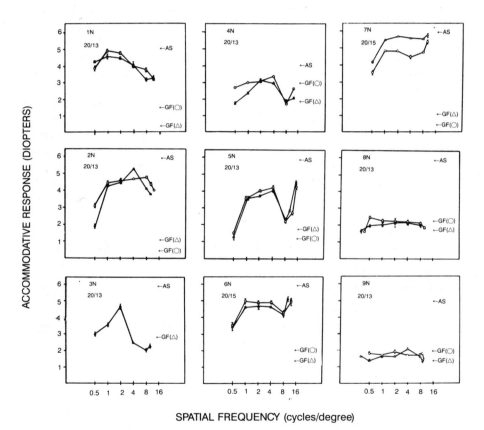

SPATIAL FREQUENCY (cycles/degree)

Figure 6.15 *Steady-state accommodation as a function of spatial frequency of a high-contrast (∼80%), vertical sinusoidal grating in nine normal (N) subjects. Spatial frequency dependence of accommodation is evident in most subjects in each eye. Open circles represent the nondominant eye, open triangles represent the dominant eye, and AS is the accommodative stimulus level; the arrows indicate the average accommodative response to a uniform green field (i.e., the tonic accommodation level); visual acuity of the dominant eye is denoted by the Snellen fraction. Data values represent X̄ ± 1 SD. (Reprinted, with permission, from Ciuffreda and Hokoda 1983.)*

thus resulting in the reduced accommodative responses found for square-wave target configurations? Does orthoptic therapy improve the spatial frequency accommodative response profile? Ciuffreda and colleagues (Ciuffreda and Hokoda 1983, Selenow and Ciuffreda 1986) recently sought to obtain answers to these questions, which bear major importance in understanding the neurologic control of accommodation in amblyopic eyes. They used a static optometer and measured steady-state accommodative responses as amblyopic subjects monocularly viewed high-contrast ($\sim 80\%$), simple, vertically oriented sinusoidal gratings (0.5 to 12.0 cycles per degree) that were randomly presented at high target vergence levels (~ 5 diopters). The results in amblyopes, as well as in normal controls, are described below (Ciuffreda and Hokoda 1983).

The results in normal individuals are presented in Figure 6.15. Responses fell into four groups, with spatial frequency dependence or specificity being the rule. Some subjects (*1N* to *3N*) exhibited maximum accommodative responses over the middle spatial frequency range, in support of Owens (1980), with a decrease of accommodative responses toward the tonic accommodative level for the lower and higher spatial frequencies as the stimulus effectiveness (i.e., the optimal contrast gradient) decreased. The accommodative response spatial frequency profile was similar in each eye. Other subjects (*4N* to *6N*) showed similar response profiles except at the highest spatial frequency; here the accommodative response once again increased, frequently exceeding the accommodative level found over the middle and low spatial frequencies. These data would support neither hypothesis. A third normal variation was found in one subject (*7N*). The accommodative response was minimum for the lowest spatial frequency, maximum for the highest spatial frequency, and high but relatively constant over the middle spatial frequency range, in support of Charman and Tucker (1977). The accommodative response profile was similar in each eye but reduced by 0.5 to 1.0 diopter in the nondominant eye. Responses in two other subjects (*8N*, *9N*) showed little evidence of spatial frequency specificity, especially in the nondominant eye, where the accommodative responses simply appeared to exhibit random variation about the tonic accommodative level; thus the simple sinusoidal gratings proved to be a poor accommodative stimulus in each eye of these two normal subjects. Further, these two subjects' subjective evaluations of the stimulus were consistent with the low accommodative measures; they saw either a uniform green field or a very low contrast sinusoidal grating, which is to be expected with several diopters of retinal defocus present.

The results in amblyopes are presented in Figure 6.16. The dominant and amblyopic eyes of all subjects demonstrated spatial frequency specificity, with variation in response patterns similar to those found in our normal subjects and accommodative responses falling off toward the tonic accommodative level as stimulus effectiveness decreased. However, with only one exception (*2A*), accommodative responses in the amblyopic eyes were generally reduced, frequently by several diopters, as compared with the fellow dominant eye, over the tested spatial frequency spectrum. These reduced accommodative responses were found in both anisometropic (*5A*, *6A*) and strabismic (*1A* to *4A*, *7A*, *FA*)

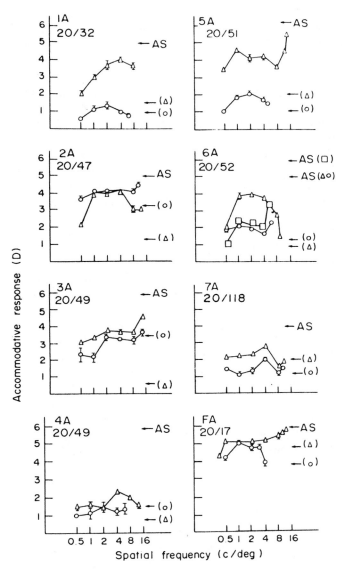

Figure 6.16 *Steady-state accommodation as a function of spatial frequency of a high-contrast (~80%), vertical sinusoidal grating in seven amblyopic (A) and one formerly amblyopic (FA) subject. As was true for normal subjects, spatial frequency dependence of accommodation is evident in most subjects in each eye, although the average response level is typically reduced in the amblyopic eyes. Open circles represent the amblyopic eye, open triangles represent the dominant eye, and AS is the accommodative stimulus; the arrows indicate the average accommodative response to a uniform green field (i.e., the tonic accommodative level); visual acuity in the amblyopic eye is denoted by the Snellen fraction. Data values represent $\bar{X} \pm 1$ SD. (Reprinted, with permission, from Ciuffreda and Hokoda 1983.)*

amblyopes. There was generally no consistent difference in accommodative response variability between the amblyopic and fellow dominant eye (except for subjects *3A* and *4A*), although all subjects reported the task to be more difficult with the amblyopic eye. There was a difference in the general shape of the accommodative response profile between the amblyopic and fellow dominant eye in many of the subjects (*2A, 4A* to *6A, FA*).

The results of this investigation clearly demonstrate the spatial frequency dependence of accommodative responses in amblyopic eyes. Similar response dependence was found in this investigation and in others (Heath 1956, Phillips 1974, Charman and Tucker 1977, Charman and Heron 1979, Owens 1980, Bour 1981) in visually normal subjects. Absence of an appreciable change in mean accommodative response level in each eye of two normal subjects (*8N, 9N*) does not necessarily imply lack of spatial frequency dependence, but rather failure of the grating to provide an adequate accommodative stimulus, resulting in random variability about the tonic accommodative level. If the grating provided an adequate accommodative stimulus in the absence of spatial frequency dependence, one would expect the relatively stable mean accommodative response level to be somewhat higher than the tonic or resting level of accommodation and to approximate the accommodative stimulus level (Ciuffreda and Hokoda 1985). Thus, when the sinusoidal gratings provided an adequate accommodative stimulus, dependence of the accommodative response on the spatial frequency composition of the target appeared to be a general phenomenon, occurring even in amblyopic individuals who have had prolonged periods of abnormal visual experience. The presence of such spatial frequency dependence of the accommodative response, in the absence of obvious gaps or notches in the profile, suggests that the amblyopic eye visual sensory system contains the normal complement of spatial frequency channels, at least over the spatial frequency spectrum tested. However, the reduction of accommodative response magnitude in the amblyopic eye suggests an overall gain loss in the accommodation system (Hung et al. 1981, 1983b, Ciuffreda and Kenyon 1983, Ciuffreda et al. 1983). Such a sensory loss may be attributed to decreased responsiveness of the individual neural elements in the amblyopic eye's afferent visual pathways involved in processing spatial contrast information. In addition, the response output and/or the number of neurons per channel may be reduced. Electrophysiologic studies in visually deprived animals are needed to determine the site(s) of such abnormal function in the visual pathways and to characterize the response properties of the involved neurons. (Also see the next section on contrast.)

These experimental findings using simple sinusoidal, high-contrast gratings are consistent with recent experimental (Ciuffreda and Kenyon 1983, Ciuffreda et al. 1983, Ciuffreda et al. 1987) and modeling (Hung et al. 1981, 1983b) studies that also showed reduced static accommodative responses in amblyopic eyes to high-contrast, broadband stimuli such as Snellen letters (see earlier sections of this chapter for details). In these previous studies (Ciuffreda and Kenyon 1983, Ciuffreda et al. 1983, Hung et al. 1981, 1983b), experimental determination of three model parameter values was sufficient to describe quantitatively the static accommodation system of the amblyopic eye (see Figure 6.7). It was demonstrated that the accommodative controller gain, which determines most of the accommodative response magnitude at high stimulus levels (Hung and Semmlow 1980) (as used in the present experiment) was primarily responsible for the decreased accommodative responses found, which was typically reduced in the amblyopic eye (Ciuffreda and Kenyon 1983, Ciuffreda et al. 1983, Hung et al. 1981, 1983b). In the present experiment, reduced accommodative controller gain in the amblyopic eye would be reflected by reduced accommodative responses over the entire spatial frequency range. In general, this appeared to be true.

Pre- and postorthoptic therapy results are presented in the one adult (29-year-old) amblyope (Figure 6.17). Following 7 months of intensive orthoptic therapy, which included much accommodation training (Liu et al. 1979) and resulted in improved visual acuity in the amblyopic eye (20/120 to 20/75), the accommodative response profile markedly improved in the amblyopic eye. Further, this now clearly supported the fine focus control rather than the contrast control hypothesis (as it did before therapy). Maximum accommodative response was now at 16.0 cycles per degree. There was a significant increase over the pretherapy results with respect to both response magnitude and high spatial frequency range that elicited an accommodative response.

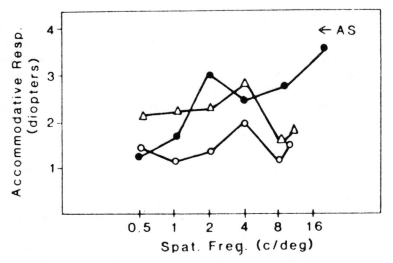

Figure 6.17 *Steady-state accommodation as a function of spatial frequency of a high-contrast (~80%), vertical sinusoidal grating in a 29-year-old strabismic amblyope before and after intensive orthoptic therapy. Spatial frequency dependence of accommodative responses is evident. Accommodative response level increased dramatically in the amblyopic eye following therapy. Open circles represent the amblyopic eye before therapy (20/118), open triangles represent the dominant eye before therapy (20/14), and closed circles represent the amblyopic eye after therapy (20/75). (Reprinted, with permission, from Selenow and Ciuffreda 1986.)*

EFFECT OF CONTRAST

When an object is defocused, its retinal-image contrast gradient and amplitude decrease (Fry 1955, Alpern 1958, Fujii et al. 1970). If the amount of defocus is sufficient to exceed the depth of focus, the subject reports blur of the fixated object. Presence of such a blurred retinal image typically elicits a change in accommodation, having a "reflex" component in response to small blur magnitudes (up to 1.25 diopters or so) with addition of a "voluntary" component for larger amounts of blur (Fincham 1951). The goal of the accommodative response is to maximize foveal retinal-image contrast to render small details visible (Heath 1956).

However, while reduction of retinal-image contrast sufficient to produce the perception of blur under such conditions is undoubtedly a primary stimulus to accommodation (Phillips and Stark 1977), until recently, relatively few investigations have focused on this topic in normal individuals. Heath (1956) showed that steady-state accommodation for intermediate and high stimulus levels reduced only moderately when targets were blurred (by means of interposed lenses and/or ground glass) to about the 20/300 level, with accommodation markedly decreasing when the target was further degraded. Thus the accommodation system is relatively robust to degraded retinal-image contrast. Fujii et al. (1970) found that when small amounts of retinal defocus were introduced, the contrast gradient information was used to reduce the error; however, when large amounts of retinal defocus were introduced, the more robust contrast amplitude information was used to initiate and guide the large error-reducing accommodative response. In a preliminary investigation, Phillips (1974) found that the contrast of sine-wave gratings of intermediate spatial frequencies (3 to 15 cycles per degree) could be reduced by a remarkable amount (from 63% to 2.6%) before the accommodative response was reduced, while this effect was immediate for lower and higher spatial frequencies. These results suggest that the sine-wave grating gradient for intermediate spatial frequencies is optimal with respect to generation of a blur signal; for the lower spatial frequencies, the gradient is too shallow, while for the higher spatial frequencies, it is too steep. Lastly, Bour (1981) found that the accommodative response to a very high contrast sine-wave grating decreased slightly and regularly as contrast was initially reduced and then continued to decrease, at times precipitously, as it was reduced further ($\sim 30\%$), to the point where the accommodative response now approached the tonic accommodation level.

Thus, based on the preceding findings, a clearer picture is beginning to emerge with respect to the role and effects of contrast on accommodation in visually normal individuals. However, until recently (Ciuffreda and Rumpf 1985), this remained unexplored in amblyopes. The results of such an investigation provide insight into the effects of early abnormal visual experience on the neurosensory pathways involved in processing spatial contrast information for use in the control of accommodation in amblyopic eyes.

In the study by Ciuffreda and Rumpf (1985), the experimental apparatus, paradigm, and types of subjects tested were similar to those described earlier in the chapter involving the effect of grating spatial frequency on accommodation. However, now grating contrast rather than spatial frequency was the variable. Starting with a base contrast of 80% (0 dB; decibel units), possible randomly presented target grating contrast values (− dB/% contrast) were 2/63.5, 4/50.5, 6/40.1, 8/31.8, 10/25.3, 15/14.2, 20/8.0, 25/4.5, 30/2.5, 40/0.8, 50/0.25, 60/0.08, and 70/0.025.

The results for a representative visually normal subject (*N3*) are presented in Figure 6.18 for sine- and square-wave stimuli in the dominant (left) eye (determined by a sighting test) and nondominant (right) eye. In either eye, (1) the difference in average accommodative level for the sine- and square-wave stimuli decreased as the grating spatial frequency increased, with essentially overlapping contrast response profiles occurring at about 2.0 to 4.0 cycles per degree, (2) the accommodative error could be as large as 2.5 diopters, especially for the low spatial frequency sine-wave grating with moderate contrast reduction (− 10 dB), and (3) the steady-state accommodative response either remained relatively constant, decreased, or even slightly *increased* as contrast was reduced, until the spatial frequency dependent contrast cutoff value (− 20 to − 30 dB) was reached, where the contrast was now insufficient to drive and maintain accommodation near the stimulus level, thus resulting in a large reduction of accommodation to its tonic level. Of interest is the slight asymmetry in amplitude and contrast cutoff between the two eyes for both types of gratings in this subject; response amplitude was greater in the nondominant eye, while the contrast cutoff was larger in the dominant eye. Such interocular asymmetries were sometimes present in other subjects but were of smaller magnitude and less consistent.

The results of a representative adult amblyope (20/50) are presented in Figure 6.19 for sine- and square-wave stimuli in the dominant and amblyopic eye. In either eye, (1) the difference in average accommodative level for the sine- and square-wave gratings decreased as the spatial frequency increased, with essentially overlapping response profiles occurring at 2 cycles per degree in the amblyopic eye and 4 cycles per degree in the fellow dominant eye, (2) the accommodative error was frequently as large as 1.0 to 2.5 diopters, especially at the lower spatial frequencies for sine-wave stimuli, and (3) the steady-steady accommodative response level either remained relatively constant, decreased, or even *increased* as contrast was reduced, until the spatial frequency dependent contrast cutoff value was reached, where contrast was now insufficient to drive and maintain accommodation near the accommodative stimulus level, thus resulting in a large reduction of accommodation to its tonic level. *Two* primary differences between the amblyopic and fellow dominant eye were evident. First, for both sine- and square-wave stimuli, the average accommodative response level was frequently reduced by about 0.5 to 1.0 diopter in the amblyopic eye, especially for sine-wave stimuli at the lower spatial frequencies (0.5 to 2.0 cycles per degree); in other amblyopes, this interocular difference could be as large as 2 diopters. However, at the higher spatial frequencies, the average accommodative response amplitude in the amblyopic eye either approached or equaled

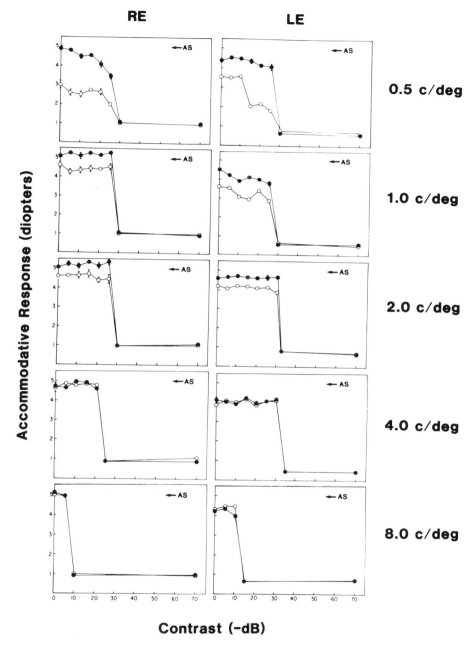

Figure 6.18   *Accommodation as a function of contrast in the right and left eye of a visually normal subject for sine-* (open circles) *and square-wave* (closed circles) *stimuli. (For Figures 6.18 to 6.20, AS = accommodative stimulus level and −70 dB represents the tonic accommodative level; plotted is X̄ ± 1 SD.) (Reprinted, with permission, from Ciuffreda and Rumpf 1985.)*

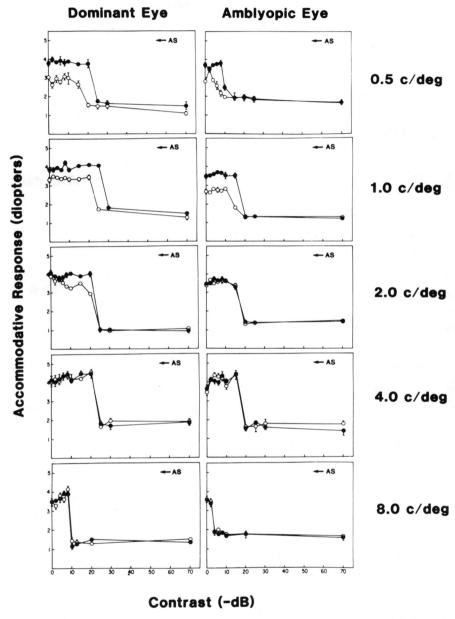

Figure 6.19 *Accommodation as a function of contrast in the amblyopic and dominant eye of a strabismic amblyope for sine-* (open circles) *and square-wave* (closed circles) *stimuli. Plotted is $\bar{X} \pm 1$ SD. (Reprinted, with permission, from Ciuffreda and Rumpf 1985.)*

that of the fellow dominant eye. Thus the amblyopic eye exhibited greater accommodative error. Second, for both sine- and square-wave stimuli, the contrast cutoff value was smaller in the amblyopic eye, with contrast differences as great as 35%, especially at the higher spatial frequencies. This was true for most amblyopic eyes at most spatial frequencies. Thus the amblyopic eye required more contrast to maintain accommodation.

The results of an adult (23-year-old) anisometropic amblyope before and after a 5-month period of intensive conventional orthoptic therapy (monocular accommodation training and direct occlusion) (Griffin 1976) to improve vision function in the amblyopic eye are presented in Figure 6.20. Measurements were taken for at least four critical points: 80% contrast, the minimum contrast that still elicited an accommodative response significantly above the tonic level, the maximum contrast that elicited an accommodative response equivalent to the tonic level (i.e., -70 dB point), and the tonic accommodative level. From this abbreviated test paradigm one can still generate a reasonably accurate accommodative contrast response profile. Several important points deserve mention. First, the pretherapy accommodative responses in the amblyopic eye were always less than in the fellow dominant eye. Second, the pretherapy contrast cutoff value in the amblyopic eye was always smaller than in the dominant eye. Third, the posttherapy accommodative response level in the amblyopic eye now equalled or slightly exceeded that found in the fellow eye. And fourth, the pre- versus posttherapy contrast cutoff value in the amblyopic eye was relatively unchanged.

The findings in visually normal subjects are consistent with those of others showing steady-state accommodation to be relatively robust to substantial decreases in target contrast (Heath 1956, Phillips 1974, Bour 1981, Ward 1987). The results are consistent with the contrast gradient/amplitude theory and the experimental findings of Fujii et al. (1970). As contrast (i.e., amplitude) of a square-wave grating is reduced (for a fixed average luminance level), the steep gradient remains constant. Thus accommodative accuracy is predicted to be, and indeed was, relatively unchanged until contrast was markedly reduced. However, with a sine-wave grating, the contrast gradient is by its nature less steep than that of a square-wave grating, and this is especially evident at low and intermediate spatial frequencies. Thus, even at high contrast levels, the contrast gradient, and in turn the accommodative accuracy, is reduced relative to the square-wave response. As sine-wave grating contrast is further reduced, this effect becomes increasingly evident. Lastly, as grating spatial frequency increased, the accommodative response contrast profiles for sine- and square-wave gratings superimposed, presumably due to the physical extent (i.e., steepness) of their contrast gradient now being more similar, as well as due to high spatial frequency filtering of the human eye. In fact, our subjects generally reported little difference between 8 cycle per degree sine- and square-wave gratings at all contrast levels tested.

The results in our amblyopes clearly demonstrate abnormal accommodative control with respect to stimulus contrast effectiveness. The two deficits specific to and occurring together in amblyopia include decreased average steady-state

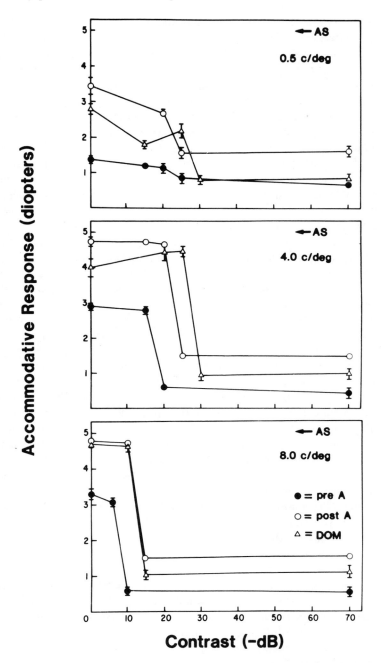

Figure 6.20   *Accommodation as a function of contrast in the dominant eye* (closed triangles), *and in the amblyopic eye before* (closed circles) *(20/50) and after* (open circles) *(20/25) intensive orthoptic therapy, in an adult anisometropic amblyope. Plotted is $\bar{X} \pm 1$ SD. (Reprinted, with permission, from Ciuffreda and Rumpf 1985.)*

accommodation *and* a reduced or smaller contrast cutoff value. This is true when compared with the fellow dominant eye, as well as either eye of visually normal subjects. Thus, when physical contrast of the grating presented to either eye of an amblyope was the same, the amblyopic eye response was less and required greater contrast to sustain accommodation than did the fellow eye. These results are consistent with other recent experimental findings (described earlier in this chapter) showing reduced accommodation in amblyopic eyes for a variety of high-contrast square- and sine-wave stimuli (Hokoda and Ciuffreda 1982, Ciuffreda and Hokoda 1983, Ciuffreda and Kenyon 1983, Ciuffreda et al. 1983, 1984, Hung et al. 1983b); further, they are in agreement with the recent modeling studies (also described earlier), Hung et al. 1983b, Ciuffreda et al. 1984) in which reduced accommodative controller gain and increased depth of focus were believed to be the primary model parameters contributing to the reduced accommodative responses in amblyopic eyes.

As discussed earlier, the reduced accommodative responses found in amblyopic eyes reflect a primary sensory loss over the central retinal region due to prolonged, early, abnormal visual experience and resulting in an overall reduced sensitivity of the eye. This agrees with numerous studies showing reduced sensory function within the central retinal region in amblyopic eyes (Feinberg 1956, Mackensen 1957, Ciuffreda et al. 1978a and b, Hess and Howell 1977, Bedell and Flom 1981). More specifically, this reduction of accommodative response magnitude in the amblyopic eye suggests a gain loss in the accommodation system (Hung et al. 1983b, Ciuffreda and Kenyon 1983; Ciuffreda et al. 1983), with presence of eccentric fixation, impaired contrast perception, and/or abnormal fixational eye movements (see detailed discussion later) having at best only relatively modest adverse effects on accommodation to a grating, especially at the lower spatial frequencies (Ciuffreda and Hokoda 1983). Further, such a sensory loss might be attributed to decreased responsiveness of the individual neural elements in the amblyopic eye's afferent visual pathways involved in processing spatial contrast information. Electrophysiologic studies in visually deprived animals are needed to determine the site(s) of such abnormal function in the visual pathways and to characterize the response properties of the involved neurons. Candidate cells for such study would include striate cortical neurons, since their overall contrast/neural response profiles bear striking resemblance to our psychophysically determined contrast/response profiles, especially for somewhat analogous test conditions in which sine-wave gratings of low spatial frequency were used (Dean 1981, Tolhurst et al. 1981, Ohzawa et al. 1982, Sclar and Freeman 1982). At very low contrasts, cortical neurons exhibited only spontaneous activity; this can be compared with our contrast region in which the accommodative response remained at the tonic level. As contrast was increased, neuronal firing rate gradually increased; this can be compared with our contrast region in which either gradual or sharp increases in accommodation were found as contrast was increased. And at 10% to 30% contrast, some saturation became evident, although modest increases in cell responsivity were clearly found as contrast was further increased to as high as 80% in some cells;

this can be compared with our contrast region in which accommodation either increased slightly or remained relatively constant as grating contrast was increased to its maximum of 80%.

The results in the adult amblyope following orthoptic therapy provide important additional insight into visual system plasticity in human amblyopia. She had not received any orthoptic therapy or optical correction until she was tested by us at age 23 years. When retested 5 months later, visual acuity improved from 20/40 to 20/25, and the accommodative response contrast profile normalized (Figure 6.20) in the amblyopic eye. These results were consistent with her own report of markedly improved target clarity and contrast in both the experimental apparatus and real-life surrounds when viewing with the amblyopic eye alone. These findings agree nicely with other recent results in several older amblyopes (ages 6½ to 29 years) (as reviewed in earlier sections of this chapter) in which steady-state accommodative accuracy to a variety of square- and sine-wave stimuli improved concurrent with improvement in numerous other vision functions such as visual acuity, contrast sensitivity, and eye movements following periods of orthoptic therapy (3 to 18 months) (see Ciuffreda et al. 1978a and b, 1979a, b, and c, 1983, 1984, Ciuffreda and Hokoda 1983, Selenow and Ciuffreda 1983, Ciuffreda 1986 for a detailed overview). Such improvements in accommodative function presumably reflect changes in those neural pathways involved in sensory processing of the blur input, with such processing including computations that result in maximizing contrast of the central retinal image.

EFFECT OF HIGHER-ORDER SPATIAL FREQUENCIES

As discussed earlier in the section on spatial frequency, those experiments were performed to determine if there was evidence for spatial frequency dependence of accommodative responses. This was clearly the case. With the accommodative stimulus level and target contrast fixed and only the (simple) sinusoidal spatial frequency of the grating varied, the steady-state accommodative responses also varied systematically, most frequently showing the maximal accommodative response for the intermediate spatial frequencies. This was true in normal individuals, as well as in amblyopes and strabismics, thus demonstrating the generality and robustness of this basic phenomenon.

Since the accommodation system responds differentially to simple sinusoids of various spatial frequencies, could the higher-order (odd-harmonic) spatial components be added algebraically to the appropriate lower spatial frequency sinusoids to approximate a square-wave grating and thus potentially provide a better accommodative stimulus? The ability of the visual system to function optimally and accurately frequently necessitates the presence of higher-order, odd-harmonic sinusoidal spatial components in the scene (Ginsburg 1981). The presence of such harmonically related sinusoidal components, summed in phase with their common fundamental or first harmonic sinusoidal component, effectively functions to "sharpen" the border between objects, thereby providing greater definition and detail. This is depicted graphically in Figure 6.14.

Although these higher-order, odd-harmonic sinusoidal spatial frequency components have been implicated in the accommodative behavior described earlier (Ciuffreda and Rumpf 1985, Charman and Tucker 1977, 1978, Ward and Charman 1985, Tucker and Charman 1986, 1987), the precise role and/or relative contribution of the individual sine-wave components to the fundamental have only recently been directly investigated (Ciuffreda et al. 1987, Dul et al. 1988). Some earlier evidence suggested that the presence of these spatial components could indeed contribute to the steady-state accommodative response, especially with respect to accuracy. Heath (1956) found that when Snellen letters were moderately to markedly degraded so that their contrast and contrast gradient were reduced, accommodative accuracy decreased. The results suggest that reduction and/or elimination of the higher (and perhaps intermediate) spatial components, which act to steepen the contrast gradient, played a role in reducing accommodative accuracy. Phillips (1974), using simple sinewaves and squarewaves of various spatial frequencies at a fixed target contrast (63%), found that steady-state accommodative responses to sine- and square-wave gratings were equivalent above about 2 cycles per degree, but lower for the sinewaves at the lower spatial frequencies (0.3 to 2.0 cycles per degree). This suggests that any odd-harmonic effect when accommodating on a complex grating would only be present when the fundamental spatial frequency is relatively low. The effect could only be present when the accommodative response to the fundamental sine wave alone yields a sufficient accommodative error that potentially could be reduced toward the more accurate square-wave level of response by addition of its harmonically related sine-wave components (Ciuffreda and Rumpf 1985). Charman and Tucker (1977, 1978) found that accommodative responses were more accurate for a square-wave-type stimulus (i.e., 20/20 Snellen line) than for any of the full range (0.4 to 30.0 cycles per degree) of high-contrast (80%), simple sine waves tested. They speculated that a "broadband" stimulus (e.g. one containing a wide range of spatial frequency components such as found in a square-wave grating) results in more accurate accommodation than the sine wave owing to the presence of low spatial frequency components providing the initial "coarse" accommodative guidance, with the high spatial frequency components providing the subsequent "fine-tuning" of the response, resulting in accurate accommodation. Owens (1980), on the other hand, found that the accommodative responses to either a high-contrast (63%) sine- (3.0 cycles per degree) or square-wave (4.3 cycles per degree) grating were equivalent. From this he concluded that "sharp edges or high spatial frequencies are not necessary for accurate accommodation." However, for either lower or higher spatial frequencies, the accommodative response was more accurate for the square-wave grating than for any of the simple sine-wave gratings. Lastly, Bour (1981), using an infrared dynamic optometer to monitor fluctuations of accommodation, found that the response variance (i.e., root mean square deviation) was much smaller for the square-wave grating than for any of the range of simple sine-wave gratings at the moderate- to high-contrast levels tested. Thus the presence of the broad spatial frequency band of the square-wave target can act to reduce small fluctuations of accommodation and thereby have a stabilizing role in dynamic accommodative control.

Recently, this critical experiment to determine directly the higher-order, odd-harmonic spatial frequency contribution to steady-state accommodation was performed in normal and amblyopic observers (Ciuffreda et al. 1987). Computer-generated stimuli consisted of either the fundamental sine-wave grating (f), the fundamental sine-wave grating with in-phase summation of its higher-order, odd-harmonic components ($f + 3f$, $f + 3f + 5f$, and so on to $15f$ in the normal individuals and to $7f$ in the amblyopes), or a square-wave grating having the same fundamental frequency as the sine. Contrast of the base fundamental sine- and square-wave gratings was either 84%, 40%, 15%, or 5%. Accommodative stimulus level was generally 5 diopters. These gratings were presented on a nearby screen for monocular viewing by the subjects.

The responses of a representative visually normal subject are presented in Figure 6.21 for the full range of fundamental spatial frequencies and contrast levels tested. While no effect of contrast was evident, the predicted odd-harmonic effect (i.e., reduction of accommodative error with addition of the higher spatial components) was clearly present at the two lower fundamental spatial frequencies. For example, at a base frequency of 0.5 cycle per degree, there was a clear reduction in accommodative error (by up to 1.5 diopters *relative* to the sine wave) as the higher spatial components were added (up to the eleventh or so), with convergence of responses (and reduction in mean response variance) to the square-wave level. Such an effect was not obvious at the higher base fundamental spatial frequencies of either 2 or 4 cycles per degree. Here, however, the average accommodative responses to the fundamental sine wave were essentially equivalent to that of the square wave. Thus, if the accommodative responses to the *least* complex waveform (i.e., simple sine-wave grating) were already accurate, addition of the *higher* spatial components could have no further impact on the accuracy of steady-state accommodation.

The responses in each eye of a representative amblyope are presented in Figure 6.22. Here the fundamental spatial frequency remained constant (0.5 cycle per degree), and the steady-state accommodative response for *each* eye was determined at each of the four contrast levels. As expected, there was considerably more response variability for a given waveform in the amblyopic eye (Ciuffreda et al. 1984). However, evidence of an odd-harmonic effect in each eye was clearly seen at the two highest contrast levels. At the two lowest contrast levels, there was increased response variability across stimuli in *each* eye, with little evidence of any systematic reduction in accommodative error as the higher spatial frequency components were added. Responses here generally showed no obvious pattern or trend. Such increased response variability was frequently

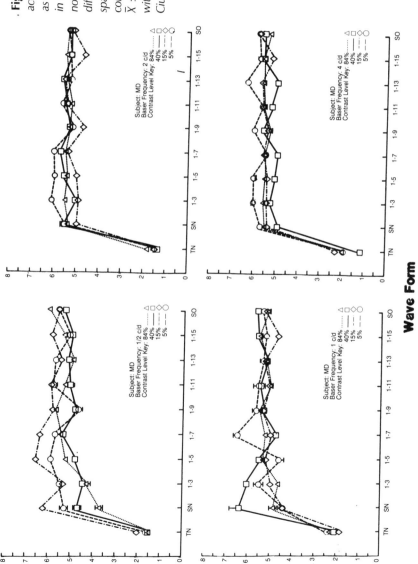

Figure 6.21 *Mean accommodative response as a function of waveform in a representative visually normal subject at four different fundamental spatial frequencies and contrast levels. Plotted is* X̄ ± 1 SD. *(Reprinted, with permission, from Ciuffreda et al. 1987.)*

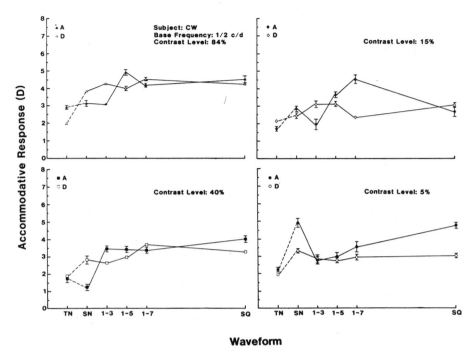

Figure 6.22   *Mean accommodative response as a function of waveform in a representative amblyopic subject at four different fundamental spatial frequencies and contrast levels. Plotted is $\overline{X} \pm 1$ SD. (Reprinted, with permission, from Ciuffreda et al. 1987.)*

found in less experienced amblyopic observers. At these lower contrast levels, accommodation can be quite difficult to maintain, requiring a high level of concentration; further, the presence of the higher spatial components is much less obvious here. Lastly, although the mean accommodative response levels were reduced in each eye relative to that typically found in visually normal subjects, there were no consistent interocular differences in this subject. However, moderate to gross (~ 1 diopter) underaccommodation relative to the dominant eye was found at the higher contrast levels in three of the five amblyopic eyes tested.

Group results are presented in Figure 6.23 for the 0.5 cycle per degree fundamental, with this being the base spatial frequency where the odd-harmonic effect was most evident. Similar but less dramatic results were found for the 1.0 cycle per degree fundamental. For the normal eyes, the dominant eye of amblyopes, and the amblyopic eye, the odd-harmonic effect was clearly present. This was confirmed by statistical analyses.

The results clearly demonstrate the presence and generality of the odd-harmonic effect with respect to steady-state accommodative accuracy. The effect was striking in the visually normal individuals, as might be predicted based

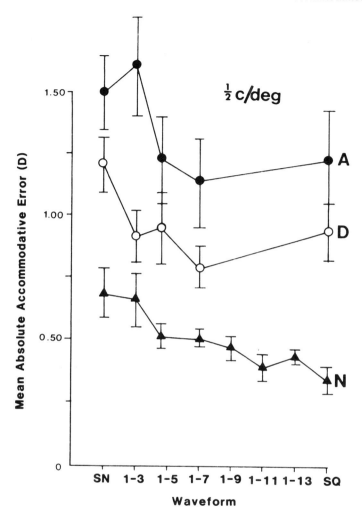

Figure 6.23 *Group mean absolute accommodative error as a function of wave form in the amblyopic eye (A), fellow dominant eye of the amblyope (D), and eyes of visually normal subjects (N). Absolute error is plotted in the graph to emphasize accommodative accuracy independent of direction of accommodation (i.e., over- or underaccommodation) relative to the stimulus level. Data are collapsed across contrast levels. Fundamental spatial frequency is 0.5 cycles per degree. Plotted is $\bar{X} \pm 1$ SEM. (Reprinted, with permission, from Ciuffreda et al. 1987.)*

on Heath's (1956) early study in which relatively crude manipulations of the higher-order spatial content of the target were made. The effect was present in each eye of both the strabismic and anisometropic amblyopes, demonstrating robustness of the phenomenon in spite of differences in early abnormal visual experience (e.g., suppression and/or monocular contrast deprivation) leading to the gradual development of functional amblyopia. Presence of the odd-harmonic effect in each eye of a strabismic without amblyopia is consistent with our earlier findings (Ciuffreda et al. 1984, Ciuffreda and Rumpf 1985), suggesting that strabismus alone has relatively little negative impact on either the overall response pattern or magnitude of accommodative response in most subjects.

The lack of any obvious odd-harmonic effect at the higher base spatial frequencies is consistent with earlier findings (Ciuffreda and Rumpf 1985, Tucker and Charman 1987) and with theoretical predictions (Fujii et al. 1970). As the base spatial frequency increased, the steady-state accommodative response to the simple sine- and square-wave gratings were essentially equal, owing to the physical extent (i.e., steepness) of their contrast gradient now being more similar, as well as to the naturally occurring high spatial frequency filtering of the human eye. Once the gratings were informally judged to be perceptually similar, sensorimotor equivalence was attained. Thus, if the accommodative response to the simple sine- and square-wave gratings are equivalent, then addition of the higher-order, odd-harmonic spatial components to the fundamental sinusoid would have little impact on steady-state accommodative accuracy. The present sine- versus square-wave grating results are consistent with and help explain the earlier findings of Phillips (1974) and Owens (1980), where the accommodative responses to simple sine- and related square-wave gratings were equal at intermediate (or higher) spatial frequencies.

The results demonstrating the effect of contrast on accommodation are also in agreement with earlier findings. When an object becomes defocused in most real-life situations and even laboratory investigations, both its contrast amplitude and its gradient are reduced; thus their respective independent contributions to accommodative control are difficult to ascertain. In the present experiment, however, contrast was manipulated independent of the contrast gradient, and thus the effect of contrast amplitude versus contrast gradient could be determined directly. The results clearly demonstrated that for most normal and amblyopic observers it was the contrast gradient that was most influential in determining accommodative response magnitude. Thus, as both theorized and demonstrated by Fujii et al. (1970) in normal individuals, the contrast gradient is most important in driving the accommodation system in the presence of relatively small amounts of defocus. However, the contrast amplitude may be more important in the presence of relatively large amounts of defocus, for here the contrast gradient would be very shallow, producing a situation somewhat akin to a contrast increment threshold task. With large amounts of retinal defocus, voluntary rather than reflex accommodation is probably the dominant initiating component (Fincham 1951). The present results are also consistent with the recent findings of Ciuffreda and Rumpf (1985), which showed that with the exception of the lowest spatial frequency (0.5 cycle per degree sine), steady-state accommodative responses in both normal and amblyopic eyes were relatively unaffected by wide variations in grating contrast, similar to that found by Bour (1981) and Ward (1987) in normal individuals.

Thus, once the contrast gradient becomes sufficiently steep, the grating becomes a highly effective accommodative stimulus, almost independent of its visible contrast range.

CONTRAST DISCRIMINATION

One of the primary driving forces of the accommodation system is contrast of the retinal image (Fry 1955, Alpern 1958, Fujii et al. 1970, Wildt et al. 1976). The goal of the accommodation system is to maximize foveal retinal-image contrast to render small details visible (Heath 1956). Impaired ability to perceive or discriminate either gradual fluctuations or rapid step changes in retinal-image contrast can clearly result in relatively large steady-state accommodative errors and reduced visibility.

It is now well established that amblyopic eyes exhibit impaired steady-state accommodation, as discussed in detail throughout this chapter. However, most relevant is the recent finding by Ciuffreda et al. (1984) of increased depth of focus in amblyopic eyes. The increased depth of focus suggests that changes in retinal-image contrast must be greater in the amblyopic than in the fellow dominant eye before the perception blur is elicited. Thus one would predict contrast discrimination to be impaired in the amblyopic eye and contribute to its increased steady-state error.

There have been only two studies in which contrast discrimination in amblyopic eyes has been assessed (Hess et al. 1983, Bradley and Ohzawa 1986). The amblyopic eyes typically required more contrast to make the discriminations at the intermediate and higher spatial frequencies. However, besides having a small number of subjects, these two studies had other problems methodologically.

Therefore, Ciuffreda and Fisher (1987) decided to perform such an experiment with most of the earlier problems corrected in their design. They used a successive, two-alternative, forced-choice procedure to measure the contrast necessary to determine that two suprathreshold gratings differed in contrast. The procedure incorporated double-interleaved staircases with a standard grating of 25% contrast and initial comparison gratings of 10% (ascending series) and 40% (descending series) briefly presented on an oscilloscope.

The group results for the amblyopes are presented in Figure 6.24. The amblyopic eye performed more poorly than the fellow dominant eye at each spatial frequency. Contrast discrimination became poorer as spatial frequency increased. Also, there was no effect of spatial frequency on the magnitude of the interocular contrast discrimination differences.

The group results for the normal individuals and for the strabismics without amblyopia are also presented in Figure 6.24. In the normal individuals, there was a significant effect of eye. Although there was a trend for better performance in the right eye for all spatial frequencies, only the interocular difference at the lowest spatial frequency was significant. There was also a significant effect

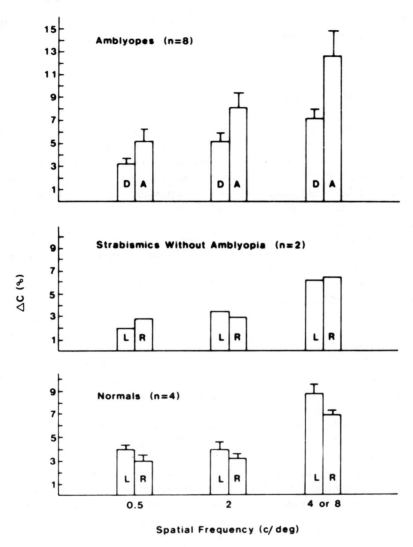

Figure 6.24 *Contrast discrimination [ΔC(%)] as a function of spatial frequency in each eye for each diagnostic group. Plotted is $\overline{X}$ ± 1 SD. (Reprinted, with permission, from Ciuffreda and Fisher 1987.)*

of spatial frequency, indicating a difference in contrast discrimination ability related to spatial frequency. There was no effect of spatial frequency on the magnitude of the interocular contrast discrimination differences.

Results for the strabismics without amblyopia were clearly within normal limits. There was little interocular difference for any spatial frequency, and contrast discrimination became progressively poorer with increased spatial frequency.

The results clearly show impairment of contrast discrimination ability in amblyopic eyes. Interocular differences in the amblyopes were about 2 to 3.5 times greater than in the normal individuals and about 2 to 25 times greater than in the strabismics without amblyopia (for the respective spatial frequencies). This deficit was present at each of the spatial frequencies tested. Such anomalous contrast discrimination in the amblyopic eyes is presumably due to the abnormal visual experience, perhaps involving visual cortical cells sensitive to contrast (Campbell and Kulikowski 1972), during the early years of life. This includes abnormal binocular interactions due to constant strabismic suppression (Burian and von Noorden 1974) and/or mild monocular form/contrast deprivation due to uncorrected anisometropia (Bradley and Freeman 1981). Apparently, the intermittent suppression experienced in the strabismics without amblyopia was not sufficient to affect contrast discrimination adversely; the periods of normal visual experience were sufficient to maintain a normal sensory status.

The abnormal contrast discrimination ability in amblyopic eyes might contribute to the increased steady-state accommodative error typically found in these subjects (Ciuffreda et al. 1984), especially when target contrast is reduced and/or target spatial frequency is increased (Ciuffreda and Rumpf 1985, Ciuffreda et al. 1987). As stated earlier, such a deficit would result in an impaired ability to perceive or discriminate small fluctuations in retinal-image contrast. If the amblyopic eye requires several times more change in contrast than normal to detect a just-noticeable difference, a larger steady-state accommodative error would be allowed to be present without any obvious adverse perceptual consequences, such as blur or reduced apparent target contrast. Thus the accommodative response for a given stimulus would be reduced as compared with normal observers or with the fellow dominant eye of the amblyope. In terms of the accommodation model parameters affected, the presence of poor contrast discrimination ability leading to reduced accommodative responses would be reflected in an increased depth of focus, as has been found experimentally and modeled using computer simulations (Hung et al. 1983b, Ciuffreda et al. 1984).

Normal contrast discrimination ability, however, was found in each eye of the strabismics without amblyopia. The slightly increased steady-state accommodative errors found in the nondominant eyes of some strabismics without amblyopia (Ciuffreda et al. 1984) is therefore probably due to factors other than contrast discrimination ability.

For all three diagnostic groups, a greater contrast difference was generally required for discrimination as spatial frequency increased [i.e., $\Delta C(\%)$ increased as a function of spatial frequency]. If spatial frequency and mean luminance of a sinusoid were held constant while its physical contrast was enhanced by increasing its amplitude, the contrast/luminance gradient effect may be occurring and be evident with lower spatial frequency gratings, thus making their contrast discrimination easier. The gradient effect, however, would probably not be apparent for higher spatial frequency sinusoidal gratings where the contrast gradient is already quite steep (Ciuffreda et al. 1987).

Three other points deserve brief mention. First, there was a trend for $\Delta C(\%)$ to increase as visual acuity in the amblyopic eye decreased, especially for the 0.5 and 2.0 cycle per degree test targets. However, a much larger sample size ($n > 30$) would be needed to determine, with confidence, the true presence and strength of such a relationship. Second, the similarity between the values obtained for the normal individuals, strabismics without amblyopia, and the dominant eyes of the amblyopes show the similarity and normalcy in contrast discrimination ability in these groups. Third, comparison of contrast discrimination ability in strabismic versus anisometropic amblyopes is difficult owing to the small sample size and visual acuity differences. However, similarity of results between a anisometropic amblyope (20/170) who had never received orthoptic therapy or optical correction and a strabismic amblyope (20/122) who had received intensive orthoptic therapy with excellent results 5 years earlier but who had regressed to his pretherapy visual acuity level suggests that monocular form/contrast deprivation in anisometropic amblyopia per se may not have a significant differential adverse effect on contrast discrimination in these two diagnostic groups. Further detailed investigation of contrast discrimination ability in a larger group of anisometropic and strabismic amblyopes, however, will be necessary to address this important question.

PERCEIVED OR EGOCENTRIC DISTANCE AS A FUNCTION OF ACCOMMODATION

The role of accommodation in visual space perception, or more specifically, perceived or egocentric absolute distance, has been one of considerable controversy. Unfortunately, previous studies have had a variety of methodologic pitfalls, including the use of poor accommodative stimuli, reliance on indirect judgments of apparent size rather than apparent distance, creation of situations in which accommodation is in conflict with other distance cues, and failure to measure accommodation (see Fisher and Ciuffreda 1988 for a review). All these factors would contribute to underestimation of the ability of accommodation to influence perceived distance.

In a study using visually normal individuals, Fisher and Ciuffreda (1988) measured perceived distance using a sliding indicator adjusted with the unseen hand and the monocular steady-state accommodative response to good accommodative stimuli presented in a Badal optical system. The results (Figure 6.25) demonstrate that apparent distance was clearly linearly related to the accommodative response. Monocular blur-driven accommodation alone has the potential to provide distance information in a lawful manner. Thus, as one increases accommodation, and presumably (correlated) accommodative effort, the apparent distance of the fixated object shifts in a predictable manner. In two amblyopes tested so far, the results are somewhat different: The perceptual range is shifted inward and is more restricted and, more importantly, the response function is curvilinear (Figure 6.25). These results presumably reflect

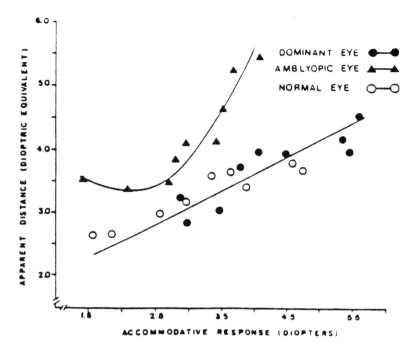

Figure 6.25 *Apparent distance as a function of mean accommodative response. (From Fisher and Ciuffreda, 1988.)*

increased accommodative effort to attain a given accommodative response level, resulting in biased and distorted perceived distance judgments. Results in the dominant eye of amblyopes were similar to those in normal subjects. Although the functions are not identical, the results clearly show that for both normal and amblyopic observers, accommodation serves as a reasonable cue to perceived distance.

ACCOMMODATIVE DYNAMICS

As discussed in detail throughout the earlier sections of this chapter, amblyopic eyes exhibit a variety of steady-state accommodative abnormalities that have been observed and documented in both clinical and laboratory situations. These include increased accommodative error, increased depth of focus, decreased maximum accommodative amplitude, increased accommodative variability, and impaired sustaining ability, all of which can be normalized to some extent by appropriate and intensive remedial therapeutic intervention. The general decrease in accommodative responsivity in the amblyopic eye has not been attributed to either abnormally low tonic innervation or a defective peripheral accommodative mechanism or "plant" (i.e., ciliary muscle/nerve, suspensory ligaments, or lens components), but rather to reduced central controller gain and decreased sensitivity of the accommodative neurosensory system. This is presumably due to the presence of early abnormal visual experience, namely, suppression in strabismus and mild monocular form deprivation in anisometropia.

While much is known about steady-state accommodation in amblyopic eyes, there have been relatively few careful clinical observations and/or subjective/ objective laboratory measures of accommodation dynamics in amblyopic eyes. Clinicians have reported and attempted to improve the overall reduced monocular accommodative response times found in such patients when tracking lens-induced step changes in the near accommodative stimulus (Smith 1950, Schapero 1970, Sherman 1970, Greenwald 1979). Ciuffreda and Kenyon (1983) presented objective responses of accommodation in each eye of a deep amblyope with anisometropia while tracking step changes in target position at near distances. Results showed markedly increased accommodative latency, decreased response amplitude, increased response variability, and impaired sustaining ability in the amblyopic eye; however, the presence of a large posterior staphalyoma in this eye may have confounded the results. Ukai et al. (1986) found decreased accommodative responses and increased variability in the amblyopic eye (as compared with the fellow dominant eye) when monocularly tracking a slow (0.3 diopter per second) ramp stimulus to determine the full range of the accommodative stimulus/response function objectively (Ciuffreda and Kenyon 1983). This provided objective confirmation and extension of the work by Ciuffreda et al. (1984). Lastly, Winn et al. (1987) presented objective recordings and related power spectra in two amblyopes while they attempted to sustain accommodation monocularly with concurrent changes in chromatic composition of the target. While overall accommodative responsivity was greater for the yellow versus either the blue or red targets, comparison with the fellow dominant eye was unfortunately not provided. Thus, while the preceding observations and studies provide some insight into accommodation dynamics in amblyopic eyes, there has been no systematic attempt to investigate basic dynamic aspects of accommodation—namely, the latency, time constant, and peak velocity/amplitude relationship—in a sufficiently large and diverse group of

Table 6.3   Mean Group Data: Latency (ms)*

Normal Individuals
  Right eye: 364
  Left eye: 354

Strabismics without Amblyopia
  Nondominant eye: 349
  Dominant eye: 331

Amblyopes
  Amblyopic eye: 372
  Dominant eye: 351

*Significant mean group interocular difference found only in amblyopes ($p < 0.05$; t test).

amblyopes. A recent study by Ciuffreda et al. (*in preparation*) has attempted to provide such basic and important information. Ciuffreda and colleagues used a high-speed, dynamic, infrared optometer to measure monocular accommodative responses to randomized step and pulse inputs at 4- and 2-diopter target vergence levels. These were physical targets in space having both blur and size inputs similar to those found in real-life situations. Adult subjects included (1) 16 amblyopes, generally of the strabismic variety, with 2 tested before and after successful conventional orthoptic therapy consisting of accommodation, eye movement, eye-hand coordination, and antisuppression "exercises," (2) 3 strabismics without amblyopia to assess the possible contribution of strabismus-related sensorimotor deficits alone on the accommodative responses of strabismic amblyopes, and (3) 3 visually normal control subjects.

Representative responses are shown in Figure 6.26. There were four abnormalities found in the amblyopic eyes. First, there was a small (21.5 ms) but significant increase in response latency or reaction time (see Table 6.3). Second, there was a 30% reduction in response amplitude (or system gain). Third, variability of response amplitude was increased. And fourth, there was impairment of the ability to sustain accommodation at the nearer test distance, which never equalled or exceeded the accommodative amplitude in the amblyopic eye. However, there were two key dynamic parameters that were within normal limits. These were the accommodative response time constant (i.e., time needed to attain 63% of the final response amplitude; see Table 6.4) and the accommodative peak velocity/amplitude relationship (i.e., "main sequence") (Schnider et al. 1984), as shown in Figure 6.27 for the amblyopic eyes. The graph in Figure 6.27*A* clearly demonstrates that there was an appropriate match between the accommodative response amplitude and its peak velocity; the vast majority of values fit within the predicted envelope for normality. The graph in Figure 6.27*B* shows that orthoptic therapy normalized accommodative responsivity, with the posttherapy average accommodative amplitude increasing the full amount of 30%. Normal main sequence values were found in the dominant eye of the amblyopes, as well as in each eye of the strabismics without amblyopia.

Table 6.4 Mean Data: Time Constant (ms)*

Normal Individuals
  Right eye: 221
  Left eye: 254

Strabismics without Amblyopia
  Nondominant eye: 193
  Dominant eye: 215

Amblyopes
  Amblyopic eye: 225
  Dominant eye: 230

*No significant mean group interocular difference was found for any of the three diagnostic groups ($p > 0.05$; t test).

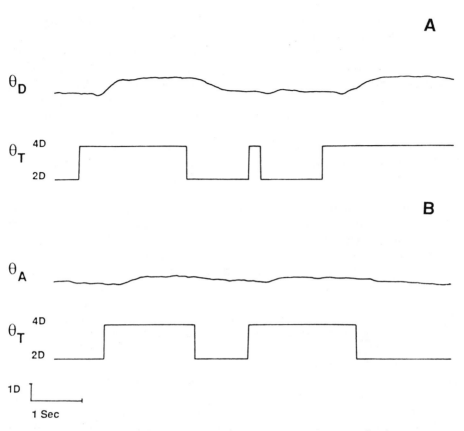

Figure 6.26   *Dynamic accommodative responses to step inputs (θ_T; 2 and 4 diopters) in an amblyope. (A) Dominant eye (θ_D). (B) Amblyopic eye (θ_A). (From Ciuffreda et al., in preparation.)*

The results have important theoretical and clinical implications, and they provide new insights into accommodative dynamics in amblyopic eyes. There were two normal findings: time constant and main sequence values. The former result suggests that the peripheral accommodative apparatus in the amblyopic eye had normal biomechanical properties, whereas the latter result suggests normal neurologic control of accommodation with regard to appropriate motoneuronal controller signals being generated centrally to drive the accommodative "plant" to reduce retinal-image blur. There were four dynamic accommodation abnormalities. The findings of reduced response amplitude, increased response variability, and impaired sustaining ability point to a loss in neurosensory sensitivity; "sensing" of the blur input was therefore compromised, presumably resulting from early abnormal visual experience (as discussed in detail earlier in this chapter). The fourth dynamic abnormality, namely, increased accommodative latency, suggests a processing delay in the afferent visual pathways, again

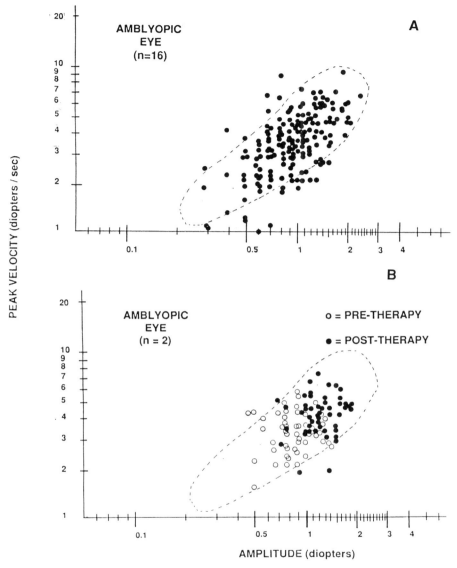

Figure 6.27 *Plots showing the accommodative amplitude/peak velocity relationship ("main sequence"). Dashed line encloses normal response range. (A) Amblyopic eye. (B) Amblyopic eyes before and after therapy. (From Ciuffreda et al., in preparation.)*

presumably as a result of early abnormal visual experience. This finding is consistent with the results of others with regard to the presence of small time delays in transmission and/or processing of visual information with the amblyopic eye alone (von Noorden and Burian 1960, Burian et al. 1962, Goldstein and

Greenstein 1971, Ciuffreda et al. 1978a and b) (Also see Chapter 2). Earlier discussions with respect to the effects of eccentric fixation, impaired contrast perception, and abnormal fixational eye movements on steady-state accommodative performance with the amblyopic eye also apply here with regard to accommodative dynamics.

FACTORS CONTRIBUTING TO REDUCED
ACCOMMODATIVE STIMULUS EFFECTIVENESS
IN AMBLYOPIC EYES

The results of the various laboratory and clinical studies demonstrate that accommodative function in amblyopic eyes is primarily distinguished by its reduced response level. This finding of reduced accommodative range in amblyopic eyes has been confirmed using objective infrared recording techniques (Hatsukawa et al. 1983, Ukai et al. 1983). The most probable cause of this reduced accommodative performance in amblyopia is a primary sensory loss over the central retinal region. (See earlier sections for detailed discussion of this related to the model and the neurophysiologic implications.) This could occur as a result of prolonged, early, abnormal visual experience due to the presence of strabismus, resulting in abnormal binocular interactions (Burian and von Noorden 1974), including neural sensory inhibition (Kirschen and Flom 1978), and/or anisometropia, resulting in mild monocular contrast deprivation (Bradley and Freeman 1981). This agrees with numerous studies showing reduced sensory function over the central retinal region in amblyopic eyes (Feinberg 1956, Mackensen 1958, Hess and Howell 1977, Ciuffreda et al. 1978a and b, Bedell and Flom 1981). In the case of the accommodation system, reduced sensitivity to either a focused or a slightly defocused (as reflected by our finding of increased depth of focus) retinal image would result in reduction of accommodative responsiveness.

Such a sensory loss also may result in markedly elevated threshold (Hess and Howell 1977) and slightly elevated suprathreshold (Hess and Bradley 1980, Loshin and Levi 1983) contrast perception. The presence of elevated threshold contrast sensitivity could result in impaired accommodative responses in two ways. First, in cases where the extent of retinal defocus is marked, the resultant low-contrast target image may simply be imperceptible. Second, when attempting to focus on normal suprathreshold stimuli, slight reductions and/or fluctuations in retinal-image contrast due to imprecise focus may not be appreciated (as suggested by the finding of slightly impaired contrast discrimination as discussed earlier). The presence of depressed suprathreshold contrast sensitivity (especially as found in anisometropic amblyopes for high spatial frequency gratings) also could result in reduction of accommodative responses. This is consistent with the finding of somewhat reduced accommodative responses in normal individuals when suprathreshold target contrast is moderately to markedly decreased (Heath 1956, Phillips 1974, Bour 1981, Ciuffreda and Rumpf 1985, Ward 1987).

Could such a suprathreshold contrast deficit, however, be *primarily* responsible for the *markedly* reduced steady-state accommodative responses found in amblyopic eyes? Probably not. Ciuffreda and Hokoda (1983) measured static accommodative responses as a function of target spatial frequency for high-contrast sinusoidal gratings in amblyopic subjects (as discussed earlier). Accommodative responses were reduced in the amblyopic as compared with the fellow dominant eye over the entire spatial frequency spectrum. In addition, using a crude contrast-matching paradigm with either low or moderate spatial frequency gratings prearranged to be approximately *focused* on the retina, little difference in perceived interocular contrast was found. Further, in some subjects in whom the physical *and* perceived contrasts were equivalent in each eye, accommodative responses were still markedly reduced in the amblyopic eye. Thus any deficit in high suprathreshold contrast perception for low and moderate spatial frequencies appears to play a relatively minor role in adversely affecting static accommodative responses in amblyopic eyes. This is consistent with subsequent, more formal studies showing only relatively slight impairment of contrast discrimination over a wide range of spatial frequencies and contrast levels (Hess et al. 1983, Bradley and Ohzawa 1986, Ciuffreda and Fisher 1988), as discussed in detail earlier. Rather, the common finding of reduced accommodative response to the various stimuli suggests the amblyopic deficit to be one of general overall reduced gain of the sensory accommodative system. However, the transient "dynamic" suprathreshold contrast loss frequently reported by amblyopes (noted as "fading" of the object), presumably due to abnormally rapid retinal-image adaptation during attempted steady fixation (Feinberg 1956, Lawwill 1968, Ciuffreda et al. 1979b, Sireteanu and Fronius 1981, Ciuffreda et al. 1984), may act to reduce the effective (i.e., perceived) target contrast, which in turn may result in additional fluctuations in the reduced accommodative responses (Heath 1956, Phillips 1974, Bour 1981, Ciuffreda and Rumpf 1985).

Several other findings suggest that these accommodative deficits found in amblyopic eyes appear to have a sensory (afferent) rather than motor (efferent) origin. First, the presence of normal accommodative function in the dominant eye of amblyopes suggests that the motor controller is unaffected (assuming a single central neural network). This is consistent with findings in other sensorimotor systems in amblyopes (Mackensen 1957, Burian and von Noorden 1974, Ciuffreda et al. 1978a and b). Second, the presence of normal consensually but not direct-driven accommodation in the amblyopic eye suggests that the accommodative deficit resides neither in the motor controller nor in the peripheral accommodative apparatus (i.e., lens, ciliary body, and suspensory zonules). And third, the presence of slightly abnormal accommodative function in the non-dominant eye of strabismics without amblyopia suggests that (intermittent) suppression alone is sufficient to have a mildly adverse effect on the accommodation system (although such effects may be reversed by orthoptic therapy) (Schnider et al. 1985). Thus, in some strabismic amblyopes, part of the reduced accommodative function in the amblyopic eye could be attributed to this strabismic-suppression component.

In addition, two other factors may act to reduce stimulus effectiveness and in turn reduce the accommodative response. The first is the eccentric fixation present in most amblyopic eyes (Brock and Givner 1952). Such nonfoveal monocular fixation with the amblyopic eye could reduce the accommodative response, since the normal closed-loop gain of the accommodation system decreases with eccentricity of the blur stimulation (Figure 6.28) (Whiteside 1957, Phillips 1974, Semmlow and Tinor 1978, Bullimore and Gilmartin 1987, Gu and Legge 1987). Results of Kirschen et al. (1981) for broadband stimuli supported this notion in amblyopic eyes (Figure 6.6), although the effect was small (~ 0.25 diopter). Further, there is a trend for the accommodative response slope (Ciuffreda et al. 1984) and the accommodative amplitude (Figure 6.11) (Ciuffreda and Kenyon 1983) to decrease as eccentric fixation increases. Recent

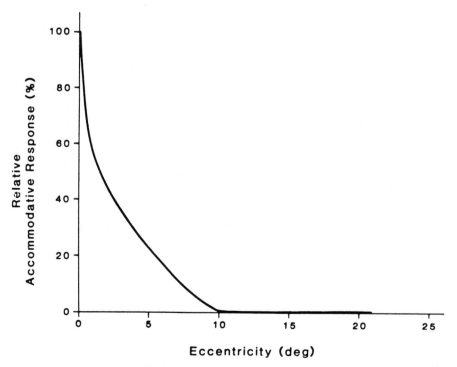

Figure 6.28   *Plot of the effectiveness of a defocused target in driving accommodation as a function of retinal eccentricity. Magnitude of the response has been calculated as a percent of the response to a centrally fixated target. Data averaged from three normal subjects. (Reprinted, with permission, from Phillips 1974.)*

preliminary data in one amblyope show reduced slope of the accommodative stimulus-response function over the central 10 degrees of retina, as compared with the fellow dominant eye (Figure 6.29) (Bullimore and Gilmartin 1987). This was especially marked over the 2-degree or so central-most portion, presumably due to stronger inhibitory effects there than over the adjacent, more peripheral regions. For the experiments with gratings, even less of an effect is predicted owing to presence of eccentric fixation. Since most amblyopes tested had less than 0.75 degrees of eccentric fixation and the grating pattern constitutes a spatially redundant target configuration, both the fovea *and* the eccentric fixation point (as well as surrounding regions) received adequate stimulation at all times. The second factor is abnormal fixational eye movements, such as occur during monocular viewing with the amblyopic eye (see Chapter 5). Abnormalities include increased drift amplitude (Matteucci 1960, Ciuffreda 1977, Schor and Hallmark 1978, Ciuffreda et al. 1979a, 1980), jerk nystagmus (Ciuffreda 1977, Ciuffreda et al. 1979a), and saccadic intrusions (Ciuffreda et al. 1979b). Increased drift amplitude and nystagmus amplitude could account for increased variability of accommodative responses in the amblyopic eye. As the eye slowly moves, the stimulus impinges over a relatively wide (~ 1 degree or so) range of cones in the fovea and near-retinal periphery. This results in a continuously

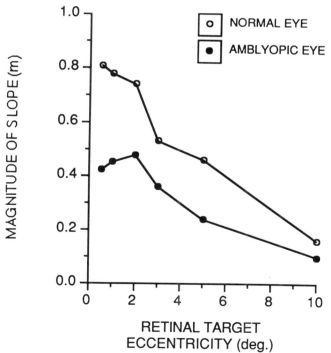

Figure 6.29   *Magnitude of the slope (m) of the stimulus-response function (stimulus range −1 to −4 diopters) as a function of retinal target eccentricity for the normal and amblyopic eyes of subject R.L. (Reprinted, with permission, from Bullimore and Gilmartin 1987.)*

changing degree of accommodative stimulus effectiveness (Figure 6.28) (White-side 1957, Phillips 1974, Semmlow and Tinor 1978, Bullimore and Gilmartin 1987, Gu and Legge 1987). The increased drift velocity and nystagmus slow-phase velocity, while probably not rapid enough to degrade visual resolution significantly ($<$ 2.5 degrees per second; Westheimer and McKee 1975, Ciuffreda et al. 1980), would "smear" the retinal image and possibly reduce its value as an accommodative stimulus. Since accommodation in normal individuals (Phillips 1974, Charman and Tucker 1977, Charman and Heron 1979, Owens 1980, Bour 1981, Ciuffreda and Hokoda 1983) and in amblyopes (Ciuffreda and Hokoda 1983) is spatial frequency dependent, loss or marked reduction in contrast of *high* and *intermediate* spatial frequency components of the retinal image by such smearing could adversely affect the accommodative response in amblyopic eyes. Since it has been speculated (Charman and Tucker 1977) and recently demonstrated (Ciuffreda et al. 1987) in both normal individuals and in amblyopes that these high and intermediate spatial frequency components are involved in "fine-tuning" of the accommodative response, degradation and/or loss of this information could result in reduced accommodative responses, especially for square-wave stimuli having a low (0.5 cycle per degree) fundamental spatial frequency (Ciuffreda et al. 1987). Saccadic intrusions (Ciuffreda et al. 1979b) probably do not adversely affect the accommodative response, since they rapidly ($\sim$ 200 ms) return the eye to the preferred fixation locus for relatively long durations (400 ms to several seconds). These 1-degree or so intrusive saccades may, in fact, be beneficial because they provide spatial and temporal modulation of the retinal image and thus counteract the abnormally rapid retinal adaptation and resultant fading (owing to the dynamic suprathreshold contrast perception abnormality) of the target frequently found in amblyopic eyes (Feinberg 1956, Lawwill 1968, Hess et al. 1977, Ciuffreda et al. 1979b, Sireteanu and Fronius 1981). Such variations in perceived contrast may be responsible for the increased variability and impaired accommodative sustaining ability found in amblyopic eyes (Ciuffreda et al. 1983, 1984, Ciuffreda and Kenyon 1983).

SUMMARY

The results presented in this chapter clearly demonstrate several types of accommodative deficits in the amblyopic eye when attempting to focus on sine- and square-wave-type stimuli under static and dynamic test conditions. However, a common feature was the overall reduced average response level, frequently found in conjunction with increased response variance. It has been argued that the site of the accommodative dysfunction was not in the motor controller nor in the peripheral apparatus, but rather in the sensory controller. Such a sensory defect was presumed due to the early, prolonged abnormal visual experience, including suppression in strabismus and mild monocular contrast-

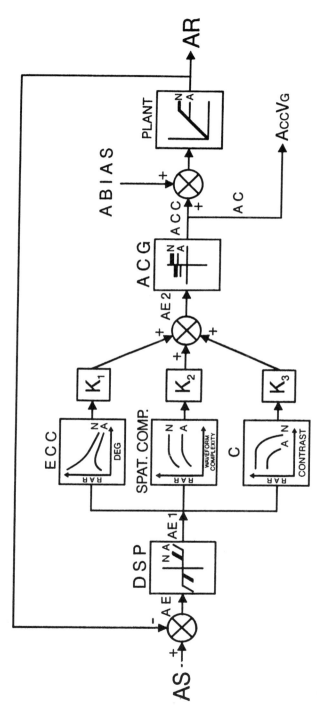

Figure 6.30 *Block diagram of the static model of the accommodative system, with inclusion of several of the sensory factors that account for much of the reduced accommodative responses found in amblyopic eyes. These include target retinal eccentricity (ECC), spatial composition of the target (SPAT. COMP.), and target contrast (C), with K_1, K_2, and K_3 being gain terms and RAR being the relative accommodative response. Accommodative error (AE) is the difference between accommodative stimulus (AS) and accommodative response (AR). Deadspace ($\pm$DSP) reflects depth of focus of eye. Output (AE1) from the deadspace operator goes into the accommodative controller, which exhibits nonlinear accommodative controller gain (ACG). Output (ACC) from the accommodative controller is summed at the summing junction ($\otimes$) and also cross-linked to the vergence system (Acc Vg) by means of gain AC. Accommodative bias (ABIAS) or tonic accommodation under the "no stimulus" (i.e., open-looped vergence and accommodation) condition is also summed here. Output from the summing junction goes through a saturation element, which reflects plant saturation of the accommodative system. N and A are normal and amblyopic eyes, respectively.*

derivation in anisometropia. In terms of the model of steady-state accommodation, the accommodative defect is primarily localized at the site of the accommodative controller gain. Thus an effect of such abnormal visual experience is to reduce the effective gain, resulting in reduced response amplitude. In addition, such factors as abnormal fixational eye movements, defective contrast perception, and/or eccentric fixation may contribute to the reduced responsivity. A steady-state model of the human accommodation system, as proposed by Hung and Semmlow (1980) (see Figure 6.7), with several of these sensory factors now incorporated to account for much of the reduced responses in amblyopic eyes is presented in Figure 6.30. Lastly, orthoptic therapy always resulted in marked improvement in accommodation, even in older amblyopes. With regard to dynamic accommodation abnormalities, this included increased latency, reduced gain, increased response variability, and poor sustaining ability. The sensory basis for these dynamic abnormalities and additional factors contributing to the deficits are the same as described above with regard to static accommodation.

REFERENCES

Abraham SV. (1961) Accommodation in the amblyopic eye. *Am. J. Ophthalmol.* 52:197–200.

Alpern M. (1958) Variability of accommodation during steady fixation at various levels of illumination. *Am. J. Ophthalmol.* 52:197–200.

Bateman WA. (1980) *Introduction to Computer Music.* New York: Wiley.

Bedell HE, Flom MC. (1981) Monocular spatial distortion in strabismic amblyopia. *Invest. Ophthalmol. Vis. Sci.* 20:263–8.

Borish IM. (1970) *Clinical Refraction*, 3d Ed. Chicago: Professional Press.

Bour LJ. (1981) The influence of the spatial distribution of a target on the dynamic response and fluctuations of the accommodation of the human eye. *Vision Res.* 21:1287–96.

Bradley A, Freeman R. (1981) Contrast sensitivity in anisometropic amblyopia. *Invest. Ophthalmol. Vis. Sci.* 21:467–76.

Bradley A, Ohzawa I. (1986) A comparison of contrast detection and discrimination. *Vision Res.* 26:991–7.

Brock FW, Givner I. (1952) Fixation anomalies in amblyopia. *Arch. Ophthalmol.* 47:775–86.

Bullimore MA, Gilmartin B. (1987) The Influence of Retinal Area Stimulated on the Accommodative Response. In Fiorentini A, Guyton DL, Siegel IM (Eds.), *Advances in Diagnostic Visual Optics*, pp. 181–5. New York: Springer-Verlag.

Burian HM, von Noorden GK. (1974) *Binocular Vision and Ocular Motility.* St. Louis: Mosby.

Burian HM, Benton AL, Lipsius RC. (1962) Visual and cognitive functions in patients with strabismus amblyopia. *Arch. Ophthalmol.* 68:785–91.

Campbell FW. (1954) The minimum quantity of light required to elicit the accommodation reflex in man. *J. Physiol.* 123:357–66.

Campbell FW. (1957) The depth of field of the human eye. *Optica Acta* 4:157–64.

Campbell FW, Kulikowski JJ. (1972) The visual evoked potential as a function of contrast of a grating pattern. *J. Physiol.* 222:345–56.

Charman WN, Heron C. (1979) Spatial frequency and the dynamics of the accommodation response. *Optica Acta.* 26:217-28.

Charman WN, Tucker J. (1977) Dependence of accommodation response on the spatial frequency spectrum of the observed object. *Vision Res.* 17:129-39.

Charman WN, Tucker J. (1978) Accommodation as a function of object form. *Am. J. Optom. Physiol. Opt.* 55:84-92.

Ciuffreda KJ. (1977) Eye Movements in Amblyopia and Strabismus. Ph.D. dissertation, School of Optometry, University of California, Berkeley.

Ciuffreda KJ. (1986) Visual System Plasticity in Human Amblyopia. In Hilfer R, Sheffield J (Eds.), *Development of Order in the Visual System.* New York: Springer-Verlag.

Ciuffreda KJ. (in press a) Accommodation and Its Anomalies. In Charman WN (ed.), *Visual Optics and Instrumentation.* London: Macmillan.

Ciuffreda KJ. (in press b) Accommodation to gratings and more naturalistic stimuli. *Optom. Vis. Sci.*

Ciuffreda KJ, Dul M, Fisher SK. (1987) Higher-order spatial frequency contribution to accommodative accuracy in normal and amblyopic observers. *Clin. Vis. Sci.* 1:219-29.

Ciuffreda KJ, Fisher SK. (1987) Impairment of contrast discrimination in amblyopic eyes. *Ophthalmic Physiol. Opt.* 7:461-7.

Ciuffreda KJ, Hokoda SC. (1983) Spatial frequency dependence of accommodative responses in amblyopic eyes. *Vision Res.* 23:1585-94.

Ciuffreda KJ, Hokoda SC. (1985) Effect of instruction and higher level control on the accommodative response spatial frequency profile. *Ophthalmic Physiol. Opt.* 5:221-3.

Ciuffreda KJ, Hokoda SC, Hung GK, Semmlow JL. (1984) Accommodative stimulus/response function in human amblyopia. *Doc. Ophthalmol.* 56:303-26.

Ciuffreda KJ, Hokoda SC, Hung GK, Semmlow JL, Selenow A. (1983) Static aspects of accommodation in human amblyopia. *Am. J. Optom. Physiol. Opt.* 60:436-49.

Ciuffreda KJ, Kenyon RV. (1983) Accommodative Vergence and Accommodation in Normals, Amblyopes, and Strabismics. In Schor CM, Ciuffreda KJ (Eds.), *Vergence Eye Movements: Basic and Clinical Aspects.* Boston: Butterworth.

Ciuffreda KJ, Kenyon RV, Stark L. (1978a) Processing delays in amblyopic eyes: evidence from saccadic latencies. *Am. J. Optom. Physiol. Opt.* 55:187-96.

Ciuffreda KJ, Kenyon RV, Stark L. (1978b) Increased saccadic latencies in amblyopic eyes. *Invest. Ophthalmol. Vis. Sci.* 17:697-702.

Ciuffreda KJ, Kenyon RV, Stark L. (1979a) Fixational eye movements in amblyopia and strabismus. *J. Am. Optom. Assoc.* 50:1251-8.

Ciuffreda KJ, Kenyon RV, Stark L. (1979b) Saccadic intrusions in strabismus. *Arch. Ophthalmol.* 97:1673-9.

Ciuffreda KJ, Kenyon RV, Stark L. (1979c) Different rates of functional recovery of eye movements during orthoptics treatment in an adult amblyope. *Invest. Ophthalmol. Vis. Sci.* 18:213-19.

Ciuffreda KJ, Kenyon RV, Stark L. (1980) Increased drift in amblyopic eyes. *Br. J. Ophthalmol.* 64:7-14.

Ciuffreda KJ, Kruger PB. (1988) Dynamics of human voluntary accommodation. *Am. J. Optom. Physiol. Opt.* 65:365-370.

Ciuffreda KJ, Rumpf D. (1985) Contrast and accommodation in amblyopia. *Vision Res.* 25:1445-57.

Ciuffreda KJ, Schnider CM, Mathews S, Selenow A. Accommodative dynamics in amblyopic eyes (in preparation).

Dean AF. (1981) The relationship between response amplitude and contrast for cat striate cortical neurones. *J. Physiol.* 318:413–27.

Dul M, Ciuffreda KJ, Fisher SK. (1988) Accommodative accuracy to harmonically related complex gratings and their components. *Ophthalmic Physiol. Opt.* 8:146–52.

Feinberg I. (1956) Critical flicker frequency in amblyopia exanopsia. *Am. J. Ophthalmol.* 42:472–81.

Fincham EF. (1951) The accommodation reflex and its stimulus. *Br. J. Ophthalmol.* 35:381–93.

Fincham EF, Walton J. (1957) Reciprocal action of accommodation and convergence. *J. Physiol.* 137:488–508.

Fisher SK, Ciuffreda KJ. (1988) Accommodation and apparent distance. *Perception* 17:609–621.

Fry GA. (1955) *Blur of the Retinal Image.* Columbus: Ohio State University Press.

Fujii K, Kondo K, Kasai T. (1970) An analysis of the human eye accommodation system. *Osaka University Technical Report No. 925,* 20:221–36.

Ginsburg AP. (1981) Spatial Filtering and Vision: Implications for Normal and Abnormal Vision. In Proenza LM, Enoch JM, Jampolsky A (Eds.), *Clinical Applications of Visual Psychophysics,* pp. 70–166. Cambridge, England: Cambridge University Press.

Goldstein JH, Greenstein F. (1971) Eye-Hand Coordination in Strabismus. In Fells P (Ed.), *The First Congress of The International Strabismological Association.* St. Louis: Mosby.

Green DG, Powers MK, Banks MS. (1980) Depth of focus, eye size, and visual acuity. *Vision Res.* 20:827–35.

Greenwald I. (1979) *Effective Strabismus Therapy,* pp. 80–84. Duncan, Oklahoma: Optometric Extension Program Foundation.

Griffin JR. (1976) Binocular anomalies: procedures for vision therapy. Professional Press, Chicago.

Gu Y, Legge GE. (1987) Accommodation to stimuli in peripheral vision. *J. Opt. Soc. Am. [A]* 8:1681–7.

Hatsukawa Y, Murai Y, Kawanishi T, Nagao N, Nakao Y, Otori T. (1983) A new method for the determination of the range of accommodation in amblyopic patients. *Folia Ophthalmol. Jpn.* 34:1030–6.

Heath GG. (1956) The influence of visual acuity on accommodative response of the eye. *Am. J. Optom. Arch. Am. Acad. Optom.* 33:513–24.

Hennessy RT, Leibowitz HW. (1971) The effect of a peripheral stimulus on accommodation. *Percept. Psychophys.* 10:129–32.

Hess RF, Bradley A. (1980) Contrast perception above threshold is only minimally impaired in human amblyopia. *Nature* 287:463–4.

Hess RF, Howell ER. (1977) The threshold contrast sensitivity function in strabismic amblyopia: Evidence for a two-type classification. *Vision Res.* 17:1049–55.

Hess RF, Bradley A, Piotrowski L. (1983) Contrast coding in amblyopia: I. Differences in the neural basis of human amblyopia. *Proc. R. Soc. Lond.* B217:309–30.

Hess RF, Campbell FW, Greenhalgh T. (1977) On the nature of the neural abnormality in human amblyopia: Neural aberrations and neural sensitivity loss. *Pflugers Arch.* 377:201–7.

Hokoda SC, Ciuffreda KJ. (1982) Measurement of accommodative amplitude in amblyopia. *Ophthalmic Physiol. Opt.* 2:205–12.

Hokoda SC, Ciuffreda KJ. (1986) Different rates and amounts of vision function recovery during orthoptic therapy in an older strabismic amblyope. *Ophthalmic Physiol. Opt.* 6:213–20.

Hung GK, Semmlow JL. (1980) Static behavior of accommodation and vergence: Computer simulation of an interactive dual-feedback system. *IEEE Trans. Biomed. Eng.* 27:439–47.

Hung GK, Ciuffreda KJ, Semmlow JL. (1981) Modeling of Human Near Response Disorders. In *Proceedings of the Ninth Annual Northeast Biomedical Engineering Conference, Rutgers University*, pp. 192–7. New York: Plenum Press.

Hung GK, Ciuffreda KJ, Semmlow JL, Hokoda SC. (1983b) Model of static accommodative behavior in human amblyopia. *IEEE Trans. Biomed. Eng.* 30:665–71.

Hung GK, Semmlow JL, Ciuffreda KJ. (1983a) Identification of accommodative vergence contribution to the near response using response variance. *Invest. Ophthalmol. Vis. Sci.* 24:772–7.

Ittelson WH, Ames AA. (1950) Accommodation, convergence, and their relation to apparent distance. *J. Psychol.* 30:43–62.

Kiorpes L, Boothe RG. (1984) Accommodative range in amblyopic monkeys. *Vision Res.* 24:1829–34.

Kirschen DK, Flom MC. (1978) Visual acuity at different retinal loci of eccentrically fixating functional amblyopes. *Am. J. Optom. Physiol. Opt.* 55:144–50.

Kirschen DG, Kendall JH, Riesen KS. (1981) An evaluation of the accommodative response in amblyopic eyes. *Am. J. Optom. Physiol. Opt.* 58:597–602.

Krishnan VV, Phillips S, Stark L. (1973) Frequency analysis of accommodation, accommodative vergence and disparity vergence. *Vision Res.* 13:1545–1554.

Kruger PB, Pola J. (1985) Changing target size is a stimulus for accommodation. *J. Opt. Soc. Am. [A]* 2:1832–5.

Kruger PB, Pola J. (1986) Stimuli for accommodation: Blur, chromatic aberration, and size. *Vision Res.* 26:957–71.

Lawwill T. (1968) Local adaptation in functional amblyopia. *Am. J. Ophthalmol.* 58:597–602.

Liu JS, Lee M, Jang J, Ciuffreda KJ, Wong JH, Grisham D, Stark L. (1979) Objective assessment of accommodation orthoptics: I. Dynamic insufficiency. *Am. J. Optom. Physiol. Opt.* 56:285–94.

Longhurst RS. (1967) *Geometrical and Physical Optics.* London: Longman.

Loshin DS, Levi DM. (1983) Suprathreshold contrast perception in functional amblyopia. *Doc. Ophthalmol.* 55:213–36.

Mackensen G. (1957) Reaktionszeitmessungen bei Amblyopie. *Arch. Klin. Exp. Ophthalmol.* 159:636–42.

Matteucci P. (1960) Strabismic amblyopia. *Br. J. Ophthalmol.* 44:577–82.

McLin LN, Schor CM, Kruger PB. (1988) Changing size (looming) as a stimulus to accommodation and vergence. *Vision Res.* 28:883–98.

Morgan MW. (1944a) Analysis of clinical data. *Am. J. Optom. Arch. Am. Acad. Optom.* 21:477–91.

Morgan MW. (1944b) Clinical measurements of accommodation and convergence. *Am. J. Optom. Arch. Am. Acad. Optom.* 21:301–21.

Morgan MW. (1968) Accommodation and vergence. *Am. J. Optom. Arch. Am. Acad. Optom.* 45:417–54.

Ohzawa I, Sclar G, Freeman RD. (1982) Contrast gain control in the cat visual cortex. *Nature* 298:266–8.

Otto J, Graemiger A. (1967) Uber Unzweckmabige Akkommodation Amblyoper Augenmit Exzentrisher Fixation. *Arch. Klin. Exp. Ophthalmol.* 173:125–40.

Otto J, Safra D. (1974) Uber das Akkommodation verhalten Hochradig Amblyoper Augen. *Klin. Monatsbl. Augenheild.* 165:175–9.

Otto J, Safra D. (1976) Methods and Results of Quantitative Determination of Accommodation in Amblyopia and Strabismus. In Moore S, Mein J, Stockbridge L (Eds.), *Orthoptics: Past, Present, Future.* New York: Stratton.

Owens DA. (1980) A comparison of accommodative responsiveness and contrast sensitivity for sinusoidal gratings. *Vision Res.* 20:159–67.

Owens DA, Leibowitz HW. (1983) Perceptual and Motor Consequences of Tonic Vergence. In Schor CM, Ciuffreda KJ (Eds.), *Vergence Eye Movements: Basic and Clinical Aspects.* Boston: Butterworth.

Owens DA, Mohindra I, Held R. (1980) The effectiveness of the retinoscopic beam as an accommodative stimulus. *Invest. Ophthalmol. Vis. Sci.* 19:942–9.

Phillips SR. (1974) Ocular Neurological Control Systems: Accommodation and the Near Response Triad. Ph.D. dissertation, Department of Mechanical Engineering, University of California, Berkeley, 1974.

Phillips SR, Stark L. (1977) Blur: A sufficient accommodative stimulus. *Doc. Ophthalmol.* 43:65–89.

Saladin JJ, Stark L. (1975) Presbyopia: New evidence from impedance cyclography supporting the Hess-Gullstrand theory. *Vision Res.* 15:537–41.

Schapero M. (1971) *Amblyopia*, pp. 243–244, 261–263. Radnor, Penn.: Chilton.

Schnider CM, Ciuffreda KJ, Selenow A. (1985) Orthoptic effects on accommodation and related vision functions in an adult alternating esotrope. *Ophthalmic Physiol. Opt.* 5:425–33.

Schnider CM, Ciuffreda KJ, Cooper J, Kruger PB. (1984) Accommodation dynamics in divergence excess exotropia. *Invest. Ophthalmol. Vis. Sci.* 25:414–18.

Schor CM, Hallmark W. (1978) Slow control of eye position in strabismic amblyopia. *Invest. Ophthalmol. Vis. Sci.* 17:577–81.

Sclar G, Freeman RD. (1982) Orientation selectivity in the cat's striate cortex is invariant with stimulus contrast. *Exp. Brian Res.* 46:457–61.

Selenow A, Ciuffreda KJ. (1983) Vision function recovery during orthoptic therapy in an exotropic amblyope with high unilateral myopia. *Am. J. Optom. Physiol. Opt.* 60:659–66.

Selenow A, Ciuffreda KJ. (1986) Vision function recovery during orthoptic therapy in an adult strabismic amblyope. *J. Am. Optom. Assoc.* 57:132–40.

Semmlow JL, Jaeger R. (1972) Modeling the Visual Motor Triad: An Example of a Multiple Input-Output Biocontrol System. In *Proceedings of the 25th Symposium of the Association of Engineers in Biology and Medicine. Bal Harbor, Florida.*

Semmlow JL, Tinor T. (1978) Accommodative convergence response to off-foveal retinal images. *J. Opt. Soc. Am.* 68:1497–1501.

Sherman A. (1970) Some recent clinical observations and training procedures in functionally amblyopic patients. *J. Am. Opt. Assoc.* 41:624–6.

Sireteanu R, Fronius M. (1981) Nasotemporal asymmetries in human amblyopia: Consequence of long-term interocular suppression. *Vision Res.* 21:647–56.

Smith W. (1950) *Clinical Orthoptic Procedure*, pp. 75, 218–219. St. Louis: Mosby.

Stark L, Ciuffreda KJ, Kenyon RV. (1982) Abnormal Eye Movements in Strabismus and Amblyopia. In Lennerstrand G, Zee DS, Keller E (Eds.), *Functional Basis of Ocular Motility Disorders.* Oxford: Pergamon Press.

Toates FM. (1972) Accommodation function of the human eye. *Physiol. Rev.* 52:828–63.

Tolhurst DJ, Movshon JA, Thompson ID. (1981) The dependence of response amplitude and variance of cat visual cortical neurones on stimulus contrast. *Exp. Brian Res.* 41:414–19.

Travers T. (1938) Suppression of vision in squint and its association with retinal correspondence and amblyopia. *Br. J. Ophthalmol.* 22:577–604.

Troelstra A, Zuber BL, Miller D, Stark L. (1964) Accommodative tracking: A trial-and-error function. *Vision Res.* 4:585–94.

Tucker J, Charman WN. (1985) Depth of focus and accommodation for sinusoidal gratings as a function of luminance. *Am. J. Optom. Physiol. Opt.* 63:58–70.

Tucker J, Charman WN. (1987) Effect of target content at higher spatial frequencies on the accuracy of the accommodation response. *Ophthalmic Physiol. Opt.* 7:137–47.

Turner MJ. (1958) Observations on the normal subjective amplitude of accommodation. *Br. J. Physiol. Opt.* 15:70–100.

Ukai K, Ishii M, Ishikawa S. (1986) A quasi-static study of accommodation in amblyopia. *Ophthalmic Physiol. Opt.* 6:287–95.

Ukai K, Tanemoto Y, Ishikawa S. (1983) Direct Recording of Accommodative Response versus Accommodative Stimulus. In Breinin GM, Siegel I (Eds.), *Advances in Diagnostic Visual Optics*, pp. 61–8. New York: Springer-Verlag.

Urist MJ. (1950) Primary and secondary deviation in comitant squint. *Am. J. Ophthalmol.* 48:647–56.

van der Wildt GJ, Keemiink CJ, van der Brink G. (1976) Gradient detection and contrast transfer by the human eye. *Vision Res.* 16:1047–53.

von Noorden GK, Burian HM. (1960) Perceptual blanking in normal and amblyopic eyes. *Arch. Ophthalmol.* 64:817–22.

Ward PA, Charman WN. (1985) Effect of pupil size on steady-state accommodation. *Vision Res.* 25:1317–26.

Ward PA. (1987) The effect of stimulus contrast on the accommodation response. *Ophthalmic Physiol. Opt.* 7:9–15.

Westheimer G, McKee SP. (1975) Visual acuity in the presence of retinal-image motion. *J. Opt. Soc. Am.* 65:847–50.

Whiteside TCD. (1957) *The Problems of Vision in Flight at High Altitude.* London: Butterworth.

Wick B, Grisham JD. (1980) Visual therapy for anisometropic amblyopia. *Rev. Optom.* 117:37–8.

Winn B, Heron G, Pugh JR, Eadie AS. (1987) Amblyopia, accommodation and color. *Ophthalmic Physiol. Opt.* 7:365–72.

Wold RM. (1967) The spectacle amplitude of accommodation of children aged six to ten. *Am. J. Optom.* 44:642–64.

Wood ICJ, Tomlinson A. (1974) The accommodative response in amblyopia. *Am. J. Optom. Physiol. Opt.* 52:243–47.

Chapter 7

The Pupillary System

Study of the pupil in amblyopia, especially with respect to the light reflex, represents somewhat of a departure neurologically. Most studies involve investigation of the integrity of cortically related neural pathways. However, the pupillary system is regarded as primarily noncortical in origin (Guyton 1966, Zinn 1972) (Figure 7.1), although higher-level cortical centers can have an influence (usually to inhibit constriction) (Davson 1969). In this chapter we will review clinical and laboratory investigations of the pupillary light reflex in human amblyopia, including the effects of orthoptic therapy.

CLINICAL INVESTIGATION OF THE PUPIL IN AMBLYOPIA

To the busy clinician, useful tests of visual system dysfunction should be easy to administer, accurate, and should yield reliable information regarding the integrity of the neural pathways under investigation. In amblyopia, the presence of an afferent pupillary defect, such as a Marcus-Gunn pupil, which suggests neurologic dysfunction (i.e., optic neuritis), may lead to much initial concern as well as additional unnecessary testing and expense. However, if pupillary abnormalities are indeed part of the functional amblyopia "syndrome," then they simply become one of the anticipated abnormal findings in the complete test armamentarium used in the diagnosis, prognosis, and treatment of amblyopia.

There are four primary clinical studies that clearly show that *subtle* afferent pupillary defects are quite commonly found in amblyopic eyes, and these may be quantifiable by the observant clinician. One of the earliest investigations was by Harms (1937). He used a pupilloscopic system to observe changes in pupillary diameter in response to central and peripheral light stimuli. In his visually normal subjects, pupillary responses were larger for the central stimuli. In contrast, in a group of strabismics with moderate to deep amblyopia, the reverse was true when the amblyopic eye was tested, thus suggesting a central sensory deficit in the amblyopic eye. Later, Kruger (1961) used the "pseudo-anisocoria test of Kestenbaum" (Kestenbaum 1946) as an indicator of pupillary sensitivity.

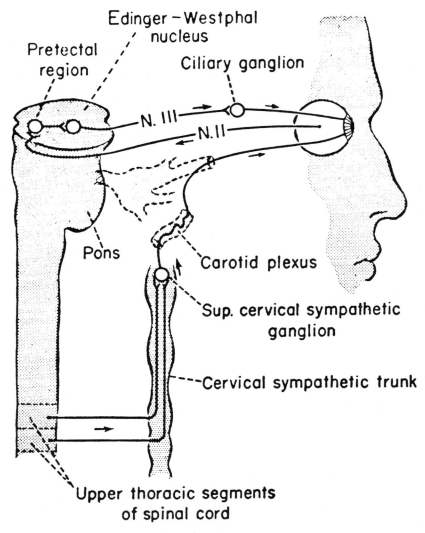

Figure 7.1 *Neural pathways for pupillary light and accommodative responses. (Reprinted, with permission of the publisher, from Guyton 1966.)*

He found abnormal responses in 93 of the 100 functional amblyopes tested. None of Kruger's visually normal control subjects, nor any of his patients having strabismus without amblyopia, showed abnormal findings, thus suggesting that the abnormal responses were specifically related to the presence of the amblyopia. In a recent well-controlled study, Portnoy et al. (1983) tested 55 patients with functional amblyopia who were between the ages of 8 and 54 years. They used the swinging flashlight test with neutral density filters (Thompson et al.

1981) to compare and quantify the direct and consensual pupillary responses to light stimulation. None of the amblyopic patients exhibited an afferent pupillary defect in the dominant eye. In contrast, 45 of the 55 patients ($\sim 80\%$) demonstrated an afferent pupillary defect in the amblyopic eye. Such defects were no greater than 0.6 log units, with a mean of about 0.25. There was no relationship between magnitude of the pupillary defect and either etiology or depth of the amblyopia. Further, neither color-vision test results nor visual-evoked responses were predictive of the presence and/or magnitude of the subtle afferent pupillary defect in the amblyopic eye. Based on these results, the authors believed that only in amblyopic patients with an afferent pupillary defect of greater than 0.6 log units should factors other than functional amblyopia be sought to explain the pupillary abnormality. Thus their results (1) are similar to those of Kruger (1961, as described earlier) and Urist (1961), (2) agree in concept but not frequency with those of Greenwald and Folk (1983), who found the presence of a similar afferent pupillary defect using the swinging flashlight test but only in about 10% of the 45 amblyopic patients tested, and (3) are consistent with the case report of Merritt (1977), whose young anisometropic patient had a Marcus-Gunn pupil and myelinated nerve fibers in the amblyopic eye in the absence of any evidence of neurologic disease.

LABORATORY INVESTIGATION OF THE PUPIL IN AMBLYOPIA

While clinical investigation of the pupil in amblyopia provides important insight into dysfunction of the underlying neural substrate and perhaps even provides an estimate of the magnitude of the defect, laboratory studies allow for more careful, quantitative, objective investigation. Further, laboratory studies allow for breakdown of the abnormality into its constituent dynamic component contribution, such as response latency, amplitude, and velocity.

To date, there are three primary laboratory studies, with two of them clearly demonstrating subtle afferent pupillary defects in the amblyopic eye consistent with those found in the previously described clinical investigations. Morone and Matteucci (1958) used an objective pupillographic system to monitor changes in pupillary response amplitude to light stimuli in 11 surgically corrected strabismic amblyopes (with and without eccentric fixation). They found no significant difference in monocular response amplitude between the amblyopic and fellow dominant eye. Later, Trimarchi et al. (1976) used a fast-sampling (every 20 ms) computerized electronic TV pupillocampimeter to assess changes in pupillary diameter for a variety of light stimuli in older (over 6 years of age) strabismics with deep amblyopia who had no previous history of orthoptic therapy. In the first experiment ($n = 18$), the authors compared pupillary responses to diffuse light (i.e., the entire perimeter changed color) that was either red, yellow, or blue. They found reduced responses in the amblyopic versus fellow dominant eye for the red light. In the second experiment ($n = 15$), the authors studied responses to central versus peripheral (40 degrees) retinal stimuli (100 ms, 2 mm, white light). While there was no difference between eyes for the peripheral stimulus, there was a reduction of response in the amblyopic eye for the central stimulus, suggesting [as did the early experiment of Harms (1937)] the presence of a central sensory deficit in the amblyopic eye. Trimarchi et al. believed their results provided evidence for a pregeniculate defect in the amblyopic eye, perhaps in the retina itself or in the related pupillary-light neural pathways. They further speculated that the defect also may have an efferent component; fibers from the mesencephalic region may provide inhibition to retinal amacrine cells. More recently, Kase et al. (1984) used a sophisticated fast-sampling (every 16.7 ms) infrared pupillometer to assess latency of the pupillary light reflex in strabismic and anisometropic amblyopes aged 8 to 51 years. Visual acuity in the amblyopic eye was 20/40 or worse. Diffuse light stimulation of 500-ms duration was used, and the direct and consensual responses were recorded. Dynamic pupillary parameters investigated included latency, amplitude, and maximum velocity. In 10 of the 15 amblyopes, the direct *and* consensual pupillary latencies were greater in the amblyopic eye than in the fellow dominant eye by about 30 ms (Figure 7.2), with this increase being about the same as found in some amblyopic eyes using the visual-evoked response (Yinon et al. 1974). This latency defect was found with about equal frequency in the strabismic and anisometropic amblyopes. There were no significant differences between the eyes for the two other parameters tested. Kase and colleagues believed that their results suggested the presence of slowed processing in the afferent pupillary pathway, although the consensual abnormality suggests efferent involvement. These pupil studies, in conjunction with other recent studies showing increased latency for saccadic initiation (Ciuffreda et al. 1978a and b) and eye-hand responses (Hamasaki and Flynn 1981) in amblyopic eyes, suggest a rather pervasive abnormality of temporal processing in the afferent visual pathways in most amblyopic eyes. Lastly, lack of correlation between the depth of amblyopia and pupillary response latency suggests differences in the mechanism and/or sites of these two defects, as well as their susceptibility to the affects of early abnormal visual experience leading to amblyopia.

ORTHOPTIC EFFECTS

There is some direct and indirect evidence indicating that orthoptic therapy can improve certain aspects of the abnormal pupillary light responses found in many amblyopic eyes. Dolenek et al. (1962) made cinematographic pupillographic measurements of the pupillary light responses in seven children aged 8 to 12 years before and after successful orthoptic therapy. Dynamic pupillary parameters investigated included latency, speed, and amplitude of the direct and consensual responses. They found that the direct response latency became normal (i.e., decreased significantly, from 240 to 180 ms) in the amblyopic eye following therapy; other parameters remained the same. Greenwald and Folk

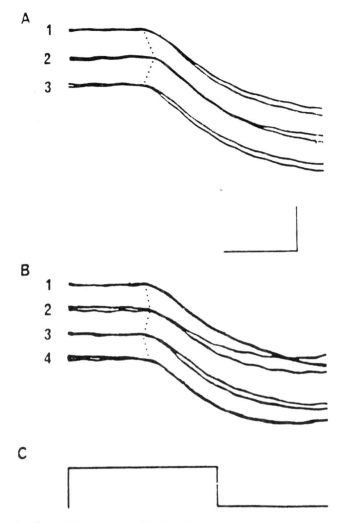

Figure 7.2 *Pupillographic patterns of light reflexes in two patients: a 24-year-old anisometropic (A) and a 25-year-old strabismic amblyope (B). Two responses of each reflex were superimposed with onset of stimulus aligned. (1 = direct reflex of normal eye; 2 = direct reflex of amblyopic eye; 3 = consensual reflex of the pupil of the amblyopic eye when the normal eye was stimulated; 4 = consensual reflex of the normal eye when the amblyopic eye was stimulated.) Dotted lines indicate the onset of contraction in each reflex. Upward step in (C) denotes stimulation of light. Calibration represents 250 ms and 10 mm². (Reprinted, with permission of the publisher, from Kase et al. 1984.)*

(1983) noted that the afferent pupillary defect measured with the swinging flashlight test became noticably reduced during the course of successful orthoptic therapy in one amblyopic child 8 years of age. Lastly, Kase et al. (1984), using a sophisticated dynamic infrared pupillometer system, found no significant difference in the latency of the pupillary light response between eyes in eight children (ages 8 to 12 years; pretreatment visual acuity range 0.03 to 0.6 and posttreatment visual acuity range 0.8 to 1.2) who had recovered fully following orthoptic therapy for remediation of their amblyopia. The results of these three investigations provide evidence suggesting plasticity in this noncortical "reflex" pupillary neural pathway in response to more controlled and increased visual stimulation to the amblyopic eye by the orthoptic therapy, although improved fixation ability following successful therapy also could result in greater effectiveness of the light stimuli. If these findings can be confirmed and expanded in additional controlled studies, the results would suggest that both noncortical and cortical pathways may exhibit reversible deficits in the amblyopic eye following appropriate intensive therapy.

SUMMARY

The results of the clinical and laboratory investigations of the pupillary light reflex clearly demonstrate the presence of a subtle afferent pupillary defect in many amblyopic eyes. This is manifested in the form of reduced pupillary response amplitude reflecting diminished sensitivity and increased pupillary response latency reflecting slowed processing. However, the abnormal consensual response suggests an efferent-pathway abnormality. Orthoptic therapy appeared to normalize pupillomotor function, although these results must be regarded with caution and as preliminary in nature. More comprehensive studies with appropriate controls must be conducted. The orthoptic results suggest the presence of a reversible afferent defect of primarily noncortical origin. While additional studies are needed to expand on our present knowledge with respect to effectiveness of additional types of light and patterned stimuli (i.e., pulses, sinusoids, and white noise), an important area that has been neglected is the pupillary-accommodation pathway in amblyopes. Such studies would dovetail nicely into ongoing research on accommodation in amblyopia, as well as expand our insight into the pervasive nature of the visual system dysfunction in human amblyopia. Further, since study of this system would include (contrary to the pupillary light reflex) neural signals "shaped" by the abnormal accommodation pathways (see Chapter 6), one would anticipate finding more defective pupillary drive for accommodative rather than for simple diffuse light stimuli.

REFERENCES

Ciuffreda KJ, Kenyon RV, Stark L. (1978a) Increased saccadic latencies in amblyopic eyes. *Invest. Ophthalmol. Vis. Sci.* 17:697–702.

Ciuffreda KJ, Kenyon RV, Stark L. (1978b) Processing delays in amblyopic eyes: Evidence from saccadic latencies. *Am. J. Optom. Physiol. Opt.* 55:187-96.

Davson H. (1969) *The Eye*, Vol. 3. New York: Academic Press.

Dolenek, VA, Kristek A, Nemee J, Komenda S. (1962) Uber Veranderungen der Pupillenreaktion nach erfolgreicher amblyopiebe-handlung. *Klin. Monatsbl. Augenheilkd.* 141:353-7.

Greenwald MJ, Folk ER. (1983) Afferent pupillary defects in amblyopia. *J. Pediatr. Ophthalmol. Strabismus* 20:63-7.

Guyton AC. (1966) *Textbook of Medical Physiology*, 3d Ed. Philadelphia: Saunders.

Hamasaki DI, Flynn JT. (1981) Amblyopic eyes have longer reaction times. *Invest. Ophthalmol. Vis. Sci.* 21:846-53.

Harms H. (1937) Ort und Wesen der Bildhemmung bei Schielenden. *Arch. Ophthalmol.* 138:149-210.

Kase M, Nagata R, Yoshida A, Hanada I. (1984) Pupillary light reflex in amblyopia. *Invest. Ophthalmol. Vis. Sci.* 25:467-71.

Kestenbaum A. (1946) *Clinical Methods of Neuro-Ophthalmologic Examination.* New York: Grune & Stratton.

Kruger KE. (1961) Pupillenstorungen und Amblyopie. *Z. Dtsch. Ophthalmol. Ges.* 63:275-8.

Merritt JC. (1977) Myelinated nerve fibers associated with afferent pupillary defect and amblyopia. *J. Pediatr. Ophthalmol. Strabismus* 14:139-40.

Morone G, Matteucci P. (1958) Studio sull'inibizione nell'occhio affetto da ambliopia strabica. *Ras. Ital. D'Ottalmol.* 27:161-8.

Portnoy JZ, Thompson HS, Lennarson L, Corbett JJ. (1983) Pupillary defects in amblyopia. *Am. J. Ophthalmol.* 96:609-14.

Thompson HS, Corbett JJ, Cox TA. (1981) How to measure the relative afferent pupillary defect. *Surv. Ophthalmol.* 26:39-42.

Trimarchi F, Casali G, Franchini F, Gilardi E. (1976) Pupillographic Responses in Patients with Untreated Strabismic Amblyopia. In Moore S, Mein J, Stockbridge L. (Eds.), *Orthoptics: Past, Present, Future.* New York: Stratton.

Urist MJ. (1961) Fixation anomalies in amblyopia ex anopsia. *Am. J. Ophthalmol.* 52:19-28.

Yinon U, Jakoboritz L, Auerbach E. (1974) The visual evoked response to stationary checkerboard patterns in children with strabismus amblyopia. *Invest. Ophthalmol.* 13:293-6.

Zinn KM. (1972) *The Pupil.* Springfield, Ill.: Thomas.

Chapter 8

Clinical Diagnosis and Prognosis of Amblyopia

In recent years it has become more apparent that functional amblyopia can no longer be regarded simply as an impairment of visual acuity alone. An ever-growing body of literature now supports the clinical observation that some amblyopic eyes perform much worse than an ametropic eye (with equal visual acuity loss) on many visual tasks (Leibowitz et al. 1955, Stigmar 1971, Winterson and Steinman 1978, Post and Liebowitz 1980, Williams et al. 1984). This has been attributed to a variety of sensory/motor/perceptual deficits that occur in the amblyopic visual system. We shall discuss the clinically observable effects of amblyopia on five areas: visual acuity, fixation and eye movements, accommodation, monocular sensory perception, and binocular function.

It is important to obtain as accurate a measure as possible in these five areas for the following reasons:

1. To monitor the degree of success of vision therapy. Improvement is thought to occur more rapidly if training in all five of these areas is done (Francois and James 1955, Callahan and Berry 1968).
2. To know when the patient is ready for dismissal. It may not be sufficient to dismiss a patient based on their visual acuity improvement alone.
3. To detect regression at its earliest stage. It has been our experience that visual acuity regression follows eye movement and/or accommodation regression. To maintain the visual acuity improvement, one must either establish some degree of stereopsis, teach the patient to alternate freely, or have the patient on a retainer patching regimen (Priestley et al. 1959) (see also Chapter 10).

The clinician's task at this time is to determine the etiology of the amblyopia (refer to classification section in Chapter 1), rule out any organic contributions to the visual acuity loss (see definition section in Chapter 1), determine the

315

prognosis and the probability for success (see this chapter), and organize a comprehensive monocular and binocular treatment strategy (see case studies in Chapter 10).

Table 8.1 summarizes the diagnostic procedures that need to be performed to accomplish these four tasks. Figure 8.1 includes a diagnostic and treatment flowchart. The discussion of a diagnostic amblyopia battery will be preceded by a brief description of the important clinical questions specific to amblyopia that need to be addressed in the case history.

HISTORY TAKING

When faced with a new patient having amblyopia, there are four important questions the clinician needs to ask and have answered fully:

1. When was the amblyogenic anomaly (i.e., strabismus, anisometropia, etc.) first noted?
2. When was treatment first initiated?
3. What did this treatment consist of?
4. What was the extent of compliance?

Table 8.1   Summary of Diagnostic Procedures

Tests to determine etiology:
  History
  Cover test
  Objective refraction
  Visuoscopy
Tests to rule out organic amblyopia:
  History
  Anterior and posterior segment evaluation
  Pupils
  Color vision
  Neutral-density test
  Threshold visual fields
  Visual-evoked potentials
Tests to determine prognosis:
  History
  Visual acuity
  Laser interferometry
  Visuoscopy
Tests to determine treatment plan:
  Visual acuity
  Accommodation
  Fixation and eye movements
  Monocular sensory perception
  Binocular evaluation

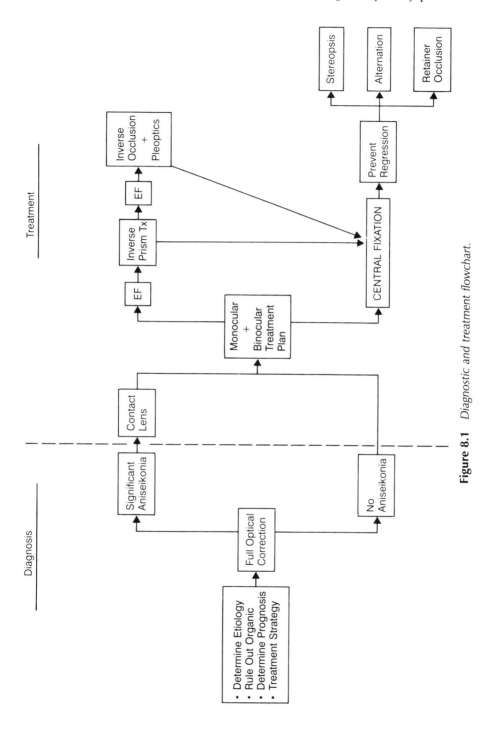

Figure 8.1 *Diagnostic and treatment flowchart.*

The answers to these four questions will help the clinician make a more edu-
cated prognosis. A prognostic guide based on the four factors mentioned above
is provided in Table 8.2.

When Did the Amblyogenic Anomaly Begin?

The later the onset of the anomaly, the better is the prognosis. Unfortunately,
the age of onset, which can be anywhere from birth to 7 years of age, is often
difficult to ascertain. Parents are more likely to recall the onset of amblyopia
secondary to strabismus rather than to anisometropia. The anisometropic amblyope is typically first detected during a vision screening, the child's first eye
examination, or by a parent who notes a behavioral change upon accidental
occlusion of the child's fellow eye. It is amazing how frequently one sees a high
unilateral myopic amblyope with little or no strabismus whose visual deficit was
not discovered until *after* the child was in school.

Regardless of how deep the amblyopia, if one knows that the vision anomaly
occurred *after* age 4 years, the prognosis for significant acuity improvement is
excellent. Obtaining the results of the earliest vision examination is helpful in
determining when the amblyogenic anomaly began. An exact time is not critical.
Early photographs of the child may help pinpoint the age of onset of any strabismus
and thus provide a rough guide as to time of development of the amblyopia.

Table 8.2 Primary Factors Related to Prognosis in Amblyopia

	Poor to Fair	*Fair to Good*	*Good to Excellent*
Onset of amblyogenic anomaly	Birth to age 2 years	2 to 4 years	4 to 7 years
Treatment onset minus anomaly onset	> 3 years	1 to 3 years	≤ 1 year
Extent and success of initial treatment	Optical correction Minimum VA improvement	Optical correction and patching Moderate VA improvement	Full optical correction Proper patching Significant VA improvement Accommodation, eye-hand coordination, and fixation training Stereopsis or alternation established
Compliance	None to poor	Fair to good	Good to excellent

When Was Treatment Initiated?

This question is much easier to answer. However, one must obtain specifics as to when each of the possible forms of remediation began (optical correction, patching, and/or orthoptic therapy). Here the clinician is trying to determine the amount of time elapsed between the age of onset of the amblyopia and the initial attempt at remediation. If the uncorrected anomaly has existed for less than 1 year, the prognosis for success is much better. Examples of this can be seen in the studies on the reversal of occlusion amblyopia (Thomas et al. 1978, Awaya 1973, Levi 1976). One may say, "If the therapy began soon after the onset of the anomaly, then the patient must now have very mild amblyopia." This is not always the case, since after the initial successful therapy, regression may have caused a significant decrease in visual acuity (Wild 1961, Kivlin and Flynn 1981). The following is an example:

- Right constant unilateral esotropia with age of onset at 2 years.
- Visual acuity at age 3 years of 20/200 (due to development of amblyopia).
- Patching instituted at age 3 years for 1 year.
- Patching successful.
- By age 4, visual acuity 20/20, but the strabismus remains unchanged and patching discontinued.
- Arrives at age 10 years with constant right unilateral esotropia and 20/100 visual acuity.

It has been our clinical experience that there is no drastic difference in prognosis once the nontreated amblyogenic anomaly has existed for greater than 5 years (i.e., 5 years versus 8 years versus 15 years of amblyopia have similar prognosis). In addition, if the amblyopia is not treated before the age of 6 years when plasticity is greatest, there may not be any significant advantage to treatment at that time as compared with waiting until a later date (Gould et al. 1970).

What Did the Treatment Consist of and How
Successful Was It?

In answering this question, the important points are

1. Was the full optical correction implemented?
2. Was an appropriate patching regimen used?
3. What type of orthoptic exercises, if any, were used?
4. To what extent did visual acuity improve?
5. Was either stereopsis or alternation of fixation established once therapy was discontinued?

An amblyope left without either stereopsis or alternation of fixation after treatment is likely to demonstrate some regression in recovered vision function, especially visual acuity (Schapero 1971, von Noorden 1980).

What Was the Extent of Compliance?

This is the most difficult question for which to obtain an accurate answer. A child is going to peek from behind a patch whenever possible. Most formerly patched adults will tell you that they rarely *fully* complied with their patching regiment. This is one reason why many clinicians favor more carefully controlled and monitored part-time occlusion with intensive vision therapy over relatively unmonitored full-time occlusion.

Other important general questions to ask are

1. Any history of trauma? This must be ruled out.
2. Is there a family history of amblyopia or strabismus? Strabismus is present in about 4% of the general population (Grutzner et al. 1970). The frequency of inherited strabismus as reported in the literature varies from 22% to 66% (Francois 1961). The frequency of esotropia among siblings of affected individuals when neither parent is affected is 15%. If one parent also has esotropia, the frequency increases to 40% (Czellitzer 1923). This does not help with the prognosis but is of value for the offspring.
3. Any diplopia? If the answer is yes, it suggests that the amblyopia is either of recent onset or not very severe.
4. Is the patient or parent (for young children) motivated? Without motivation, *there will be little or no success.*

VISUAL ACUITY

The standard Snellen chart has been used to measure clinical visual acuity since 1862 (Snellen, 1868). These measurements are reliable in nonamblyopic eyes (Borish 1970). However, there are several reasons why it is difficult to measure visual acuity accurately and reliably in an amblyopic eye using a Snellen chart.

An important consideration is contour interaction, which is responsible for the "crowding phenomenon" (Irvine 1948, Stuart and Burian 1962, Flom et al. 1963a, b). This occurs when neighboring contours impair the resolution of a centrally fixated letter. In 1963, Flom et al. described and quantified this phenomenon in normal and amblyopic eyes. They had their subjects monocularly view a Landolt C and determined the viewing distance where letter orientation could be correctly identified 80% of the time. The Landolt C was then surrounded with four black bars that were gradually moved inward (Figure 8.2). Measurements of visual resolution were repeated as a function of distance *d* of

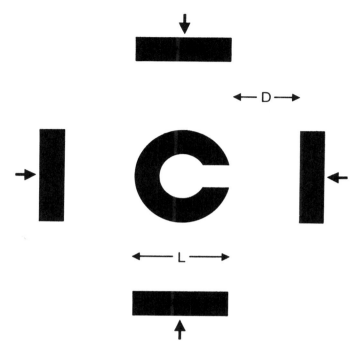

Figure 8.2   *The effect of contour interaction on visual resolution determined by evaluating the influence of the surrounding black bars on visibility of the Landolt C. (D = linear separation between Landolt C and interacting bars, and L = width of Landolt C.) (Reprinted, with permission of the publisher, from Flom et al. 1963b.)*

the bars from the outer extent of the Landolt C (Figure 8.3). Resolution remained unimpaired, until the bars were located at a distance equivalent to one letter diameter (D = L) (Figure 8.2) from the Landolt C. Detection of the "gap" in the C was maximally affected when the bars were 0.4 of a letter diameter away from the periphery of the Landolt C (D = 0.4L) and became somewhat less affected with still closer distances.

It is often stated that amblyopic eyes are much more affected by contour interaction than normal eyes. This is not really true. Actually, the effect is approximately equal at *threshold visual acuity levels for both normal and amblyopic eyes.* However, when testing nonamblyopic eyes, 20/20 is considered normal visual acuity, but crowding is not experienced because threshold is between 20/15 and 20/10 in normal eyes. Even when the nonamblyopic patient is presented with a 20/15 or smaller line of letters, the separation of the letters at these acuity levels is still greater than two letter diameters (see Figure 8.4). Contour interaction does not begin at greater than one letter diameter separation. On the other hand, the threshold acuity level in the amblyopic eye is typically

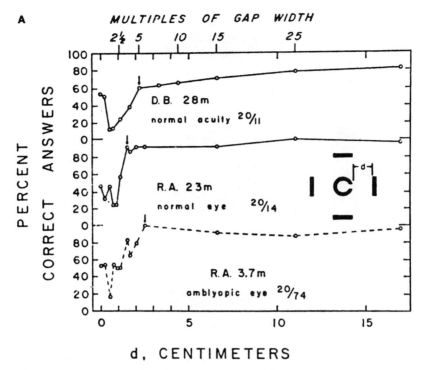

Figure 8.3   (A) *The percent correct responses plotted as a function of the linear separation (d) between the Landolt C and the surrounding bars. Viewing distance is disregarded in this plot, and the bar separations are thus represented as multiples of gap width. The arrow specifies the maximum bar separation affording interaction. The similarity between the curves for the amblyopic and normal eyes is evident in the plot.*

between 20/200 and 20/50. The interletter separations on the Snellen chart for this range of acuities are *all* less than one letter size (see Figure 8.4). Consequently, the amblyopic eye appears to show an effectively greater decrease in visual acuity due to the presence of increased contour interaction effects when tested using a Snellen chart over this range than is present over the range tested in the fellow dominant eye.

Another problem with the Snellen chart is that it does not provide control for contour interaction owing to the variable number and spacing of the letters leading to greater variability of visual acuity in the amblyopic eye (Flom 1966). Amblyopes typically find it easier to read the first and last letters on a line because there are less interacting contours surrounding them. The use of a fixed aperture in the projector to isolate single lines and single letters provides no additional control, since contour interaction will vary with letter size. In addition, the rectangular aperture may itself spatially interact with the isolated letters; 20/20 letters will not be close enough to the edge of the aperture to reach

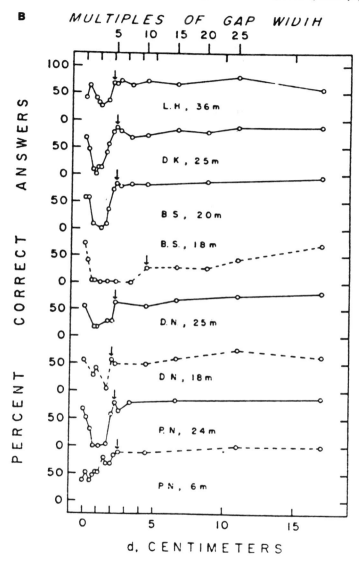

Figure 8.3   (B) *Same graphical representation as (A) for an additional five normal (solid lines) and three amblyopic (broken lines) eyes. Each circle represents the percent correct responses for 32 or more presentations of the four-position Landolt C; percentages have been adjusted for one chance in four of guessing correctly. (Reprinted, with permission of the publishers, from Flom et al. 1963b.)*

the critical separation, but the 20/80 letters certainly will. Therefore, the typical finding of single-letter acuity being better than single-line or whole-chart acuity cannot necessarily be attributed wholly to the elimination of contour interaction

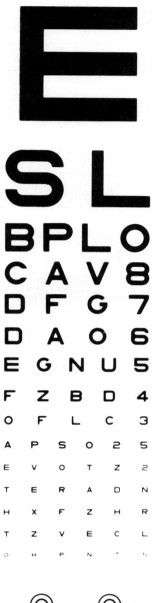

Figure 8.4 *Typical Snellen chart. Note variable interletter separations and number of letters on each line.*

with this clinical procedure. The presence of abnormal monocular fixation with the amblyopic eye may actually be a primary reason for obtaining better acuity with the aperture arrangement, since it provides a restricted field with fewer letters present to confuse the amblyopic eye whose "aiming" ability is indeed impaired (Figure 8.5).

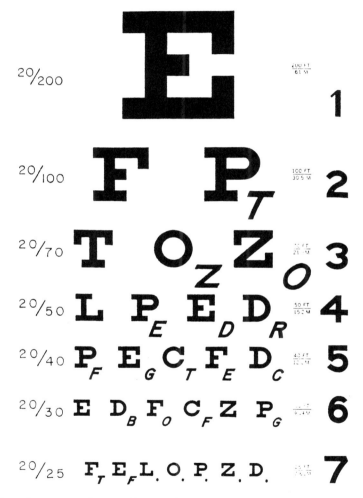

Figure 8.5 *Responses of an amblyope when tested with a conventional Snellen visual acuity chart. Errors are indicated by the slanted letters or dots (no response) drawn to the lower right of the test letters. Test letters without these markings were correctly identified. As is characteristic of amblyopes, this subject's miscalls often agree with adjacent test letters. Note that although he missed one of the two letters on the 20/100 row, he correctly identified two of the six letters on the 20/30 row. (Reprinted, with permission of the publisher, from Flom 1966.)*

Moreover , when presented with an entire Snellen chart, the amblyopic eye will characteristically resolve a few letters per line across a broad range of acuity values with no clear cutoff point to define threshold (Flom 1966) (see Figure 8.5). Similarly, even when using a visual acuity chart that controls for contour interaction (Figure 8.6), a broad range of correct responses is found (Figure 8.7). If the percent correct responses is plotted as a function of letter size, the difference between the normal and amblyopic eyes is at once apparent (see Figure 8.7). The normal eye will generate a curve with a steep slope, demonstrating a sharp dropoff in the ability to resolve Snellen letters across a very narrow range of acuity values. The amblyopic eye, on the other hand, will generate a sigmoid, or S-shaped, curve with a more gradual decrease in resolution across a wide range of acuity values. This greater range of uncertainty makes the typical Snellen visual acuity determination in the clinic unreliable, especially at low acuity levels (Wick and Schor 1984).

The visual acuity levels on the Snellen chart at the low end are 20/400, 20/200, and 20/100. These large gaps between acuity levels can cause either gross over- or underestimations of acuity in moderate to severe amblyopes. A true

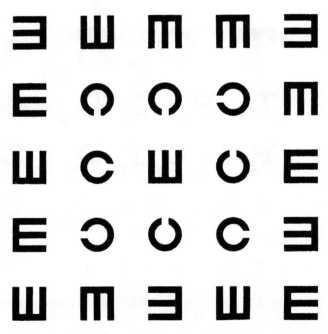

Figure 8.6 *Flom's visual acuity test slide. The eight randomly arranged Landolt C's are the test letters, and the E's provide additional controlled contour interaction. Twenty-one slides of this target configuration cover the letter sizes from 20/277 to 20/9, with interletter spacing on all being equal to one letter diameter. (Reprinted, with permission of the publisher, from Flom 1966.)*

20/120 amblyope would show a Snellen acuity of 20/200 ⁺, since there are no test targets between 20/200 and 20/100. In addition, the determination of visual acuity is based only on one or two letters per line at these acuity levels (see Figure 8.4). Use of a Clason projector with its continuously variable magnification would be of benefit in these cases (Borish 1970).

Each Snellen line contains letters with different degrees of difficulty (Borish 1970). When presented with the more difficult optotypes, the visual acuity of an amblyopic eye is decreased significantly more than that of a normal eye. In a group of 15 amblyopes, the mean visual acuity of the amblyopic eye was 20/225 using "difficult" optotypes and 20/138 with "easy" optotypes (Jagerman 1970) (see Figure 8.8).

Frequent retesting of the visual acuity of amblyopes to assess the effectiveness of vision therapy can result in contamination of the results by memorization. In the more severe, younger amblyopes, it is not uncommon during therapy to get a response of "E" (20/400) or "SL" (20/200) when monitoring visual acuity behind the phoropter even with *both* phoropter occluders in place (an obvious case of patient memorization to please the examiner).

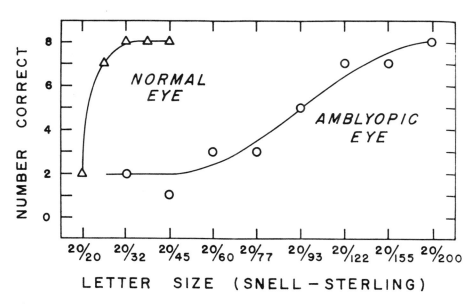

Figure 8.7 *Plot of visual acuity responses for both eyes of an amblyope as tested with Flom's test slides. Corrected for a guessing error of two letters, a correct response for seven of the eight letters corresponds to approximately 80% correct and five correct responses corresponds to approximately 50% correct. The 80% and 50% threshold acuities obtained from the fitted curve for the amblyopic eye are about 20/135 and 20/93, respectively, and for the normal eye about 20/26 and 20/21, respectively. The flatter curve for the amblyopic eye reflects the marked variability in acuity responses. (Reprinted, with permission of the publisher, from Flom 1966.)*

	"Easy" Chart	"Difficult" Chart
20/300	T O L	F H B
20/300	U Z T	M R X
20/200	I A O C Z	Y S N B M
20/100	I U L T A	X H Y N F
20/80	I D V L C	R M Y S Q
20/60	Z T V I U	B S X F R
20/40	D O L C V	H Q F B M
20/30	A U T Z I	X R N Y Q
20/25	D L C V U	B M H S X
20/20	T O C Z A	N R Y F H
20/15	L A D U V	B F Q N S

Figure 8.8 *Two visual acuity charts varying in letter difficulty. (Left) "Easy" chart containing optotypes that are less difficult for the amblyopic eye to discern. (Right) "Difficult" chart containing optotypes that are more difficult for the amblyopic eye to discern. (Reprinted, with permission of the publisher, from Jagerman 1970.)*

These five factors cause standard clinical Snellen visual acuity measurements to be unreliable in amblyopic eyes. However, Snellen whole-chart (WC), whole-line (WL), and single-letter (SL) acuities should still be taken in conjunction with S-chart visual acuity. A large discrepancy between whole-chart and single-letter acuity may indicate a more favorable prognosis for visual acuity improvement (especially when fixation and eye-movement training are emphasized). The prognostic value of single-letter visual acuity has been supported by some researchers (Schlossman 1961, Stuart and Burian 1962) but denied by others (Cibis et al. 1968). However, we feel that if presented with two amblyopes having equal whole-line acuities but unequal single-letter acuities, the one with the better single-letter acuity has a slightly better prognosis. In addition, the reliability of Snellen visual acuity improves dramatically in the 20/50 and better acuity range (Wick and Schor 1984). However, S-chart visual acuities are still needed here, especially to establish an accurate and reliable baseline value.

Flom designed a visual acuity test specifically for the evaluation of amblyopic eyes (Flom 1966).* The test consists of a series of 21 slides that span a range of visual acuity values from 20/277 to 20/9 (see Table 8.3). Each slide contains a series of eight Landolt C's, and the patient is asked to identify the orientation of the gap in each C (up, down, left, right) (see Figure 8.6). At each of the 21 acuity

*Available from the Alumni Association, The School of Optometry, University of California, Berkeley, CA 94720.

Table 8.3 Progression of Target Sizes Used in the Psychophysical Test Sequence

Card No.	Foot-Letter Size	20-foot Snellen Equivalent	Snell-Sterling
1	4.5	20/9	110
2	7.5	20/15	105
3	10	20/20	100
4	13	20/26	95
5	16	20/32	90
6	19	20/38	85
7	22.5	20/45	80
8	26	20/52	75
9	30	20/60	70
10	34	20/68	65
11	38.5	20/77	60
12	43.5	20/87	55
13	48.5	20/97	50
14	54.5	20/109	45
15	61	20/122	40
16	68.5	20/137	35
17	77.5	20/155	30
18	87.5	20/175	25
19	100	20/200	20
20	116	20/232	15
21	138.5	20/277	10

levels, the interletter spacing is equal to the letter diameter, and every test letter is surrounded by an equal number of contours. Thus at each acuity level the amount of contour interaction is *constant*. The determination of visual acuity uses a psychometric analysis. The number of correct responses is plotted against letter size, yielding the characteristic sigmoidal, or S-shaped, curve (see Figure 8.7). Where the curve crosses the five of eight correct response level (50% corrected for guessing) is the recorded clinical visual acuity [in the research laboratory, probit analysis (Finney 1971) is used to determine the visual acuity level more accurately]. The 21 slides, each representing a 5% change on the Snell-Sterling scale of visual efficiency (Snell and Sterling 1925), provide a more precise measurement than the conventional Snellen chart. This design bypasses all five of the previously discussed inadequacies with standard Snellen determination of visual acuity in amblyopic eyes.

A modification of the S-chart was designed and used by Davidson and Eskridge (1977). This E chart (Figure 8.9) increases contour interaction by reducing interletter spacing to half the test-letter size (instead of the one letter size used with the S-chart). Since only letter E's are present, this chart is easier and less confusing to use with children than the S-chart.[†]

[†]Available from Michael Wesson, O.D., M.S., University of Alabama, School of Optometry, Birmingham, AL 35294.

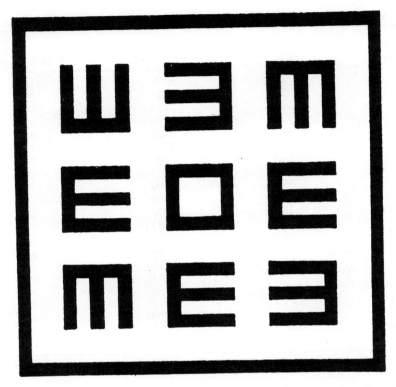

Figure 8.9 *E-chart with interletter spacing of one-half test-letter size. (Reprinted, with permission of the publisher, from Davidson and Eskridge 1977.)*

There are several "tricks" that the patient may attempt during visual acuity testing with the amblyopic eye to improve resolution of letters near threshold:

1. *Slow blinking.* Amblyopes report a reduction in letter "fading" if the amblyopic eye is briefly closed just before attempting to fixate a letter.
2. *Looking away.* Similarly, amblyopes report that "fading" is minimized if they quickly look away just before they attempt to fixate a letter.
3. *Pressing a finger over the closed lid of the dominant eye.* Amblyopes report that the dominant eye does not "interfere" with the amblyopic eye when using this more "total" form of occlusion. This is important to remember when testing an amblyope wearing a patch or being occluded behind the phoropter. The dominant eye still gets some stimulation through light leaks in the lid margins, edge of the patch, and/or sides of the phoropter. Such binocular neural inhibition of the dominant eye over the amblyopic eye persists unless most of the stimulation to the dominant eye is abolished.

Telescopic Acuity

Amblyopic distance visual acuity through a focusable telescope has been reported to be helpful in the differential diagnosis between organic and functional amblyopia (Feldman and Taylor 1942) (Figure 8.10). There are conflicting philosophies, however, as to the value of telescopic acuity in amblyopia (Press 1983). Some of these are (1) that any improvement in acuity through a telescope indicates a functional amblyopia (Feldman and Taylor 1942), (2) that telescopic acuity greater than predicted by the magnification of the telescope indicates a functional amblyopia with good prognosis (Smith 1972), and (3) that the pretherapy acuity through the telescope is the predicted acuity following successful therapy (Press 1983). In a review of the literature, Press (1983) reported that "information on the subject of telescopes as an aid in prognosis or therapy for amblyopia reveals contradictions, poorly controlled studies, and clinical folklore."

We feel that there are three main explanations for the apparent prognostic value of telescopic visual acuity in amblyopic eyes. First, a telescope reduces the field of view, which, in turn, effectively allows for more accurate localization and fixation. This is similar to the effect found for single-letter versus whole-chart acuity (Press 1983). As previously noted, improvement in amblyopic visual acuity with letter isolation indicates a fixation anomaly and indeed is a good prognostic indicator. Second, by having the ability to focus the telescope, an amblyope can compensate in part for any inaccuracies of accommodation and/or refractive error (which is quite common). Therefore, an amblyope can optically

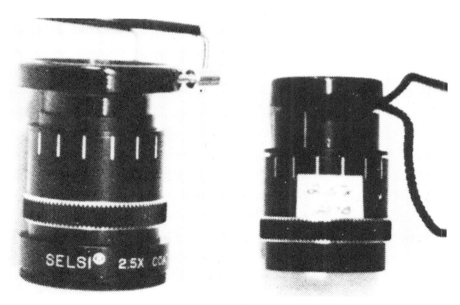

Figure 8.10 *Selsi 2.5× telescope.* (Left) *Clip-on model.* (Right) *Hand-held model.*

accomplish what he or she cannot do naturally with the amblyopic eye, namely, reduce any residual defocus blur. Third, the most significant cause of an exaggerated telescopic visual acuity in amblyopia is secondary to the use of a Snellen chart where there are large resolution intervals between lines at the lower acuity levels. We measured Snellen and S-chart visual acuity both with and without a telescope in several amblyopes (see Table 8.4). A noteworthy example is patient 1, whose Snellen acuities without and with a 2.2× telescope were 20/200 and 20/50, respectively. This fourfold acuity increase with a telescope is much greater than the expected 2.2-fold increase based on optical magnification, thus suggesting to some clinicians an excellent prognosis. However, the more accurate S-chart acuities of the *same* patient were 20/122 and 20/52, respectively, without and with the same 2.2× telescope. This change is approximately the increase predicted by the optics of the telescope. Therefore, since this patient's true acuity fell in the large Snellen gap between 20/200 and 20/100, the nontelescopic Snellen acuity was grossly underestimated. On the other hand, telescopic Snellen acuity was accurate, since acuity levels are more finely graded in the 20/70 and better range. Therefore, it appears that inaccurate nontelescopic Snellen acuities are the primary cause for exaggerated telescopic acuities (at least in deeper amblyopes), and thus we have *not* found telescopic visual acuities to be either a reliable or helpful prognostic indicator. However, we do find that the focusable telescope is useful in the treatment of severe amblyopes (see Chapter 10).

Table 8.4   Comparison of Visual Acuity in the Amblyopic Eye with and without the 2.2× Telescope

Patient No. (Age in Years)	Etiology of Amblyopia	Snellen Visual Acuity	S-Chart Visual Acuity	2.2× Snellen Visual Acuity	Increase Based on Snellen Visual Acuity	Increase Based on S-Chart Visual Acuity
1 (6)	Aniso	20/200	20/109	20/50	4×	2.2×
2 (7)	ET	20/200	20/122	20/50	4×	2.4×
3 (5)	Aniso	20/200	20/232	20/100	2×	2.3×
4 (29)	Aniso	20/200	20/109	20/60	3.3×	1.8×
5 (10)	ET and aniso	20/200	20/195	20/100	2×	2×
6 (10)	ET and aniso	20/200	20/175	20/60	3.3×	2.9×
7 (29)	ET	20/200	20/109	20/60	3.3×	1.8×
8 (10)	Aniso	20/200	20/120	20/40	5×	3×
9 (9)	ET	20/200	20/250	20/100	2.5×	2.5×
10 (6)	Aniso	20/70	20/45	20/30	2.3×	1.5×
11 (14)	Aniso	20/60	20/52	20/25	2.4×	2.1×
12 (22)	XT and aniso	20/60	20/58	20/30	2×	1.9×
13 (6)	ET and aniso	20/50	20/45	20/25	2×	1.8×
14 (9)	Aniso	20/50	20/62	20/20	2.5×	3.1×
15 (11)	Aniso	20/40	20/28	20/15	2.7×	1.9×
				Average	2.8×	2.2×

LASER INTERFEROMETRY

The laser interferometer is another useful way of assessing the visual acuity of an amblyopic eye (see Figure 8.11). Gstalder and Green (1971) reported that laser interferometrically determined assessment of visual acuity in amblyopic eyes resulted in gross overestimation when compared with standard Snellen measures. Recently, Selenow et al. (1986) compared pretherapy laser visual acuity with pre- and posttherapy clinical measures of visual acuity in a group of 37 patients with functional amblyopia. Their results showed that most of the amblyopic eyes achieved a *final* Snellen and/or S-chart visual acuity level that was very close to their *pretherapy laser* interferometric visual acuity. In 90% of the eyes in which therapy was completed, the pretherapy laser and posttherapy Snellen and/or S-chart visual acuity levels were within two lines of each other, while in about 75% of the eyes the difference was one line or less (Figure 8.12 and Table 8.5).

There are several characteristics of the laser target that make it an optimal pattern for resolution tasks, especially with an amblyopic eye:

1. *Laser-generated interference pattern.* Retinal defocus caused by large errors and/ or fluctuations of accommodation, as commonly found in amblyopic eyes (Ciuffreda and Kenyon 1983), has no effect on laser interferometric grating resolution.
2. *High contrast pattern.* Threshold (Hess and Howell 1977) and suprathreshold (Hess and Bradley 1980, Loshin and Levi 1983, Hess et al. 1983) contrast abnormalities, including target "fading" (Lawwill 1968), as typically found in amblyopic eyes, would have little adverse consequences on resolution capability. With the laser target, retinal contrast is 100%.
3. *Spatially redundant pattern.* Eye-position error due to fixational abnormalities (Ciuffreda et al. 1979b) and eccentric fixation (Brock and Givner 1952), which is typically found in amblyopic eyes, would have minimal effect for such tasks with unlimited viewing time. The 3-degree grating field would overlap the fovea *and* eccentric fixation point most of the time in the vast majority of amblyopic eyes.
4. *Simpler identification.* The resolution of grating orientation with only four possible positions and the presence of multiple gaps to make such a judgement is a simpler task than identifying Snellen letters, which entails resolution of individual component parts with subsequent integration of them into the perception of a recognizable form (Borish 1970). In addition, presence of monocular spatial distortion in amblyopic eyes (Bedell and Flom 1981) would have much less adverse effect on a spatially-redundant target than a complex Snellen letter.

Therefore, the optimal nature of the laser optics and target configuration minimizes the influence of the amblyopic eye's sensory and motor deficits on resolution ability, thus allowing for accurate pretherapy prediction of the posttherapy visual acuity outcome. The basic neural resolution capability of the afferent visual pathway is therefore directly tested with the laser interferometer.

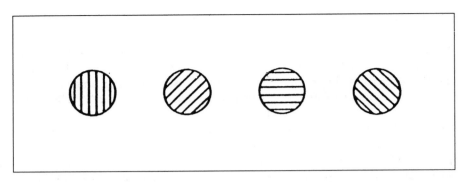

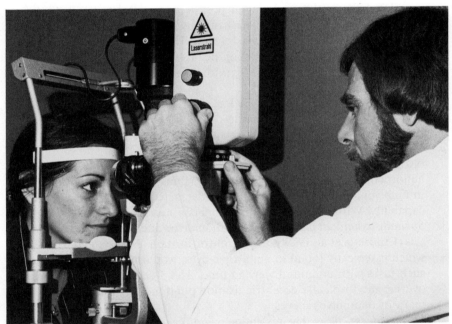

Figure 8.11 *Laser interferometer. (Above) Four possible grating orientations. (Below) Rodenstock model. The Retinometer is switched on by means of the toggle switch on the side opposite the rotating knob. It is ready to operate at once. During long breaks between measurements, the instrument should be switched off. The rotating knob serves for changing the density of the interference fringes in steps, corresponding to values of the retinal visual acuity from 0.03 to 1.0. With the knurled ring underneath the housing, the orientation of the interference-fringe patterns can be adjusted to vertical (90 degrees), horizontal (180 degrees), and two oblique (45 and 135 degrees) settings. With the small rotating knob, the performance of the laser beam can be varied by means of two filters.*

Table 8.5 Summary of Patient Data Comparing Snellen, S-Chart, and Laser Visual Acuity before and after Therapy in a Group of Amblyopes

Patient Number	Etiology of the Amblyopia	Age (yrs)	Snellen Pre	Snellen Post	S-Chart Pre	S-Chart Post	Laser Pre	Laser Post	Fixation Pre	Fixation Post	Additional Comments
1	Aniso(+)c XT	13	600	600			660		UT	UT	
2	Aniso(+)c ET	14	400	400	550	460	660	660	UN	UN	
3	Aniso(−)c ET	6	400	150			100		UN	UN	
4	Aniso(−)c XT	18	300	100			100		UT	UC	
5	Aniso(−)c ET	10	200	80	232	70	100	40	UC	UC	
6	ET	13	200	80		60	60	60	UC	UC	
7	Aniso(AST)c XT	16	200	80			60	60	UT	UC	
8	Aniso(−)c ET	10	200	100	137		60		UN	UN	Partial organic (retrolental fibroplasia)
9	ET	12	200	200			160		UN	UN	
10	Aniso(−)	9	200	60			50	50	US	UC	
11	Aniso(−)c XT	7	200	30	109	32	40	30	UT	SC	
12	Refractive(+)	7	200	60			25		UC		
13	Aniso(−)	6	200	150			100		UC	UC	
14	Refractive(+)	7	200	80			60		UC		
15	Aniso(+)c ET	10	200	60	180	62	50	30	USu	USu	
16	Aniso(−)c ET	13	200	80			70		UC	UC	
17	Aniso(−)c XT	11	200	100	175	72	60	60	UT	UT	
18	Microtropia	29	150	30	119	62	30	25	SN	UC	
19	Aniso(+)c ET	9	150	40			40	30	SN	UC	
20	Microtropia	9	150	25			30	25	SN	SC	
21	Refractive(+)	9	150	40	120	50	60	30	UC	SC	
22	Secondary XT	18	125	50			40	40	UC	UC	
23	Refractive(+)	9	125	40	109	49	30	20	UC	SC	
24	Aniso(−)	10	100	25	128		25		UC	SC	
25	Microtropia	8	100	20			25	20	SSu	SC	
26	Aniso(+) Microtropia	16	70	40	77	30	25		SN	UC	
27	Aniso(AST)c XT	21	70	40			30	30	UT	UC	Partial organic (ocular albinism)
28	ET	8	70	40	70	41	30	30	UN	UC	
29	Aniso(−)	9	70	70	70	60	60	60	UC	SC	
30	Aniso(−)	9	70	40	77	50	50		UC	SC	
31	Aniso(−)	17	70	30	85		25		SN	CSu	
32	Aniso(Ast)	9	60	30	52	38	40		UC	SC	
33	Refractive(+)c ET	10	50	30			25		UC	SC	
34	Aniso(Ast)	31	50	25			25		UC	CSu	
35	Aniso(+)	9	50	25			25	25	UN	SC	
36	ET	13	50	30	50	42	40		UN	UC	
37	Aniso(−)	7	50	25	38	26	25		UC	SC	
38	Aniso(+)	10	50	40	48	40	30		UC	UC	
39	Aniso(+)	13	40	40	45	45	30	30	UN	UN	

Key: XT = exotropia; ET = esotropia; AST = astigmatism (greater than 2 D); aniso = anisometropia; (−) = myopia; (+) = hyperopia; c = with; U = unsteady; S = steady; N = nasal; T = temporal; Su = superior; C = central.

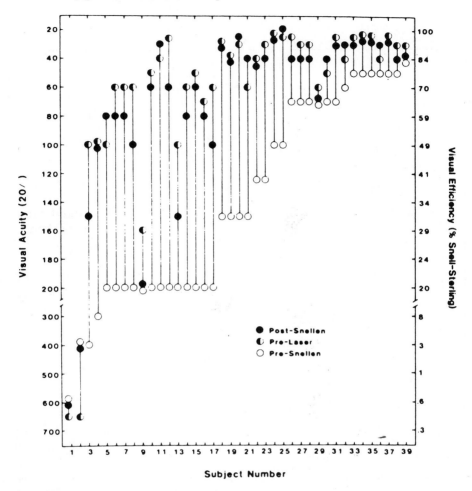

Figure 8.12   *Visual acuity in the amblyopic eye before and after therapy. In most patients, pretherapy laser visual acuity markedly overestimated pretherapy Snellen visual acuity but accurately predicted posttherapy Snellen visual acuity. Eyes 8 and 27 had a combined functional/organic amblyopic component. (Reprinted, with permission of the publisher, from Selenow et al. 1986.)*

NEUTRAL DENSITY FILTER

In 1921, Ammann measured visual acuity both with and without dark glasses that were of sufficient density to decrease visual acuity several lines in a group of visually normal patients. He was surprised to find that these patients showed a ratio of 1.0:0.4 between nonfiltered and filtered visual acuity such that

$$\frac{\text{Vision without filter} = 20/20 = 1.0}{\text{Vision with filter} = 20/50 = 0.4} = 1{:}0.4$$

Table 8.6   Average Change in Visual Acuity through Neutral-Density Filter

Normal Individuals	Strabismic Amblyopia	Organic Amblyopia
A. Ratio of Snellen fraction in decimals:		
1:0.48	1:1.01	1:0.24
	1:0.95*	
B. A.M.A. visual efficiency (Snell-Sterling) scale:		
19.3% decrease	0.2% increase	36.2% decrease
	1.7% decrease*	

*Data for amblyope with significant acuity increase are omitted.

while another group with functional amblyopia showed no reduction in visual acuity through the same filters. In addition, a third group of patients with organically based amblyopia (central retinal lesions and glaucoma) demonstrated a marked acuity loss through the same filters.

In 1959(a), von Noorden and Burian studied this phenomenon in more detail. They first measured Snellen visual acuity (no mention was made as to whether single-letter or single-line acuities were used) in each eye of 20 strabismic amblyopes and in 10 eyes with amblyopia due to organic lesions (macular degeneration, optic nerve atrophy, or chorioretinitis). The measurements were repeated through a Kodak Wratten neutral-density filter (no. 96, N.D. 3.0) after 2 minutes of adaptation to the filters. The measured change in visual acuity was expressed as a ratio as described above. Normal eyes had ratios of 1:0.4 to 1:0.5, with a mean of 1:0.48. Of the 20 amblyopic eyes, 6 showed a slight visual acuity reduction from 1:0.7 to 1:0.9, 10 showed no change (1:1), and 4 showed *slight apparent improvement* under the reduced illumination conditions (from 1:1.1 to 1:2). In contrast, those with organic lesions consistently demonstrated a marked reduction in visual acuity with the filter (1:0.1 to 1:0.05, with a mean of 1:0.24) (see Table 8.6). However, of the four amblyopes who demonstrated apparently better acuity through the filter, only one had a *substantial* improvement, going from 20/200 without the filter to 20/100 with the filter. The other three improvements were small: 20/200 to 20/200+1, 20/100−1 to 20/100, and 20/82 to 20/70. If the first patient is disregarded, then overall the functional amblyopic group showed a slight visual acuity *reduction*, with a ratio of 1:0.95, as was true for the other functional amblyopes tested in the study.

In an analysis of this study, Caloroso and Flom (1969) had several comments. First, changes in visual acuity expressed on the Snell-Sterling visual efficiency scale (Snell and Sterling 1925) provide a much more meaningful number (see Table 8.6). After converting von Noorden and Burian's results into Snell-Sterling percentages, the difference between the three groups became less dramatic. Second, in no instance did the measured visual acuity of the normal eye with the filter in place fall *below* that of the amblyopic eye. And finally, these authors questioned whether the apparent improvement in filtered visual acuity in four of the amblyopic eyes may have been due to test-measurement variability and thus did not represent a true change in visual acuity.

In the second part of their investigation, von Noorden and Burian (1959b) studied the change in visual acuity with a change in luminance in 10 normal individuals, 10 strabismic amblyopes with central fixation and mild amblyopia (20/25 to 20/60), and 10 organic amblyopes (20/20 to 20/400). They presented a single letter E in an illuminated box at a full range of luminance levels. Results showed that "the eyes with strabismic amblyopia showed an increase in visual acuity at the same or at lower levels of illumination than the normal eyes" (see Figure 8.13). von Noorden and Burian interpreted these findings to indicate that the strabismic amblyopes reached their maximum visual acuity level when the normal eye had not even reached one-half of its final visual acuity. In contrast, patients with organic amblyopia showed a significant early reduction in visual acuity as the illumination decreased. However, we feel that another interpretation of the graph may be that as target luminance increased, visual acuity in the amblyopic eye plateaued at its lower acuity value. Actually, the normal and amblyopic eyes' curves are identical, with visual acuity being the limiting factor.

In analyzing this study further, Caloroso and Flom (1969) noted the following problems. First, only amblyopes with mild to moderate visual-acuity reduction

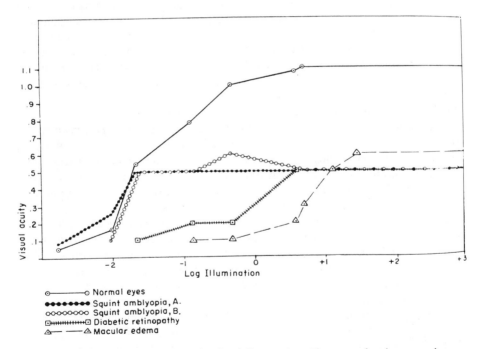

Figure 8.13 *Visual acuity with 10 levels of illumination. The curve for the normal eyes represents the average of the measurements in 10 normal eyes. The curves for strabismic and organic amblyopia represent individual cases. (Symbols: ⊙————⊙ = normal eyes; ●●●●●● = squint amblyopia A; ○○○○○○○ = squint amblyopia B; ☐+++++☐ = diabetic retinopathy; and △----△ = macular edema.) (Reprinted, with permission of the publisher, from von Noorden and Burian 1959.)*

(20/25 to 20/60) were tested. Second, Caloroso and Flom objected to the general statement that at low levels of illumination, the strabismic amblyopic eye performed *as well as or better* than the normal fellow eye. They noted that at the three lowest luminance levels, seven subjects had better acuities in the amblyopic eye, eight had equal acuities, and eight had acuities that were better in the normal eye. Thus there was much variability in the results. And finally, a contributing factor to the finding of better acuity in the amblyopic eye at low luminance levels may be the testing protocol. The large acuity gaps at these levels (20/80, 20/100, 20/200, 20/250) can lead to increased variability of repeated measurements (Wick and Schor 1984). In addition, response criteria were not set, and this factor is extremely important when dealing with the amblyopic eye's variable visual acuity responses.

Thus Caloroso and Flom (1969) conducted their own study. They measured visual acuity psychometrically at six luminance levels in four strabismic amblyopes and four normal individuals (see Figure 8.14). Their results showed that *visual acuity of both the normal and amblyopic eyes declined as luminance levels were reduced.* At essentially all luminance levels, visual acuity in the amblyopic eye was *less* than that of the normal eye, with acuities being similar at the lowest luminance levels.

In response to Caloroso and Flom (1969), von Noorden (1980) argued that the point of the neutral-density filter test was totally missed. He believed that the data of both studies made clear the *relative increase* in mesopic visual acuity of eyes with functional amblyopia. On the other hand, organic amblyopes demonstrate a dramatic and sudden loss of vision with neutral-density filters.

We believe that the following conclusions can be made regarding these two studies:

1. As luminance levels decreased, the *difference* in visual acuity between the normal and amblyopic eyes decreased.
2. At the lowest illumination levels, the amblyopic and normal eyes' acuities were similar.
3. In contrast, visual acuity in eyes with organic amblyopia suddenly and dramatically decreased.
4. Functionally based amblyopic visual acuity *did not* improve when going from photopsia to mesopia, but rather simply *decreased* less than that of the normal eye, since this amblyopic eye starts at a lower level but ends up at the same visual acuity level as the normal eye owing to normal physiologic retinocortical resolution constraints.

Clinically, we use the neutral-density filter test when presented with a patient who has decreased visual acuity, no observable pathology, and absence of any amblyogenic etiologic factors. If visual acuity with the neutral-density filter decreases dramatically, then a nonobservable pathology is suspected and electrodiagnostic testing is indicated. Fortunately, the controversy revolves around the amblyopic versus normal eye response. However, the clinician does not need the test for this purpose, since one knows that the patient in the examination chair during an amblyopic workup does *not* have two normal eyes. On the other hand, all

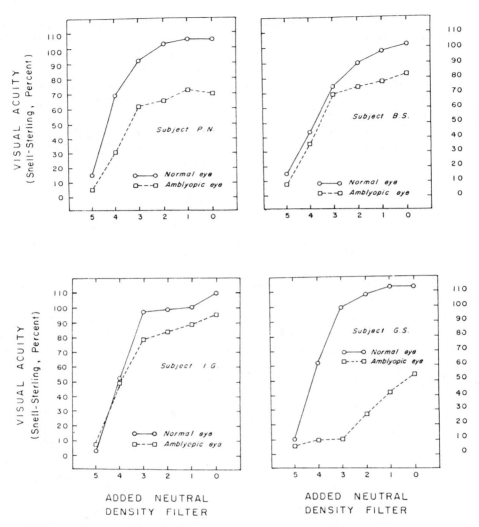

Figure 8.14 *Acuity changes in normal and amblyopic eyes as a function of luminance. Acuity was tested with an array of four-position Landolt C's and was determined by psychometric analysis using the 50% threshold corrected for guessing. With no filter in front of the projector, the test field luminance was 100 foot-Lamberts. (Reprinted, with permission of the publisher, from Caloroso and Flom 1969.)*

sides seem to agree that an organic amblyope shows a drastic loss in visual acuity with neutral-density filters, and this is precisely when one should use the test. However, one should be careful in making conclusions based on this test alone, since there is evidence that anisometropic amblyopes also may show considerable acuity loss through filters (Hess et al. 1980). We have found the following test protocol to be most useful:

1. Preadapt the good eye for 5 minutes with the polarized filters oriented 90 degrees apart (see Figure 8.15). The patient should not be able to see any light. Clinicians frequently do not preadapt the eye. However, the whole basis of the test revolves around the eye being in the mesopic state.

2. Expose an S-chart at a visual acuity value of 20/42. Slowly rotate the polarizers until the patient can just begin to resolve the direction of the gap in at least five of the eight Landolt C's.

3. Now similarly preadapt the amblyopic eye for 5 minutes, and then quickly introduce the filter that allowed the good eye to resolve the 20/42 letters.

4. Measure visual acuity of the amblyopic eye through this filter, and compare this with its acuity without the filter.

5. If visual acuity is reduced considerably more in the amblyopic eye than in the good eye (e.g., greater than a 50% Snell-Sterling difference in reduction), then organic amblyopia should be suspected. This is extrapolated from von Noorden and Burian's (1959a) data, where a filter that reduces the normal eyes' acuity from 20/20 to 20/40 (15% decrease in Snell-Sterling) reduces an organic amblyopic eye from 20/36 to 20/200 (65% decrease in Snell-Sterling), with the difference between the two being 50%.

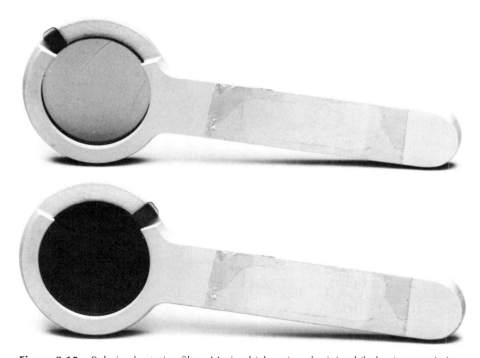

Figure 8.15   *Polarized rotating filter. Maximal (above) and minimal (below) transmission through the device.*

CLINICAL ASPECTS OF ACCOMMODATION

There are several steady-state aspects of accommodation that are abnormal in human amblyopic eyes (see Chapter 6 for details). Some of these are (1) reduced accommodative amplitude, (2) reduced slope of the accommodative stimulus-response curve, (3) increased depth of focus, and (4) increased variability of accommodative responses.These abnormalities can be attributed to the frequent presence of one or more of the following factors in amblyopic eyes.

Reduced Threshold and Suprathreshold Contrast Sensitivity   This has an adverse effect on blur detection, involving contrast and spatial frequency content of the target, especially for middle and high spatial frequencies. This may account for the reduced accommodative response amplitude and increased accommodative error found in amblyopic eyes. A greater amount of retinal defocus must be present before the perception of blur is elicited.

Target "Fading"   Many amblyopes report a suprathreshold contrast abnormality of "fading" of the target during extended monocular fixation with the amblyopic eye. This phenomenon may adversely affect the amblyopic eyes' ability to sustain accommodation, since effective target contrast is transiently reduced by considerable and continuously variable amounts.

Eccentric Fixation   One may expect a greater reduction of accommodative response in an eccentric fixator than in a central fixator. This can be explained by the difference in the number of cones, receptive field size, and overall anatomic organization between foveal and nonfoveal retinal areas.

Abnormal Fixational Eye Movements   Increased drift and jerk nystagmus can account for some of the increased variability of accommodative responses, since these movements would "smear" the retinal image, thereby effectively reducing the contrast of the retinal image especially at high spatial frequencies, resulting in less drive to the accommodative system (Ciuffreda and Goldrich 1983; Ciuffreda et al. 1983, 1987) (see Chapter 5 for details).

Vision training has a positive effect on static aspects of accommodation, although slightly abnormal accommodation may still be found in some formerly amblyopic eyes after termination of successful orthoptic therapy (Ciuffreda 1986), especially if binocular vision has not been established. In addition, regression of accommodation tends to precede regression of visual acuity once therapy has been discontinued. This suggests that accommodation may be a more sensitive measure of overall amblyopic vision function recovery and regression than visual acuity. Therefore, the clinician should obtain as accurate a baseline measure of accommodative function as possible and monitor progress throughout (and well beyond, that is, for 1 to 5 years) the therapy program.

Clinically, the best methods of measuring accommodative responses in amblyopic eyes are the minus lens and dynamic pushup retinoscopy techniques (Hokoda and Ciuffreda 1982; also see Chapter 6 for procedural details). Dynamic retinoscopy is the only clinical method of measuring accommodative responses objectively. Owing to the amblyopic eyes' increased depth of focus and abnormal accommodative stimulus-response curve, the subjective pushup technique is not a reliable measure of accommodation in amblyopic eyes. Thus the objective dynamic retinoscopy technique is preferred by the authors. The clinician also will note a reduction in accommodative dynamics when tested monocularly with plus and minus lens flippers. Clinically, near-point retinoscopy must be performed during lens flipper testing to measure the true accommodative response. Once an accurate measure of accommodation has been determined in the dominant and amblyopic eye with the subjective minus lens and objective dynamic retinoscopy techniques, the clinician will be able to monitor improvement and/or regression throughout the course of therapy with greater assurance. Ciuffreda et al. (*in preparation*, but see Chapter 6) found a slight increase in latency, a reduction in amplitude with normal peak velocities, and poor sustaining ability in the amblyopic eye when measuring accommodative dynamics objectively in the laboratory.

VISUAL ACUITY, FIXATION, AND DIRECTION SENSE

Visual Acuity across the Normal Retina

The importance of knowing how visual acuity in a normal eye changes as a function of retinal eccentricity becomes obvious when attempting to understand and deal with the phenomenon of eccentric fixation typically found in amblyopic eyes. There were several early attempts to measure visual acuity across the central retina in normal individuals. In 1949, Feinberg measured visual acuity at different retinal eccentricities (see Table 8.7). His results showed that visual acuity decreased at a fairly constant rate as retinal eccentricity increased. This loss with eccentricity was more dramatic when peripheral acuity was expressed in terms of central acuity (Borish 1970). In 1958, Weymouth also studied the rate of change of visual acuity as a function of retinal eccentricity. His data showed that when visual acuity was specified in minutes of arc rather than in a Snellen fraction, there was a linear relationship

Table 8.7 Visual Acuity Findings of Feinberg (1949)

Eccentricity (degrees)	Visual Acuity	Percent Acuity of Fovea
1	20/30	65
2	20/35	58
3	20/50	41
4	20/60	35
5	20/70	29

between visual acuity and retinal ecentricity (Figure 8.16). A similar linear relationship was found when Wertheim's data (1894) were replotted by Weymouth (1958) (Table 8.8 and Figure 8.17). Schapero (1971) averaged peripheral visual acuity values from the preceding studies to approximate the expected visual acuity for different degrees of retinal eccentricity in visually normal individuals. Table 8.9 shows the expected visual acuities for different degrees of retinal eccentricity.

In 1961, Flom and Weymouth studied the eccentricity of Maxwell's spot in both normal and amblyopic eyes. Since Maxwell's spot is a macular entoptic phenomenon, its perceived position in relation to the fixation point was used as a measure of eccentric fixation and retinal eccentricity. These authors reported that monocular visual acuity in the amblyopic eye at the point of (eccentric) fixation was the same as that found in normal eyes at the same eccentricity. Therefore, according to this study, *all* the amblyopic eye's decreased visual acuity could be simply accounted for on the basis of the *normal* visual acuity found in the peripheral retina for that specific eccentric retinal locus. Flom and Weymouth (1961) used the following equation to calculate the expected visual acuity at different retinal eccentricities:

$$MAR = E + 1$$

Table 8.8   Visual Acuity Findings of Weymouth (1958) and Wertheim (1894)

	Visual Acuity	
Eccentricity (degrees)	*Wertheim*	*Weymouth*
1	20/33	20/30
2	20/40	20/50
5	20/67	20/95
10	20/100	20/160
20	20/180	20/300

Table 8.9   Visual Acuity Findings of Schapero (1971) and Flom and Weymouth (1961)

	Visual Acuity	
Eccentricity (degrees)	*Schapero*	*Flom and Weymouth*
1	20/30	20/55
2	20/40 to 20/50	20/90
3	20/50 to 20/60	20/125
4	20/60 to 20/70	20/160
5	20/70 to 20/100	20/195
10	20/100 to 20/160	20/370
20	20/180 to 20/300	20/720

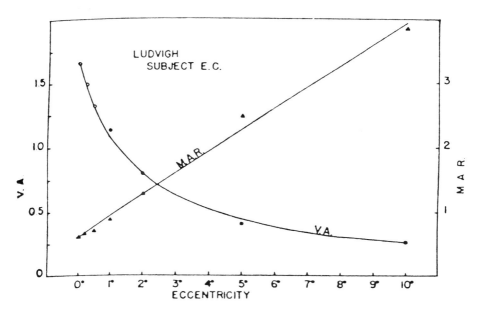

Figure 8.16 *Visual acuity as a function of degrees of retinal eccentricity. (Reprinted, with permission of the publisher, from Weymouth 1958.)*

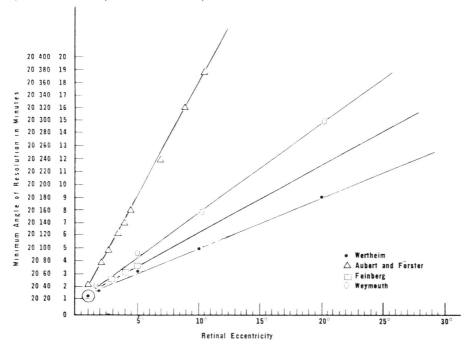

Figure 8.17 *Visual acuity for different degrees of retinal eccentricity for the various researchers listed. (Reprinted, with permission of the publisher, from Shapero 1971.)*

where *MAR* is the minimum angle of resolution in minutes of arc, *E* is the amount of eccentric fixation in prism diopters, and 1 is a constant. However, this basic finding has not been replicated (Alpern et al. 1967, Hess and Jacobs 1979), having an apparent error of about a factor of 2.

Table 8.9 compares Schapero's (1971) and Flom and Weymouth's (1961) visual acuity expecteds for different degrees of retinal eccentricity. As can be seen from the table, there is considerable discrepancy. From a clinical standpoint, it appears that Schapero's results are more realistic. For example, with 2 degrees of eccentric fixation, the best expected visual acuity predicted by Flom and Weymouth would be 20/90; however, it is not uncommon to examine an amblyope with 2 degrees of eccentric fixation having visual acuity in the amblyopic eye considerably better than 20/90. Further, their results disagree with other basic and clinical studies on visual acuity across the retina (see Borish 1970 for a review). If one substitutes degrees for prism diopters in the formula $MAR = E + 1$, then Flom and Weymouth's visual acuity values become similar to Schapero's (Levi et al. 1986). Schapero's table will therefore be used for all further clinic discussion.

There have been several other studies over the past 25 years in which visual acuity across the central retina has been investigated to establish the point of maximum visual acuity in eccentric fixators (see Flom 1978 for a review). The results have varied considerably, with almost all possibilities being observed. Some have found visual acuity to be greatest (1) at the point of eccentric fixation and not the fovea (Prince 1962), (2) at the point of fixation (either the fovea *or* eccentric fixation point) (Avetisov, translated by Kirschen et al. 1979, Hess and Jacobs 1979, Sireteanu and Fronius 1981) for treated large-angle esotropes, (3) at the fovea (Schor 1972, Kirschen and Flom 1978, Flom et al. 1980, Bedell and Flom 1981, 1983, Bedell 1982), or (4) at some point other than the fovea or eccentric fixation point (Sireteanu and Fronius 1981 for small-angle esotropes). In general, the visual acuity profile in the amblyopic eye is reduced and flattened with respect to the fellow dominant eye, with hemifield asymmetries sometimes noted (Figure 8.18).

However, many of these studies are plagued by serious methodologic deficiencies, such as lack of control of horizontal and vertical eye position and therefore not knowing precisely the retinal locus of stimulus delivery, minimal clinical data, unaccounted for practice effects, and very small sample size. Perhaps the best study to date has been by Kirschen and Flom (1978). All experimental testing was preceded by careful clinical examination and extensive practice (5 to 10 hours) at the task; further, monocular horizontal eye position was controlled and monitored during the test periods (unfortunately, vertical position was neither controlled nor monitored). For both esotropic and exotropic functional amblyopes, visual acuity in the amblyopic eye was *always* found to be highest at the fovea. Thus the presence of eccentric fixation could not be attributed to having greatest resolution at the

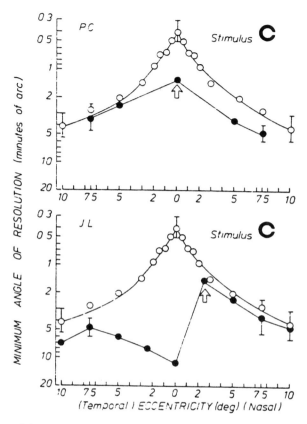

Figure 8.18 *Landolt ring acuity (P = 0.5) across the horizontal visual field is compared for amblyopes (closed circles) PC and JL with that exhibited by four normal subjects (open circles). Arrows indicate the functional fixation point and error bars represent ± 1 SE. (Reprinted, with permission, from Hess and Jacobs 1979.)*

eccentric fixation point, as predicted by Worth (1943) and Chavasse (1939). Rather, this eccentric point with its acquisition of primary visual direction dominates in all tasks involving direction sense (Ciuffreda et al. 1979a, b, Bedell 1981).

There are three factors that can limit the visual acuity of an amblyopic eye. These factors include retinal eccentricity, sensory loss, and steadiness of fixation. By knowing the maximum visual acuity potential at the point of eccentric fixation, one automatically knows the percentage of amblyopia due to the other two factors combined. Therefore, if presented with the following two patients, both of whom have 2 degrees of nasal eccentric fixation, one can see that the treatment strategies would be quite different (see Table 8.10). In patient A, the

Table 8.10   Comparison of Two Patients with Identical Fixation

	Patient A	*Patient B*
Fixation status:	2 degrees nasal	2 degrees nasal
Pretherapy visual acuity:	20/200	20/50
Expected acuity based on retinal eccentricity:	20/50	20/50
Percent of acuity loss due to eccentric fixation:	< 30%	~ 100%

initial thrust would be to "break down" the inhibition of the dominant eye over the amblyopic eye with emphasis on direct patching. If successful, one would expect an acuity improvement from 20/200 to 20/50, with the residual loss (20/50 to 20/20) the result of *normal* visual acuity characteristics for that eccentric retinal locus. In patient B, on the other hand, the clinical bias would be to "break down" the eccentric fixation with emphasis on fine fixation tasks under controlled conditions (MIT, after-image transfer, and so on; see Chapter 10), since all of the amblyopia (20/50) can be accounted for by the degree of eccentricity (2 degrees). Peripheral visual acuity profiles not only help determine the initial treatment strategy, but also can guide the therapeutic regimen during the course of orthoptic therapy (see Chapter 10).

Theories of Eccentric Fixation

There are four main theories to explain the pathophysiology of eccentric fixation: the suppression theory of Bangerter, Cupper's anomalous correspondence theory, the motor theory, and our own sensorimotor theory. Although none of these theories *fully* explains the *development* of eccentric fixation, all contribute toward an understanding of why a nonfoveal area may be used by an individual for fixation (Baldwin 1962).

Suppression Theory of Bangerter

The suppression theory of Bangerter (1953) is based on the earlier ideas of Claude Worth (1943), who proposed that amblyopia was the result of an inhibition of visual acuity limited to the central retina. Worth and Bangerter both felt that foveal visual acuity was depressed *below* that of the adjacent eccentric retinal regions. To achieve better resolution, the amblyopic eye therefore fixated with this eccentric site that provided the highest level of visual acuity (see Figure 8.19).

There are two objections to this theory. First, as discussed earlier, recent experiments in strabismic amblyopes show visual acuity to be better at the fovea than either at the eccentric fixation point or anywhere else over the central retina. Second, since there are probably annular isoacuity regions surrounding

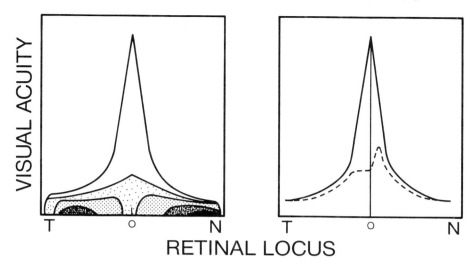

Figure 8.19 *Changes in visual acuity with retinal eccentricity. (Left) Normal eye with central fixation and amblyopic eyes with various degrees of central retinal inhibition as per Worth and Chavasse. Note loss of foveal superiority for lowermost curves. (Right) Similar plot showing a nasal bias. (Symbols: N = nasal; T = temporal; and O = fovea.)*

the depressed central foveal area, many eccentric fixators would be expected to use *multiple* acuity-equivalent points rather than one specific point for fixation if visual acuity rather than visual direction were the sole criterion for selection of a fixation point (Figure 8.19). They may even be expected to switch between nasal and temporal areas of fixation having equal visual acuity. However, clinically and experimentally we know that eccentric fixation is typically limited to one specific retinal point or relatively small locus.

Anomalous Correspondence Theory
of Chavasse and Cuppers

Chavasse (1939) and Cuppers (1956) proposed that the eccentric fixation represented a monocular sensory shift of primary visual direction that occurred secondary to the development of anomalous correspondence. In anomalous correspondence, there is a nonfoveal area in the strabismic eye that corresponds directionally to the fovea of the fixating eye under binocular viewing conditions. According to Cuppers, this nonfoveal area assumes the principal visual direction under monocular conditions as well. Therefore, this theory predicts that the objective angle and the angle of anomaly must coincide with the angle of eccentric fixation. The major objection to this theory is that most eccentric fixators have an angle of anomaly that is *much greater* than the angle of eccentricity (von Noorden 1970). However, this theory does provide a possible explanation for the development of eccentric fixation in microtropia, although it is a difficult one to test, since the difference in angles to be tested approaches the measurement limits of the clinical test procedures.

Motor Theory

The motor theory suggests that long-term strabismus leads to an afterdischarge or potentiation of the agonist muscle in the strabismic eye when the dominant eye is covered (Schor 1978). Since the sensitivity of the amblyopic eye is reduced, the resultant position error would not be detected, and monocular nonfoveal fixation results. Therefore, this theory predicts that esotropes would have nasal eccentric fixation and exotropes temporal eccentric fixation. However, there are some nonsurgically altered esotropes with temporal eccentric fixation. Also, some preoperative esotropes with nasal eccentric fixation continue to fixate nasally following postoperative overcorrection. Further, eye position errors as small as 0.6 degree can be sensed and responded to in amblyopic eyes (Ciuffreda et al. 1979a, b). Lastly, if this theory were accurate, then eccentric fixation in most strabismic amblyopes should be "cured" after no more than a few weeks of constant direct occlusion alone; however, this is clearly not the case in the vast majority of amblyopes.

Sensorimotor Theory

Eccentric fixation has been defined as "an anomaly of monocular vision in which the time-average position of the fovea is off the object of regard" (M. C. Flom, personal communication, 1977) (also see next section). While this definition is considerably better than what has been used in the past by many and takes into account the notion of variance in the measurement, it has a major deficiency—it does not separate the pure sensory visual direction disturbance or shift from the pure motor disturbance. Thus we are proposing an additional way to think about eccentric fixation and the components contributing to its measurement:

1. *Sensory-based eccentric fixation.* This refers to the time-average position of the fovea relative to the object in the total *absence* of any motor abnormality such as nystagmus or saccadic intrusions (Figure 8.20*A*). Thus the eccentric fixation would be due *solely* to a true sensory shift in the zero or foveal spatial value, probably related to the impaired direction sense found over the central retina of amblyopic eyes. This "pure" sensory variety of eccentric fixation is primarily found in anisometropic amblyopes, as well as in those strabismic amblyopes who do not have any oculomotor defect. The oculomotor drift frequently found in these amblyopic eyes therefore has a pure sensory basis.

2. *Motor-based eccentric fixation.* This refers to the time-average position of the fovea relative to the object of regard in the *presence* of an oculomotor abnormality such as jerk nystagmus and assumed *absence* of any true sensory shift in spatial values (Figure 8.20*B*). This would include the relatively small

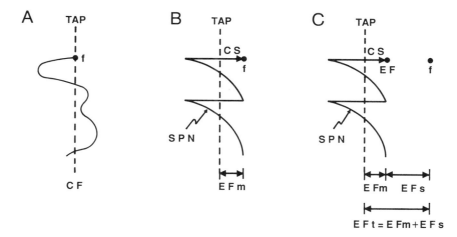

Figure 8.20 *Fixation patterns showing sensory and motor contributions to eccentric fixation. (Symbols: f = fovea; TAP = time-average position; EF$_m$ = motor component to eccentric fixation; EF$_s$ = sensory component to eccentric fixation; EF$_t$ = total amount of eccentric fixation combining the sensory and motor contributions; CS = nystagmus-correcting saccade; and SPN = slow phase of nystagmus.)*

eccentric fixation (e.g., several minutes of arc) found in the dominant eye of *some* strabismic amblyopes, since they frequently have *bilateral*, small-amplitude jerk nystagmus, and the congenital nystagmats having 70 seconds or so of stereopsis and no discernible strabismus. Thus any nystagmus patient who does not have strabismus and amblyopia *will* have such a motor-based eccentric fixation. The nystagmus slow phase drives the fovea away from the target, while the fast saccadic phase of the nystagmus attempts to realign the fovea with the target. Therefore, based on the accepted notion of time-average foveal position, the fovea and target *are not* coincident and eccentric fixation by definition must be present. If the nystagmus or other related motor disturbances were to be *symmetric* with respect to the fovea, so that, on average, the fovea and target were coincident, this *would* be classified as central (unsteady). However, this is probably *never* the case.

   3.   *Combined sensorimotor-based eccentric fixation.* This refers to the time-average position of the fovea not being coincident with the object of regard in the presence of nystagmus *and* a spatial shift in the sensory zero point (Figure 8.20C). This would typically be found in strabismic amblyopes with jerk nystagmus. Thus the measured eccentric fixation would reflect the motor anomaly (i.e., jerk nystagmus) *as well as* the sensory spatial direction shift or bias. One can think of this variety as having the motor component superimposed and adding to the sensory component, resulting in a relatively large magnitude of (total) eccentric fixation.

Assessment of Fixation

Since the type of fixation will have an impact on the prognosis, therapeutic approach, and degree of success, it is important to obtain as accurate an estimate of fixation as possible (Priestly et al. 1959, Griffin 1982). Ideally, the following information should be recorded:

1. Centricity of fixation (central versus eccentric)
2. Magnitude of eccentric fixation (point *e* in degrees)
3. Quality of fixation (steady versus unsteady)
4. Pattern of fixation (drift, saccades, nystagmus)
5. Percent foveation (30-second visuoscopy)
6. Directional bias (nasal, temporal, inferior, superior)
7. Subjective localization of primary visual direction
8. Zero retinomotor point

Before the more commonly used methods of assessing fixation are reviewed, four terms related to eccentric fixation need to be defined:

1. *Primary visual direction*—that point or area on the retina which is subjectively associated with the straight-ahead egocentric visual direction under monocular viewing conditions.
2. *Zero retinomotor point*—the retinal point to which the eye makes a reflex saccadic refixation movement when presented with a target in the retinal periphery.

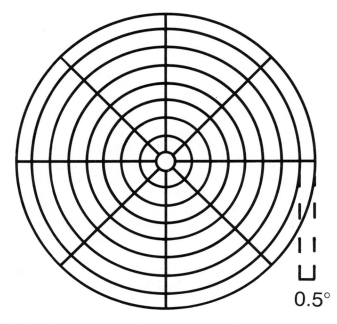

Figure 8.21 *Neitz euthoscope fixation target with 0.5-degree concentric rings.*

3. *Eccentric fixation*—an anomaly of monocular vision in which the time-average position of the object of regard is not coincident with the fovea.
4. *Point e*—the mean point on the retina that the object of regard falls on during monocular viewing by an eccentric fixator; the angular difference between the fovea and point *e* represents the magnitude of eccentric fixation.

Typically, in an amblyope with eccentric fixation, the primary visual direction and zero retinomotor point coincide with the eccentric point. The steadier the eccentric fixation, the more likely that this is the case. It is extremely rare for a true eccentric fixator to have the primary visual direction associated with any point other than this eccentric retinal point or locus. However, this may occur during therapy while in the process of breaking down the eccentric fixation (Selenow and Ciuffreda 1986).

Tests for Eccentric Fixation

Ophthalmoscopy

There are several available ophthalmoscopes that have been adapted for the evaluation of fixation status. For example, the Neitz euthoscope has a target with nine concentric circles at 0.5-degree intervals (see Figure 8.21), while the Welch Allen ophthalmoscope has about a 1.2-degree circle with notches spaced at 0.5-degree intervals (Figure 8.22). Regardless of the type of instrument, the patient is initially

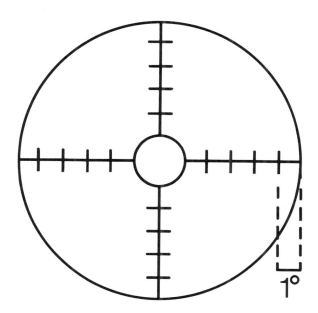

Figure 8.22 *Welch Allen ophthalmoscope fixation target.*

asked to fixate the center of the target monocularly with the dominant eye. This allows the patient to become familiar with the requirements of the test.

After assessing the fixation status of the dominant eye, monocular fixation in the amblyopic eye is tested. The patient is asked to look directly at the center of the target. The examiner notes the location of the foveal reflex in relation to the center of the fixation target. If the fixation is basically central, then only the degree of steadiness needs to be noted. Otherwise, the following information is needed:

1.   *Magnitude of eccentric fixation (EF)*. This is the distance in degrees between point *e* and the fovea. That is, the time-average position of the foveal reflex to the center of the grid represents the magnitude of eccentric fixation. This is difficult to determine when point *e* is more an area or locus of points than a single relatively fixed point. A careful mental average will give a good approximation; however, a description and diagram of the pattern of fixation are most valuable in this case.

2.   *Percent foveation*. The 30-second low-light visuoscopy procedure has been the most helpful. While observing the relationship of the foveal reflex to the center of the fixation target, the examiner counts off 30 seconds and estimates the percent time of foveation, if any. This allows a more accurate and consistent means of monitoring improvement of fixation, and perhaps visual acuity and/or changes in direction sense, during therapy. It is extremely important to set the rheostat of the ophthalmoscope to the lowest level and then gradually increase the illumination to a level where the retinal structures and foveal reflex are *just visible*. If the light is too bright, it may dazzle the patient and thus decrease the visibility of the fixation target, resulting in iatrogenically induced exaggerated fixational unsteadiness (Lawwill 1966).

3.   *Directional bias*. This is simple to determine when the eccentric fixation is reasonably steady. Determining the directional bias can be helpful in the differential diagnosis of uncomplicated amblyopic drift versus latent nystagmus, wherein the slow phase of the jerk nystagmus (which can be confused with amblyopic drift) is *always* toward the nose regardless of the eye used for monocular fixation (Ciuffreda et al. 1979b).

4.   *Pattern of fixation*. At times there is a discernible pattern of abnormal fixation. The following three abnormal fixational eye movement patterns are commonly found when performing visuoscopy in eccentric fixators: fixational drift followed by a corrective saccade or saccades (if repetitive, i.e., one to four times per second, it could represent jerklike nystagmus), two-point fixation preference interspersed by a saccade [this "saccadic intrusion" pattern is frequently found in strabismics with or without amblyopia (Ciuffreda et al. 1979b) and at least theoretically reflects a repetitive and transient increase in eccentric fixation], and random saccadic movements about multiple fixation points reflecting grossly unsteady fixation (this is frequently found in amblyopic eyes manifesting large eccentric fixation, i.e., several degrees). The following are some typical descriptions of fixation patterns that may occur in the amblyopic eye:

- 2-degree steady nasal EF
- 1/2-degree nasal and 1-degree superior unsteady EF (foveal drift followed by corrective saccade)
- 1- to 2-degree nasal unsteady EF (saccadic intrusions)
- 4- to 6-degree temporal and 5-degree inferior unsteady EF (random saccadic movements about area)
- Unsteady 75% central with nasal bias (nasal drift followed by corrective saccade)
- Unsteady 25% central (random 1-degree saccadic movements about the fovea)

5. *Primary visual direction (PVD).* After the patient with eccentric fixation is told to look at the center of the fixation target, he or she is asked whether the target appears to be straight ahead. If not, the target (with the eye maintained *fixed*) is moved in the appropriate direction until it *appears* to be straight ahead. This retinal location is noted.

6. *Zero retinomotor point (ZRM).* The fixation target is placed on a peripheral retinal area, and the patient is instructed to fixate the target rapidly. The examiner notes the retinal point *initially* used in the fixation reflex (von Noorden 1960). In most eccentric fixators, the eccentric point has functionally taken the place of the fovea as the zero retinomotor point. Thus, ideally, one would observe a single refixation saccade to place the fixation target coincident with the eccentric retinal locus. Eccentric viewers (such as found in adults with discrete foveal diseases or trauma), on the other hand, retain the fovea as the zero retinomotor point and therefore initially attempt to fixate with the "blind" fovea before their final refixation with the "seeing" eccentric point (see Figure 8.23).

Haidinger's Brush

This is a retinal foveal entoptic phenomenon that is observed only when blue polarized light is viewed (Griffin 1982). The patient sees a pair of brushlike shapes that appear to radiate from the point of fixation. Since the phenomenon is believed to be due to double refraction by the radially oriented fibers of Henle around the fovea (Hallden 1957), the fibers can be seen only by the foveal area under the proper conditions (see Figure 8.24). Therefore, the center of the preceived pattern represents the center of the fovea.

The macular intergrity tester-trainer (MIT) is a motor-driven rotating Polaroid filter (Griffin 1982) (see Figure 8.24). The patient wears a blue filter over the tested eye and, while looking at a fixation spot, is asked whether he or she sees a propeller or brushes rotating either clockwise or counterclockwise. A central fixator sees the brush superimposed over the fixation point (Figure 8.24*A*). An eccentric fixator will not perceive the center of the brushes to be coincident with the fixation point (Figure 8.24*B*). Unfortunately, the subjective nature of this test allows younger amblyopes to make up responses to please the examiner. To prevent this, one should *not* test the good eye first for demonstration purposes, since the child will know what is supposed to be seen with the

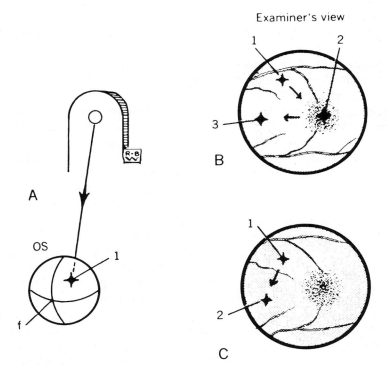

Figure 8.23   (A) *To determine whether eccentric viewing or eccentric fixation is present in the left amblyopic eye, the examiner projects the visuoscope asterisk onto the paramacular retinal region (1) of the patient. The sound eye is occluded. (B) The patient is requested to look directly at the asterisk (1) while the examiner observes the fundus through the visuoscope. First, the patient responds with an eye movement that will place the image of the fixation target on the fovea (2), where it is only dimly seen by the patient because of reduced foveal function (scotoma, organic lesion). Second, the eye will move in such a manner as to place the image from the fovea onto paramacular retinal elements (3), where visual acuity may be better than in the fovea. Eccentric viewing is present. (C) The first eye movement displaces the asterisk directly from (1) to (2), thus excluding the fovea from the act of fixation. The fixation reflex has adapted itself to paramacular nasal retinal elements. Eccentric fixation is present. (Reprinted, with permission of the publisher, from von Noorden 1977.)*

amblyopic eye. In addition, the perceived rotation of the brushes can be reversed by placing a quarter-wave plate over the eye or target (some clear plastic wrappers work well) to prevent such responses.

Again, the direction, degree, and stability of fixation are ascertained. The patient is asked to place the top of a pointer on the fixation target while fixation on the target is maintained. If this is done smoothly and without hesitation by an eccentric fixator, the primary visual direction and zero retinomotor value are probably associated with the eccentric point. The patient should then be asked

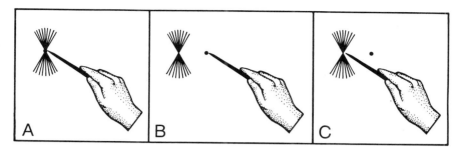

Figure 8.24 *Pointing task with Haidinger brush. Patient is instructed to align the pointer (P) with the Haidinger brush (HB) superimposed on the fixation point (F). (A) Central fixator with brush, pointer, and fixation point all aligned. (B) Eccentric fixator with the primary visual direction at the eccentric point. HB, which represents the fovea, is not superimposed with the fixation point, which represents the eccentric fixation point. (C) Scenario that may occur midtherapy during the process of disrupting the eccentric fixation. P and HB are aligned and appear to be straight ahead to the patient; however, fixation is still eccentric.*

if the fixation target and pointer tip appear to be straight ahead. If they do, the PVD is at the eccentric point. If the pointer tip initially misses the target, the ZRM point is not at the eccentric point. It is extremely rare for a true eccentric fixator (brushes and fixation point never overlap) to have the PVD at the fovea. However, this can occur during therapy while in the process of "breaking down" eccentric fixation (Figure 8.24C) (Selenow and Ciuffreda 1986). Pointing should be tested with both the dominant and nondominant hands, since there is often a discrepancy in the quality of the response. If the quality of the response is less when pointing with the nondominant hand, this should be noted, since this will be a starting point for breaking down the eccentric fixation.

Maxwell's Spot

This entoptic phenomenon is seen as a dark-purple spot corresponding to the fovea when the eye is exposed to a diffuse blue or purple field (Walls and Matthaws 1952). As with the Haidinger's brush (Figure 8.25), the spot represents a projection of the fovea into visual space and is similarly used to assess fixation status. This is difficult for many to visualize.

Goldrich Contour Rotator (GCR)

The GCR provides direct visual feedback regarding eye position and motion, which emerges from a slowly rotating matrix of dots including the perceptual illusion of a vividly rotating cross-shaped contour (Goldrich 1981) (Figure 8.26). Eccentric fixators report the center of the emergent cross to be off to the side of the fixation target; thus the magnitude of eccentric fixation can be determined. In addition, the GCR provides strabismic amblyopes with nystagmus an easy and

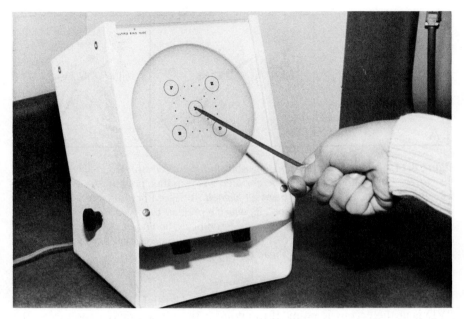

Figure 8.25   *Bernell macular integrity tester trainer (MIT) instrument with five fixation points, a perceived Haidinger brush, and patient's pointer.*

continuous means of experiencing the visual consequences of their abnormal ocular movements. The apparent movement of the cross is correlated with the eye movements, and thus for the first time the patient can "visualize" the nystagmus.

Owing to the subtle nature of some of these tests of fixation, young children may initially fail to appreciate the effect. The examiner must be persistent, and eventually after multiple exposures, the expected phenomenon can usually be seen. Sometimes it is not reported until after several weeks of vision therapy, when the amblyopic eye is more facile at figure/ground tasks.

MONOCULAR SPATIAL DISTORTION

We began this chapter by stating that functional amblyopia can no longer be simply considered an impairment of visual acuity alone. The following characteristics have led some researchers to suggest that monocular spatial distortion is the *primary* abnormality in strabismic amblyopia (Bedell et al. 1985):

1. Visual acuity itself varies according to the type of target used.
2. Regardless of the type of target used, there is no clear visual acuity cutoff point.
3. The oculomotor system is inaccurate with respect to fixation and tracking ability (Bedell and Flom 1983).

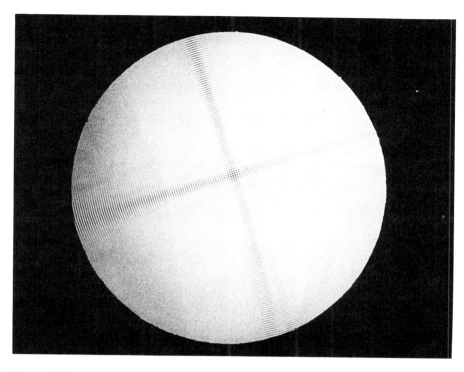

Figure 8.26 *Emergent textural contour. Center of cross represents patient's fovea. (Reprinted, with permission of the publisher, from Goldrich 1981.)*

4. The amblyopic eye has difficulty performing visually guided tasks that manifests itself as *spatial distortion* (over- and underestimation of visual space in the nasal and temporal field), *fixation directionalization errors* (offset bias), and *spatial uncertainty* (offset variability).

Bedell and Flom (1981) noted that the motor and sensory abnormalities commonly found in amblyopic eyes are difficult to explain solely on the basis of a reduction in visual acuity alone, since they cannot be produced in normal eyes when visual acuity is *artificially* lowered by decreasing luminance or introducing optical blur (Leibowitz et al. 1955, Stigmar 1971, Winterson and Steinman 1978, Post and Liebowitz 1980, Williams et al. 1984). The monocular spatial distortions occur only when both amblyopia and strabismus are present; they have not been found in amblyopes without strabismus or strabismics without amblyopia (Levi and Klein 1982, Bedell and Flom 1983). The laboratory testing and measurement of monocular spatial distortion are accomplished by the following two procedures:

1. *Spatial uncertainty and direction error.* Subjects are asked to judge the horizontal location of a small, briefly flashed, luminous vertical line with respect

to the vertical axis of an hourglass-shaped reference target (Figure 8.27). The mean alignment error and variability are greater in the amblyopic eye than in either the fellow dominant eye or each eye of visually normal individuals (Bedell and Flom 1981).

2. *Monocular distortion.* A monocular partition paradigm is used. Subjects are asked to fixate the central one of three horizontally separated luminous vertical lines (Figure 8.28*A*). The position of the right-hand line is fixed. The subject's task is to adjust the left-hand line until the space between it and the

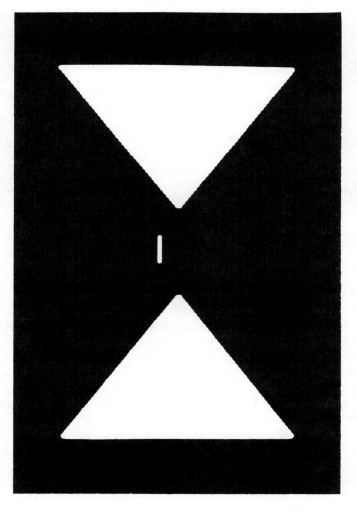

Figure 8.27 *Spatial uncertainty and directional error or bias determined by having the subject align the small vertical line with the inward-directed points of the hourglass-shaped reference target. (Reprinted, with permission of the publisher, from Bedell and Flom 1981.)*

fixation line is perceptually equal to the fixed space. This is repeated at several eccentricities, and the results for each eye are plotted and compared (Figure 8.28*B*). The amblyopic eye shows distortion over the central few degrees of visual field.

While it is true that monocular spatial distortion may be a *contributing* factor to some of the abnormal motor (e.g., saccadic tracking) and sensory (e.g., direction tasks) characteristics of the strabismic amblyope, it does not explain the amblyopic eye's deficits with respect to accommodation, contrast sensitivity, some aspects of eye movement (saccadic intrusions), and suprathreshold target fading, but most importantly, visual acuity, the hallmark sign of amblyopia. For example, if the horizontal line segments of the Snellen E are either parallel or bent and distorted, the patient should still be able to determine the E's orientation by detecting the direction of the luminance irregularities on its one side (Fry 1948). The primary overall effect of habitual binocular suppression cannot be overlooked. Further, if these distortions are the primary abnormality in amblyopia (especially strabismic), then they should reduce considerably, and perhaps be correlated with changes in visual acuity, during the course of successful orthoptic therapy. Thus far, however, this has *not* been our clinical impression.

Clinically, these patients may report spatial and contrast asymmetry when viewing a row of letters. Typically, letters falling on the nasal retina are perceived by the esotropic strabismic amblyope to appear closer together and to have less contrast than letters falling on the presumably less-affected temporal retina (Figure 8.29).

Clinically, we have used the following two procedures to obtain some insight into the amblyopic eye's abnormal direction sense:

A

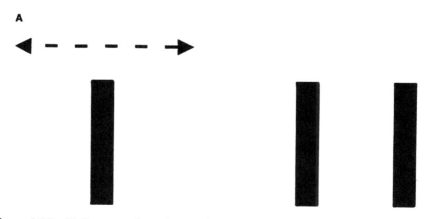

Figure 8.28 (A) *Target configuration used to measure monocular distortion. Position of the right-hand line is fixed. The subject's task is to adjust the left-hand line such that the space between it and the fixation line* (center line) *is perceptually equal to the fixed space on the right.*

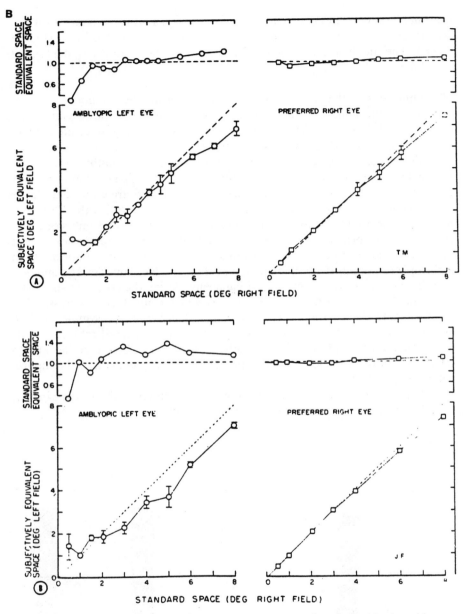

Figure 8.28   (B) *Results of monocular partitioning responses for two strabismic amblyopes. Monocular partition settings (±1 SD) are plotted as the size of the space in the left field (ordinate) that was judged equivalent to a standard space in the right field (abscissa). Shown is the ratio of the standard to the equivalent space for each standard space matched. The settings for the two amblyopic eyes reveal marked and nonuniform spatial asymmetries; settings for the preferred eyes are much closer to physical matches (indicated by the dashed lines above and below). (Reprinted, with permission of the publisher, from Bedell and Flom 1981.)*

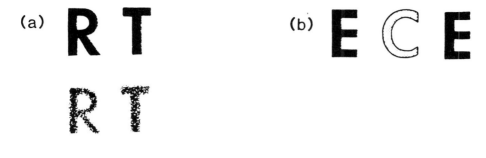

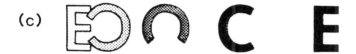

Figure 8.29   *Appearance of visual acuity test chart letters under three different conditions during monocular viewing with the amblyopic eye. (A) Sharp contours during foveal fixation (above) and diffuse contours during eccentric fixation (below). (B) Reduced perceived contrast of the fixated letter C due to presumed inhibitory interactions of the flanking letters. (C) Perceived contrast gradient and spatial asymmetry when fixating the reversed C with the eccentric point. (Reprinted, with permission of the publisher, from Selenow and Ciuffreda 1986.)*

    1.   *Amsler grid.* With the proper *near* correction over the amblyopic eye, the perception of the grid is compared between each eye monocularly. Amblyopes may report localized expansions, compressions, and bending of the parallel lines. They are asked to draw what they see (with the amblyopic eye viewing during the drawing), so that any changes in these distortions can be monitored throughout therapy and correlated with other changes in sensory (e.g., visual acuity) and motor (e.g., saccadic tracking) status of the amblyopic eye. One must be careful to rule out Amsler grid distortions secondary to maculopathy.

    2.   *Monocular disparometer.* To quantify the central offset error, the patient attempts to align the two vertical lines of the Sheedy disparameter monocularly (Figure 8.30). Twelve measurements are taken, six starting at different amounts from the right and six from the left. The two extreme values are discarded, and an average of the remaining ten is noted (in minutes of arc). Each increment on the Sheedy disparometer is 2 minutes of arc. This procedure has given us a satisfactory *clinical* measure of accuracy (degree of error) and precision (degree of variability) in some amblyopes.

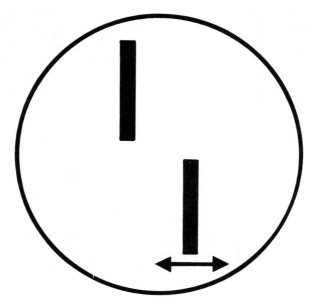

Figure 8.30 *Use of Sheedy disparometer for quantification of monocular central offset error. Patient monocularly fixates lower tip of top stationary vertical line while attempting to align vertically the bottom movable line. Offsets change in increments of 2 minutes of arc.*

BINOCULARITY

The assessment of binocularity can be divided into two major components: *motor*, which consists of the cover test at distance and near with and without various probe lenses, and *sensory*, which includes tests of stereopsis, anomalous retinal correspondence, and depth of suppression. The motor part of the evaluation of binocularity is important for determining whether or not the presence of strabismus was the cause of the amblyopia. A strabismus that is either intermittent, alternating, or periodic cannot be labeled as a cause of amblyopia. On the other hand, the sensory part of the binocular evaluation will influence one's treatment strategy of avoiding diplopia as visual acuity in the amblyopic eye improves. In addition, the sensory evaluation will help one determine what binocular state to leave the patient in, so that any regression of vision function is minimized. Hopefully, stereopsis or alternation of fixation can be achieved by the end of successful therapy.

Motor

Cover Test

It is important to perform a cover test *before* visual acuity is tested. Even a very brief period of occlusion (to perform the acuity test) can "break down" an intermittent strabismus so that it appears to be constant. The first sweep of the cover is the most critical one. Beginning with the unilateral cover test, the cover first goes over the dominant eye, while the examiner carefully observes any movement of the amblyopic eye. If there is movement, the patient has strabismus. Next, the amblyopic eye is observed as the cover is removed from the dominant eye. If it immediately moves, there is no alternation. If it does not move initially, but does so after the patient is told to blink several times, the patient is a forced alternator. If this is so, the prognosis is good for converting the patient into a natural alternator and thereby minimizing posttherapy regression of vision function. If there is no eye movement even after blinking, the patient is a true alternator. Therefore, the strabismus is not the primary cause of the amblyopia. This whole sequence is repeated several times to establish whether the strabismus is constant or intermittent at both distance and near. The high-contrast target used for fixation during the cover test should be at or just above the identification threshold level of the amblyopic eye.

Although the alternate cover test is typically used for measuring the degree of strabismus with prisms, the presence of anomalous fusional eye movements can contaminate the results (Bagolini 1967). This "eating up" of the prism (Campos and Catellani 1978), which exaggerates the amount of prism needed to neutralize the angle of strabismus, can be minimized by keeping the prism over the amblyopic eye while the dominant eye is covered. One then quickly switches the cover to the amblyopic eye, while the dominant eye is observed for any movement. If an anomalous fusional response still persists, the following sequence should be attempted. With both eyes open, the prism bar (with the estimated prismatic correction) and cover are *simultaneously* placed over the amblyopic and dominant eyes respectively, as the amblyopic eye is observed for eventual neutrality. In this way, the disparity or fusional vergence system is open looped whenever the patient is looking through a prism, thus preventing the initiation of disparity-driven anomalous fusional responses.

If there is no movement on the unilateral cover test in the presence of eccentric fixation, the diagnosis is microtropia (Helveston and von Noorden 1967). The area of ultrasmall angles of strabismus is, to say the least, a confusing one. Names such as *microstrabismus* (Irvine 1948), *retinal slip* (Pugh 1936), *fixation disparity* (Jampolsky 1956), *monofixational syndrome* (Parks 1969), and *microtropia* (Lang 1961) have been used interchangeably. The diagnostic tests and signs associated with these conditions have included various types and/or amounts of response with respect to stereopsis, anomalous retinal correspondence, four base-out test, visuoscopy, cover test, peripheral fusion, visual acuity, and central suppression. To clarify matters, Helveston and von Noorden (1967) suggested that the term *microtropia* be used for the specific case in which there is no movement on the cover test in the presence of eccentric fixation and harmonious ARC. It is our clinical impression that to make a diagnosis of microtropia, one needs to meet only *two* criteria: (1) no movement on the cover test and (2) the presence of steady eccentric fixation. Whether the patient has HARC, UHARC, or suppression does not help in making the diagnosis. In addition, we have found the four base-out test to provide very little useful or new information. A positive response means that the amblyopic eye is suppressing an image placed near the fovea when the dominant eye is not occluded. However, since we are performing the test due to the presence of monocular (obligatory) suppression (amblyopia), which is always accompanied by binocular (facultative) suppression, the test has no real diagnostic value. A positive response can be a result of any of the following diagnoses: microtropia, small-angle esotropia, macular hole, anisometropic amblyopia, or optic atrophy. Therefore, we feel that the four base-out test is not very useful as a diagnostic test. However, we do find it valuable for monitoring changes in the angular magnitude of the binocular suppression area during the course of amblyopia therapy.

Sensory

Stereopsis

This should be assessed *before* the cover test is performed, since binocularity can be easily disrupted during the cover test per se, especially when the test is repeated many times. If the patient achieves any degree of Randot stereopsis (Griffin 1982), the prognosis for absence of any posttherapy regression of vision function is excellent. The same is true if stereoscopic acuity (Titmus Stereo Test; Griffin 1982) of 70 seconds of arc or better is obtained (Simons and Reinecke 1974) owing to monocular cues. When the amount of anisometropia is greater than 2.5 diopters, stereopsis should be tested through a contact lens prescription. In addition, strabismics should be tested through full correcting prisms.

Correspondence/Suppression

There are many tests that are traditionally used to assess retinal correspondence. Table 8.11 lists eight of the most commonly used correspondence tests in approximately decreasing order of "naturalness" (i.e, normal viewing conditions). All can be used with central fixators; however, when dealing with an eccentric fixator, the following considerations need to be taken into account.

Tests 1 to 5 use a comparison of the objective angle (angle H) to the subjective angle (angle S) to assess correspondence. However, angle H is typically underestimated in strabismics with eccentric fixation (assuming the direction of eccentricity and strabismus is the same). Therefore, to obtain the true value, the degree of eccentric fixation must be added to the measured amount in order to get the true angle H. Table 8.11 summarizes the feasability of using these tests on a therapeutic basis in the office and at home. The afterimage test (no. 8) is not recommended for eccentric fixators, since it assumes that the fovea of each eye is being "tagged" with an afterimage. The bifoveal test of Cuppers (Figure 8.31) and the MIT afterimage transfer test (Figure 8.32) eliminate the

Table 8.11 Tests for Correspondence

Test	EF Accountability	Therapeutic Use	Home Use	Comments
Spontaneous diplopia	Add degree of EF to angle *H*	Good	Yes	Rare unless associated with mild amblyopia.
Bagolini striated lenses	Add degree of EF to angle *H*	Fair	Yes	If suppression occurs, add filter to dominant eye; however, this will decrease the degree of naturalness.
Vectographic presentations	Add degree of EF to angle *H*	Good	Yes	No control over suppression, since polarizing filters of each eye are equal.
Colored filters	Add degree of EF to angle *H*	Good	Yes	Good control over suppression.
Major amblyoscope	Add degree of EF to angle *H*	Good	No	Can use portable mirror stereoscope for home therapy, with red-green filters for suppression.
Bifoveal test of Cuppers	Degree of EF is accounted for	Poor	No	Requires excellent patient cooperation.
MIT afterimage transfer test	Degree of EF is accounted for	Fair	Yes	Requires excellent patient cooperation.
Hering-Bielschowsky afterimage test	Not valid with eccentric fixation	Fair	Yes	

problem of eccentric fixation by testing correspondence under *binocular* conditions. Since eccentric fixation is a monocular phenomenon, it does not affect these two binocular tests where the angle of anomaly is directly measured.

Bifoveal Test of Cuppers

The dominant eye fixates a penlight off to the side through an angled mirror or a BO prism. The examiner looks into the amblyopic eye with a visuoscope, projects the fixation target onto the fovea, and asks the patient what he or she sees. The patient must be aware of the penlight and fixation target simultaneously. If they are superimposed, the diagnosis is normal retinal correspondence (NRC). If not, the fixation target is moved in the appropriate direction until superimposition is noted by the patient. The distance between the visuoscope target location and the anatomic fovea represents the angle of anomaly

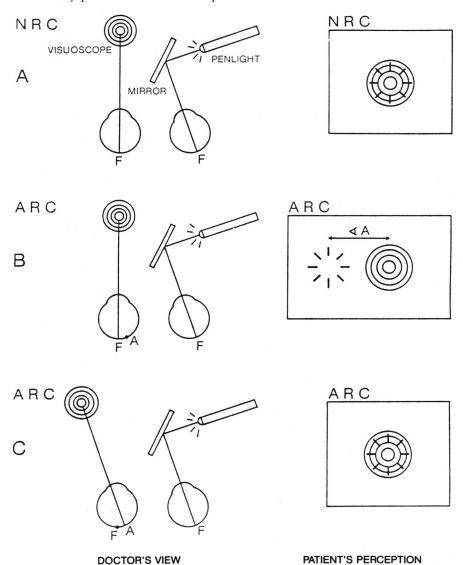

DOCTOR'S VIEW   **PATIENT'S PERCEPTION**

Figure 8.31 *Bifoveal test of Cuppers. Prism or mirror allows examiner to place visuoscope target on fovea of patient's amblyopic left eye while patient is simultaneously aware of penlight seen by dominant right eye. Left is examiner's view and right is what patient appears to be seeing (F = fovea; A = point of anomaly). (A) Left esotropic amblyope with NRC. (B) Left esotropic amblyope with ARC; visuoscopic target projected over fovea of amblyopic eye. (C) Left esotropic amblyope with ARC; visuoscopic target projected over point of anomaly.*

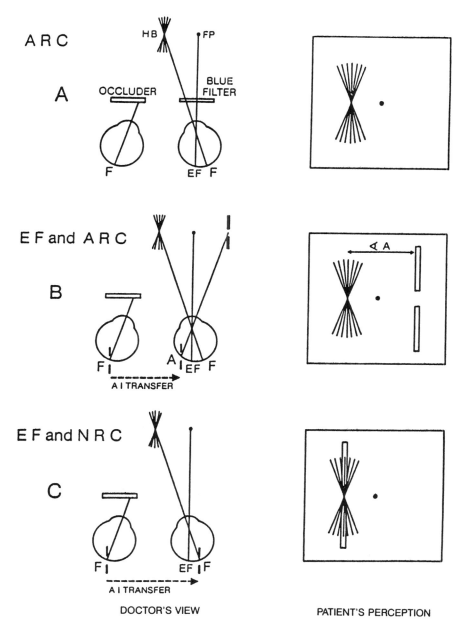

Figure 8.32 *MIT afterimage transfer test. Patient is instructed to note position of Haidinger brush (HB), transferred afterimage (AI), and fixation point (FP). (F = fovea; E = point of eccentric fixation; A = point of anomaly.) Left is examiner's view, and right is what patient appears to be seeing. (A) Use of HB to test for presence of eccentric fixation. (B) Use of HB and transferred afterimage in patient with nasal eccentric fixation and ARC. (C) Use of HB and AI in patient with nasal eccentric fixation and NRC.*

(angle *A*). This angle is measured by use of the visuoscope reticules or is estimated by comparing the angle to the width of the optic nerve head (5.5 degrees) and/or distance of the fovea to the center of the nerve head.

MIT Afterimage Transfer Test

The dominant eye is flashed with a vertical line strobe producing a vertical afterimage (A.I.). With the dominant eye occluded and a blue filter over the amblyopic eye, the patient fixates a dot on the MIT and notes the relationship between the Haidinger brush (H.B.), fixation dot, and transferred afterimage. If the Haidinger brush and afterimage are superimposed, the diagnosis is normal retinal correspondence. This distance between the Haidinger brush and afterimage is the angle of anomaly.

Clinically, diplopia testing with colored filters is the most practical way of handling problems of correspondence and/or suppression during the course of amblyopia therapy for the following reasons:

1. Suppression can be controlled by easily varying the filter density over the dominant eye.
2. Target size is simple to vary starting with large, bright targets that are easy to fuse and eventually working toward small, dim targets.
3. The setup is portable, thus allowing for daily home training.
4. The training is done in free space, which provides the patient with an opportunity to practice fusing diplopic images under natural situations. Avoiding diplopia as visual acuity in the amblyopic eye improves is a major objective.

The following diagnostic sequence will not only provide the therapist with an assessment of correspondence, but also will enable a channeling of the sensory system into a direction that will be compatible with the expected visual acuity improvement in the amblyopic eye. In addition, avoidance of fusion can be predicted, thereby avoiding intractable diplopia. This procedure is not used for measuring the subjective angle, since there are other procedures that give a more accurate measure. The patient stands approximately 20 feet from an illuminated projection visual acuity chart in a totally darkened room and is asked whether he or she sees two charts. If the patient reports diplopia, the sensory adaptation is extremely mild. Then a prism bar is gradually increased in power over the *dominant* eye until it "appears" that one chart has "slid" into the other chart. The patient is typically confused at first, not being sure whether one chart slid into the other or just disappeared (i.e., became suppressed). The examiner should not be concerned with whether there is suppression of one chart *after* the charts have become one, but must make sure that there is no suppression *before* the charts slide into one. Therefore, a positive prognostic indicator is the sliding of the diplopic images into a single binocular percept. If diplopia is *not* noticed, then a red filter is placed over the dominant eye to facilitate diplopia awareness and a prism bar is added with gradually increasing power until the charts slowly slide into one. This is repeated several times, so that the prismatic amount can be averaged and recorded as the patient's *subjective angle.* If diplopia is still not elicited, even with a red filter over the dominant eye, then a base-out prism of 15 prism diopters *greater than the objective angle* (assuming the patient is an eso-tropic amblyope) is placed over the dominant eye. The patient will report seeing two charts (one red and the other white) in crossed (heteronomous) diplopia. In effect, you have created a "sensory exotrope" (Pigassou-Albony 1976). Then have the patient concentrate on the white chart while being aware of the red one. It is easier to maintain diplopia when fixating with the nondominant eye, since sensory adaptations with fixation of the nondominant eye are milder (Greenwald 1979). The examiner then reduces the amount of base-out prism in front of the dominant eye. As this is done, the patient should notice the targets getting closer together. If one is higher, a vertical prism of the appropriate amount and direction is added over the dominant eye. Again, the examiner is looking for the amount of horizontal prism needed to allow the patient to perceive the sliding of the two targets into one. The fact that, once superim-posed, the red image of the dominant eye will be more evident and effective than the white one is of no concern at this time. All one needs to be concerned with is whether a situation can be created whereby the images of the two targets can be made to fuse slowly into one binocular percept. If one of the targets tends to disappear *before* it slides into the other, then the patient should slowly walk toward the targets while they are still near one another. This should cause the targets to appear closer and eventually slide "automatically" into one. Then have the patient slowly walk away, and the target will again become diplopic. This threshold distance for fusion and the prism amount should be recorded.

During the course of amblyopia therapy, there are three primary goals toward which the clinician can direct the binocular training phase: stereopsis, alternation, or enhancement of anomalous retinal correspondence. The binoc-ular evaluation should indicate which binocular route to choose and what state to leave the binocular system in once the amblyopic therapy has been terminated.

An amblyopia evaluation form (Table 8.12) is helpful in placing each case in the proper perspective. Once the diagnostic battery has been completed, the clinician can come up with an overall monocular and binocular treatment plan and then discuss the prognosis with the patient.

AMBLYOPIA SCREENING

There are presently no consistent screening criteria for amblyopia detection. This is mainly due to the following reason (Simons and Reinecke 1978): An ideal screening should be effective at the maximally treatable stage of amblyopia development. Studies show that treatment success is greatest when undertaken before 3 years of age (Parks and Friendly 1966, von Noorden 1973). However, studies also show that subjective screening tests are relatively unreliable in

Table 8.12   Amblyopia Evaluation

				Comments	*Prognosis*
I.	History:				
	When anomaly began	_____			
	When treatment began	_____			
	Description & success of treatment	_____			
	Compliance	_____			
II.	Visual Acuity:				
		OD		OS	
	Prescription				
	Snellen				
	(WC; WL; SL)				
	S-Chart				
	Laser				
	ND Filter (%S-S)				

III.	Accommodation:				
	Amplitude	(−)Lens	Dyn-R-Scope	(−)Lens	Dyn-R-Scope
	Facility	+ 1.5	− 1.5	+1.5	− 1.5
	(pass/fail)				

IV.	Fixation:
	Visuoscope:
	Degree + bias
	% Foveation
	Pattern
	PVD
	Haidinger brush
	Maxwell spot
V.	Spatial Distortion:
	Amsler grid
	Disparometer

VI.	Binocularity:	*Probe Lenses*	
	Cover test		
	Stereopsis	Wirt	Randot
	R-G fusion		
	Alternation		

Summary:
  Etiology
  Prognosis
  Monoc Tx plan
  Binoc Tx plan

children under the age of 3 years (Nawratski and Oliver 1972). Therefore, one is faced with the problem of not being able to screen reliably during the maximally treatable age. One way to circumvent this problem is by lowering and/or simplifying the screening criteria. However, this will lead to an increased number of false-negative results.

Several early screening strategies have been proposed. Cover-test adminis-tration by pediatricians seems to be a means of early strabismus detection. However, in a study by Kohler and Stigmar (1973), pediatricians performing the cover test did *not* detect *any* of the 44 strabismics in the study. The preferential looking technique has been used successfully to measure binocular visual acuity in infants (Teller 1979). Unfortunately, this technique is not practical for use with large screening populations because of time and cooperation require-ments. In addition, both monocular *and* binocular acuity are needed for ambly-opia detection.

It seems evident that an ideal amblyopia/strabismus screening should take place at approximately 3 years of age and involve a multiple test battery (see below), since a diagnosis based on one test alone results in a weak diagnosis.

Function Tested	Test Probe
History	Examiner's acumen
Visual acuity	Broken wheel acuity test
Ocular alignment	Cover test
Fixation status	Visuoscopy
Objective refraction	Retinoscopy
Stereopsis	Randot E test
Ocular health	Penlight/ophthalmoscopy (external/internal)

The following is a brief description of the screening procedures. See Table 8.13 for details and criteria. We have found the following test sequence to be best:

History   There are three main questions that need to be answered by parents:

1. Are there any indications of amblyopia or squint such as the report of diplopia, frequent closing of one eye, and/or observation of either eye turning in or out?
2. Is there a family history of amblyopia or strabismus? Stricter criteria with closer follow-up may be in order if there is a possible family history, thus putting the child in the "high risk" or "at risk" grouping.
3. Was there any previous therapy?

Stereopsis   Reinecke and Simons (1974) have found the random dot E test to be an accurate screening procedure for general binocular dysfunction in preschool populations. Clinically, this test is easy to administer even by nontrained personnel.

Ocular Alignment   Distance and near cover testing is needed for two main rea-sons: (1) to assess whether strabismus is the cause of an existing amblyopia, and (2) to prevent future amblyopia development by screening for intermittent squint.

Again, the use of highly skilled professional personnel is a must, since even pediatricians are likely to miss more subtle strabismus (Kohler and Stigmar 1973).

Table 8.13   Screening

Test	Pass	Fail	Administration	Test Type
Stereopsis	Four in a row correct	Less than four in a row correct	Lay personnel	Random dot E test
Monocular visual acuity	20/25 or better in each eye	20/40 or worse in either eye	Lay personnel	Broken wheel acuity test
Cover test	Heterophoria between 10 XP and 6 EP at distance and near	All strabismus; heterophoria >10 XP or >6 EP	Highly skilled examiner	Small, fine-detailed accommo-dative target at distance and near
Objective refraction	Less than indicated by criteria under "fail"	≥2 diopters hyperopia or ≥1 diopter of myopia, anisome-tropia, or astigmatism	Highly skilled examiner	Retinoscopy with lens rack viewing a distant target
Fixation	Central fixation	EF	Highly skilled examiner	Visuoscopy; auxiliary test to be performed only if fails visual acuity but passes cover test and retinoscopy

Visual Acuity   The broken wheel acuity test uses a forced-choice, nonverbal procedure to assess monocular visual acuity in preschool children (Richman et al. 1984). The authors and many others have found this test to be the most successful means of visual acuity assessment in 3-year-olds. In addition, it can be administered by nontrained personnel. Acuity levels are 20/20, 20/25, 20/30, 20/40, 20/60, 20/80, 20/100 and 20/120.

Refraction   Ingram (1977) has proposed the use of refraction as an objective screening method for amblyopia and strabismus detection. The presence of 2 or more diopters of spherical hypermetropia in both eyes or 1 or more diopters of either spherical or cylindrical anisometropia was significantly associated with that child being identified 2 years later as having either amblyopia, squint, or both. Of course, retinoscopy requires the use of highly skilled professional personnel, not the school nurse, a teacher, or a layperson.

Penlight and Ophthalmoscopy   This is used to detect external (e.g., corneal leukoma) and internal (e.g., retinal disease) structural/disease aspects that might be responsible for the presence of reduced visual acuity and/or strabismus.

Visuoscopy This test is only necessary if the child fails visual acuity but passes refraction and cover testing. In this case, one is looking for microtropia. Although it is rare for a microtrope to pass the random-dot test, visuoscopy provides the definitive diagnosis of microtropia, which then allows one to classify the patient as strabismic. As mentioned in Chapter 1, the failure to classify microtropes as strabismic amblyopes has been a problem with previous studies.

It is important that stereopsis be tested first (after case history), since the other tests are capable of disrupting binocularity, which in turn would have an adverse effect on stereopsis. Similarly, visual acuity is tested *after* the cover test, since alternate occlusion of the eyes during this test of vision is also capable of disrupting binocularity.

REFERENCES

Alpern M, Petraukas RR, Sandall GS, Vorenkamo RJ. (1967) Recent experiments on the physiology of strabismus and amblyopia. *Am. Orthopt. J.* 17:62–72.

Ammann E. (1921) Einige Beobachtunger bei den Funtion sprufungen in der Sprech-sturde: Zentrales Sehen-sehen der glaukomatosen—schen der Amblyopen. *Klin. Monatsbl. Augenheilkd.* 66:564–73.

Avetisov ES. (1979) Visual acuity and contrast sensitivity of the amblyopic eye as a function of the stimulated region of the retina. Trans. by Kirschen DG, Shlyakhov ED, Flom MC. *Am. J. Optom. Physiol. Opt.* 56:465–469.

Awaya S, Intake Y, Imaizumi Y, Shiose Y, Karda T, Komuro K. (1973) Amblyopia in man: suggestive of stimulus deprivation amblyopia. *Jpn. J. Ophthalmol.* 17:69–82.

Bagolini B. (1967) Anomalous retinal correspondence: definition and diagnostic methods. *Doc. Ophthalmol.* 23:346–98.

Bagolino P, Capobianco N. (1975) The Effect of Prisms in the Treatment of Squint (Anomalous Movements). In Moore S, Mein J, Stockbridge L (Eds.), *Orthoptics: Past, Present, Future.* New York: Intercontinental.

Baldwin WR. (1962) Pleoptics: Historical developments and overview of the literature. *Am. J. Optom.* 39:149–62.

Bangerter A. (1953) Uber pleoptik. *Wiener Klin. Wochenschr.* 65:966–982.

Bedell HE. (1982) Symmetry of acuity profiles in esotropic amblyopic eyes. *Human Neurobiol.* 1:221–4.

Bedell HE, Flom MC. (1981) Monocular spatial distortion in strabismic amblyopia. *Invest. Ophthalmol. Vis. Sci.* 20:263–8.

Bedell HE, Flom MC. (1983) Normal and abnormal space perception. *Am. J. Optom. Physiol. Opt.* 60:426–35.

Bedell HE, Flom MC, Barbeito R. (1985) Spatial aberrations and acuity in strabismus and amblyopia. *Invest. Ophthalmol. Vis. Sci.* 27:909–16.

Borish I. (1970) *Clinical Refraction*, 3d Ed. Chicago: Professional Press.

Brock FW, Givner I. (1952) Fixation anomalies in amblyopia. *Arch. Ophthalmol.* 47:1465–6.

Callahan W, Berry D. (1968) The value of visual stimulation during constant and direct occlusion. *Am. Orthopt. J.* 18:73–4.

Caloroso E, Flom MC. (1969) Influence of luminance on visual acuity in amblyopia. *Am. J. Optom.* 46:189–95.

Campos EC, Catellani T. (1978) Further evidence for the fusional nature of the compensation (or "eating up") of prisms in concomitant strabismus. *Int. Ophthalmol.* 1:57–62.

Chavasse FB. (1939) *Worth's Squint*, 7th Ed., Philadelphia, Blakiston.

Cibis L, Hurtt J, Rasicovici A. (1968) A clinical study of separation difficulty in organic and functional amblyopia. *Am. Orthopt. J.* 18:66–72.

Ciuffreda KJ. (1986) Visual System Plasticity in Human Amblyopia. In Hilfer R, Sheffield J (Eds.), *Development of Order in the Visual System.* New York: Springer-Verlag.

Ciuffreda KJ, Kenyon RV. (1983) Accommodative Vergence and Accommodation in Normals, Amblyopes, and Strabismics. In Schor CM, Ciuffreda KJ (Eds.), *Vergence Eye Movements: Basic and Clinical Aspects*, pp. 101–173. Boston: Butterworth.

Ciuffreda KJ, Goldrich SG. (1983) Oculomotor biofeedback therapy. *Int. Rehabil. Med.* 5:111–17.

Ciuffreda KJ, Kellndorfer J, Rumpf D. (1987) Contrast and Accommodation. In Stark L, Obrecht G (Eds.), *Presbyopia*, pp. 116–22. New York: Professional Press.

Ciuffreda KJ, Kenyon RV, Stark L. (1979a) Abnormal saccadic substitution during small-amplitude pursuit tracking in amblyopic eyes. *Invest. Ophthalmol. Vis. Sci.* 18:506–16.

Ciuffreda KJ, Kenyon RV, Stark L. (1979b) Fixational eye movements in amblyopia and strabismus. *J. Am. Optom. Assoc.* 50:1251–8.

Cuppers C. (1956) Moderne Schielbehandling. *Klin. Monatsbl. Augenheilkd.* 5:579–604.

Czellitzer A. (1923) Wle verebt sich Schielen. *Arch. Eassen. Ges. Biol.* 14:377–386.

Davidson DW, Eskridge JB. (1977) Reliability of visual acuity measures of amblyopic eyes. *Am. J. Optom. Physiol. Opt.* 54:756–66.

Feinberg JB. (1949) Further studies in amblyopia. *Am. J. Ophthalmol.* 32:1394–8.

Feldman JB, Taylor AF. (1942) Obstacle to squint training: Amblyopia. *Arch. Ophthalmol.* 27:851–68.

Finney DJ. (1971) *Probit Analysis*, 3d Ed. Cambridge: Cambridge University Press

Flom MC. (1966) New concepts in visual acuity. *Optom. Weekly* 57:63–8.

Flom MC. (1978) Eccentric fixation in amblyopia: Is reduced foveal acuity the cause? *Am. J. Optom. Physiol. Opt.* 55:139–43.

Flom MC, Weymouth FW. (1961) Centricity of Maxwell's spot in strabismus and amblyopia. *Arch. Ophthalmol.* 66:260–8.

Flom MC, Heath GG, Takahashi E. (1963a) Contour interaction and visual resolution: Contralateral effects. *Science* 142:979–80.

Flom MC, Kirschen DG, Bedell HE. (1980) Acuity in eccentrically fixating amblyopes (Letter). *Am. J. Optom. Physiol. Opt.* 57:191–4.

Flom MC, Weymouth FW, Kahneman D. (1963b) Visual resolution and contour interaction. *J. Opt. Soc. Am.* 53:1026–32.

Francois J. (1961) *Heredity in Ophthalmology*. St. Louis: Mosby.

Francois J, James M. (1955) Comparative study of amblyopic treatment. *Am. Orthopt. J.* 5:61–4.

Fry GA. (1948) The significance of visual acuity measurements without glasses. *Am. J. Optom. Arch. Am. Acad. Optom.* 25:199–210.

Goldrich SG. (1981) Emergent textural contours: A new technique for visual monitoring in nystagmus, oculomotor dysfunction, and accommodative disorders. *Am. J. Optom. Physiol. Opt.* 58:451–9.

Gould A, Fishkoff D, Galin M. (1970) Active visual stimulation: A method of treatment of amblyopia in the older patient. *Am. Orthopt. J.* 20:39–45.

Greenwald I. (1979) *Effective Strabismus Therapy.* Duncan, Okla.: Optometric Extension Program.

Griffin JR. (1982) *Binocular Anomalies. Procedures for Vision Therapy.* Chicago: Professional Press.

Grutzner P, Yazawa K, Spivey BE. (1970) Heredity and strabismus. *Surv. Ophthalmol.* 14:450-2.

Gstalder RJ, Green DG. (1971) Laser interferometric acuity in amblyopia. *J. Pediatr. Ophthalmol.* 8:251-6.

Hallden LI. (1957) An explanation of Haidinger's brushes. *Arch. Ophthalmol.* 57:393-9.

Helveston EM, von Noorden GK. (1967) Microtropia: A newly defined entity. *Arch. Ophthalmol.* 78:272-81.

Hess RF, Bradley A. (1980) Contrast perception above threshold is only minimally impaired in human amblyopia. *Nature* 287:463-4.

Hess RF, Howell ER. (1977) The threshold contrast sensitivity function in strabismic amblyopia: Evidence for a two-type classification. *Vision Res.* 17:1049-55.

Hess RF, Jacobs RJ. (1979) A preliminary report of acuity and contour interaction across the amblyope's visual field. *Vision Res.* 19:1403-8.

Hess RF, Bradley A, Piotrowski L. (1983) Contrast coding in amblyopia: I. Differences in the neural basis of human amblyopia. *Proc. R. Soc. Lond.* 217:309-30.

Hess RF, Campbell FW, Zimmern R. (1980) Differences in the neuronal basis of human amblyopes: The effect of mean luminance. *Vision Res.* 20:295-305.

Hokoda SC, Ciuffreda KJ. (1985) Measurements of accommodative amplitude in amblyopia. *Ophthal. Physiol. Optics* 2:205-212.

Ingram RM. (1977) Refraction as a basis for screening children for squint and amblyopia. *Br. J. Ophthalmol.* 61:8-12.

Irvine RA. (1948) Amblyopia ex anopsia: Observations on retinal inhibition, scotoma, projection, light difference, discrimination and visual acuity. *Trans. Am. Ophthalmol. Soc.* 46:527-75.

Jagerman LS. (1970) Visual acuity measured with easy and difficult optotypes in normal and amblyopic eyes. *J. Pediatr. Ophthalmol.* 7:49-54.

Jampolsky A. (1956) Differential diagnosis and management of small degree esotropia and convergent fixation disparity. *Am. J. Ophthalmol.* 41:825-33.

Kirschen DG, Flom MC. (1978) Visual acuity at different retinal loci of eccentrically fixating functional amblyopes. *Am. J. Optom. Physiol. Opt.* 55:144-50.

Kivlin JD, Flynn JT. (1981) Therapy of anisometropic amblyopia. *J. Pediatr. Ophthalmol. Strabismus* 18:47-56.

Kohler L, Stigmar G. (1973) Vision screening of 4-year old children. *Acta. Pediatr. Scand.* 62:17-21.

Lang J. (1961) Amblyopia without strabismus and with inconspicuous small angle deviation. *Ophthalmologica* 141:429-34.

Lawwill T. (1966) The fixation pattern of the light-adapted and dark-adapted amblyopic eye. *Am. J. Ophthalmol.* 61:1416-19.

Lawwill T. (1968) Local adaptation in functional amblyopia. *Am. J. Ophthalmol.* 65:903-6.

Leibowitz HW, Myers NA, Grant DA. (1955) Radial localization of a single stimulus as a function of luminance and duration of exposure. *J. Opt. Soc. Am.* 45:76-8.

Levi DM. (1976) Occlusion amblyopia. *Am. J. Optom. Physiol. Opt.* 53:16-19.

Levi DM, Klein SA, Aitsebaomo AP. (1965) Vernier acuity, crowding and cortical magnification. *Vision Res.* 25:963–977.

Levi DM, Klein S. (1982) Difference in discrimination for gratings between strabismic and anisometropic amblyopes. *Invest. Ophthalmol. Vis. Sci.* 23:398–407.

Loshin DS, Levi DM. (1983) Suprathreshold contrast perception in functional amblyopia. *Doc. Ophthalmol.* 55:213–36.

Nawratski I, Oliver M. (1972) Screening for amblyopia in children under 3-years of age. *Sight Sav. Rev.* 42:14–19.

Nicholson J. (1919) Cited by Ravel (1971).

Parks MM. (1969) The monofixational syndrome. *Trans. Am. Ophthalmol. Soc.* 67:609–657.

Parks MM, Friendly DS. (1966) Treatment of eccentric fixation in children under 4 years of age. *Am. J. Ophthalmol.* 61:395–9.

Pigassou-Albouy R. (1976) The motor disturbances of squinters: Pathogenesis and treatment. *Klin. Monatsbl. Augenheilkd.* 169:468–81.

Post RB, Liebowitz HW. (1980) Independence of radial localization from refractive errors. *J. Opt. Soc. Am.* 70:1377–9.

Press LJ. (1983) Telescopic acuity in amblyopia. *J. Am. Optom. Assoc.* 54:411–4.

Priestly BS, Byron HM, Weseley AC. (1959) Pleoptic methods in the management of amblyopia with eccentric fixation. *Am. J. Ophthalmol.* 48:490–502.

Prince JH. (1962) Visual Acuity Contours in Amblyopia. In *Transactions of the International Optical Congress*, pp. 444–55. New York: Hafner.

Pugh MA. (1936) *Squint Training* New York: Oxford University Press.

Reinecke RD, Simons K. (1974) A new stereoscopic test for amblyopia screening. *Am. J. Ophthalmol.* 78:714–21.

Richman JE, Petito GT, Cron MT. (1984) Broken wheel acuity test: a new and valid test for preschool and exceptional children. *J. Am. Optom. Assoc.* 55:561–65.

Schapero M. (1971) *Amblyopia.* Philadelphia: Chilton.

Schlossman A. (1961) Prognosis, management and results of pleoptic treatment. *Int. Ophthalmol. Clin.* 1:8–15.

Schor CM. (1972) Oculomotor and Neurosensory Analysis of Amblyopia. Ph.D. dissertation. University of California, Berkeley.

Schor CM. (1978) A motor theory for monocular eccentric fixation of amblyopic eyes. *Am. J. Optom. Physiol. Opt.* 55:183–6.

Schor CM, Flom MC. (1975) Eye Position Control and Visual Acuity in Strabismic Amblyopia. In Lennerstrand G, Bach-y-rita P (Eds.), *Basic Mechanisms in Ocular Motility and Their Clinical Implications*, Vol. 24. New York: Pergamon Press.

Selenow A, Ciuffreda KJ, Mozlin R, Rumpf D. (1986) Prognostic value of laser interferometric visual acuity in amblyopia therapy. *Invest. Ophthalmol. Vis. Sci.* 27:273–7.

Simons K, Reinecke RD. (1978) Amblyopia Screening and Stereopsis. In *Symposium on Strabismus: Transactions of New Orleans Academy of Ophthalmology*, p. 15. St. Louis: Mosby.

Simons K, Reinecke RD. (1974) A reconsideration: amblyopia screening and stereopsis. *Am. J. Ophthalmol.* 78:707–13.

Sirenteau R, Fronius M. (1981) Nasotemporal asymmetries in human amblyopia: Consequence of long-term interocular suppression. *Vision Res.* 21:1055–63.

Smith WS. (1935) A basic technique in orthoptics: Parts I–IV. *Am. J. Optom.* 12:224–31, 321–31, 394–401, 473–80.

Smith JB. (1972) Treatment of Amblyopia with Low Vision Optical Aids. In Mein J, Bierlaagh J, Brummelkamp, Dons J (Eds.), *Orthoptics: Proceedings of the 2nd International Orthoptic Congress*, pp. 211–13. Amsterdam: Excerpta Medica.

Snell AC, Sterling S. (1925) The percentage evaluation of macular vision. *Arch. Ophthalmol.* 54:443–61.

Snellen H. (1988) *Test-Types for the Determination of Acuteness of Vision.* 4th Ed. London: Williams and Norgate.

Stigmar G. (1971) Blurred visual stimuli: II. The effect of blurred visual stimuli on Vernier and stereo acuity. *Acta Ophthalmol.* 49:364–79.

Stuart JA, Burian HM. (1962) A study of separation difficulty: Its relationship to visual acuity in normal and amblyopic eyes. *Am. J. Ophthalmol.* 53:471–7.

Teller DY. (1979) The forced-choice preferential looking procedure: a psychophysical technique for use with human infants. *Infant Behav. Devel.* 2:135–53.

Thomas J, Mohindra I, Held R. (1979) Strabismic amblyopia in infants. *Am. J. Optom. Physiol. Opt.* 56:197–201.

von Noorden GK. (1960) Pathophysiology of amblyopia: diagnostic and therapeutic principles of pleoptics. *Am. Orthopt. J.* 10:7–16.

von Noorden GK. (1965) Occlusion therapy in amblyopia with eccentric fixation. *Arch. Ophthalmol.* 73:776–81.

von Noorden GK. (1970) Etiology and pathogenesis of fixation anomalies in strabismus: I. Relationships between eccentric fixation and anomalous retinal correspondence. *Am. J. Ophthalmol.* 69:210–22.

von Noorden GK. (1973) Experimental amblyopia in monkeys: Further behavioral observations and clinical correlations. *Invest. Ophthalmol.* 12:721–6.

von Noorden GK. (1977) *von Noorden-Maumenee's Atlas of Strabismus.* St. Louis: Mosby.

von Noorden GK. (1980) *Burian-von Noorden's Binocular Vision and Ocular Motility.* St. Louis: Mosby.

von Noorden GK, Burian HM. (1959a) Visual acuity in normal and amblyopic patients under reduced illumination: I. Behavior of visual acuity with and without neutral density filter. *Arch. Ophthalmol.* 61:533–5.

von Noorden GK, Burian HM. (1959b) Visual acuity in normal and amblyopic patients under reduced illumination: II. The visual acuity at various levels of illumination. *Arch. Ophthalmol.* 62:396–9.

Walls GL, Matthaws RW. (1952) *New Means of Studying Color Blindness and Normal Foveal Color Vision.* Berkeley: University of California Press.

Wertheim T. (1894) Uber die indirekte sehccharfe. *Psychol. Physiol. Sinnesorgan.* 7:172–89.

Weymouth FW. (1958) Visual sensory units and the minimal angle of resolution. *Am. J. Ophthalmol.* 46:102–13.

Wick B, Schor CM. (1984) A comparison of the Snellen chart and the S-chart for visual acuity assessment in amblyopia. *J. Am. Optom. Assoc.* 55:359–61.

Wild BW. (1961) Pleoptic techniques and visual training. *J. Am. Optom. Assoc.* 32:457–60.

Williams RA, Enoch JM, Essock EA. (1984) The resistance of selected hyperacuity configurations to retinal image degradation. *Invest. Ophthalmol. Vis. Sci.* 25:389–99.

Winterson BJ, Steinman RM. (1978) The effect of luminance on human smooth pursuit of peripheral and foveal targets. *Vision Res.* 18:1165–72.

Worth CA. (1943) *Squint: Its Causes, Pathology and Treatment*, 7th Ed. Philadelphia: Blakiston.

Chapter 9

Treatment: History and Critical Evaluation

Since occlusion for the treatment of amblyopia was first suggested by Buffon in 1743, there has been extensive and often conflicting literature pertaining to the proper treatment of amblyopia. Several questions remain: Which eye should be patched? What is the best type of patch or occluder to use? How long (hours per day, total duration of patching) should the eye be patched? Should the stimulation be passive or active? If active, what type(s) and amount(s) of stimulation are most efficacious? And, perhaps the most controversial, at what age, if any, is the amblyope too old to benefit from active therapy? A critical evaluation of the data in these areas will provide some insight into these most important questions.

DIRECT VERSUS INVERSE OCCLUSION

Eccentric fixation was first measured by von Graefe (1854), who used the Coccius ophthalmoscope and had the patient fixate the hole in its mirror. This crude method was virtually forgotten by many until Cuppers (1956) developed and introduced the visuoscope, essentially a calibrated ophthalmoscope that projected a circular grid pattern on the retina. Around the time of its development, the high prevalence of eccentric fixation ($\sim 80\%$) (Brock and Givner 1952) in amblyopic eyes became evident. This set the stage for the controversy over the use of direct versus inverse occlusion.

Duke-Elder (1949) believed that direct occlusion used with an eccentric fixator served to stabilize the anomalous eccentric fixation. Many agreed with this notion: "When fixation is eccentric, occlusion of the fixing eye is useless" (Foster 1957); "If eccentric fixation is stable, the prolonged occlusion of the other eye will only serve to increase its stability, cause no improvement in visual acuity, and make eradication of eccentric fixation more difficult, for it is obvious that the visual acuity of the eccentric spot can never become greater than is consistent with its anatomical position" (Lyle 1959). The controversy began when Wybar and Thatcher (1961) stated their objection to the use of direct occlusion in amblyopes with eccentric fixation. This prompted a rebuttal by Meakin (1961), who felt that the age of the child must be considered, since children under 5 years of age "rarely fail to produce central fixation in the squinting eye" when using direct occlusion. What followed was a number of published letters from Meakin (1961) and Giles (1961). Giles' criticism of conventional occlusion was based on a single patient whose anomalous fixation pattern was apparently "deepened" by direct patching. The age of the patient was not mentioned. Giles also stated that the amount of eccentric fixation was a determining factor in the type of occlusion to be used. Meakin disagreed. He felt strongly that direct occlusion was imperative for children under the age of 5 years and that the amount of eccentric fixation had no role in the decision. Watchurst (1961) believed that inverse occlusion was unnecessary if direct occlusion were complimented with a central training task at home: "Few cases need any more extensive treatment than fitting a light excluding occluder to the dominant eye, and simple home exercises." A typical training procedure was dotting, where the task was to place as many pencil dots as possible inside a set-diameter circle. The number of dots was recorded, and the exercise was repeated. Gradually, as vision improved, the number of dots placed within the set-size circle would increase (Revell 1971). Scully (1961) supported Watchurst's claim by directly patching 51 amblyopic children with eccentric fixation. Fifty of them achieved central fixation. Scully felt that his high success was due to (1) the young age of his patients and (2) the intensity of the occlusion. Bangerter (1952) advocated total, direct, constant occlusion of the eccentrically fixating amblyopic eye for 1 to 2 months prior to training and then inverse occlusion between training sessions thereafter. This was continued until fixation either became unsteady or steady central, and this was then followed by direct occlusion.

Although there was little evidence to support the premise that occlusion of the sound eye embeds an existing eccentric fixation, inverse occlusion became a popular treatment modality. This is somewhat surprising because the traditional method of direct occlusion, when practiced faithfully, and especially in combination with an active orthoptic program involving multidimensional sensorimotor integrative tasks, is frequently successful at improving visual acuity and fixation in the amblyopic eye.

Proponents of inverse occlusion gave two major reasons for its usefulness. The first was that the squinter's eccentric fixation point was being reinforced throughout the day with both eyes open. Therefore, to prevent this, the amblyopic eye should be patched all day. However, there is no direct and precise reinforcement in most cases, since the objective angle of the strabismus is typically much greater than the angle of the eccentric fixation. Microtropia is the only exception to this, and even here there is typically suppression of stimuli that subtend a visual angle small enough to cause much embeddedness. Consequently, there is no reason (in most cases) for an anomalous fixation pattern to be "broken up" by full-time occlusion of the squinting (amblyopic) eye. The second rationale was that during direct occlusion, the anomalous primary visual direction was reinforced. However, this would only be true for a small-angle steady eccentric fixator, since unsteady eccentric fixators do not have a distinct primary visual direction; further, when given a choice of oculocentricity versus good visual acuity, the amblyopic eye will choose the former. This is why short periods of direct occlusion, in conjunction with intense orthoptic therapy (to train and reinforce primary visual direction sense), may be necessary in some cases; however, as will be discussed in Chapter 10, the initial method of choice is generally direct occlusion.

Several other studies have demonstrated the superiority of direct over inverse occlusion. Urist (1955) used direct occlusion to treat a group of amblyopes with eccentric fixation and found that all patients with better than 20/200 initial visual acuity achieved central fixation. An example was a 7-year-old with esotropia, eccentric fixation, and 20/200 visual acuity who attained a visual acuity of 20/30 with 6 months of constant direct occlusion. The greatest improvement in vision occurred in the preschoolers. This study is exceptionally strong, since all the amblyopes had an angle of eccentric fixation *equal to* the strabismic deviation. Burian (1956) reported success with direct occlusion regardless of the type of fixation, especially in young patients. Those with eccentric fixation required a longer treatment period, with improvement being more unstable. Scully (1961) reported that all but 1 of 51 amblyopic patients achieved central fixation with direct occlusion.

In partial support of inverse occlusion, Barnard (1962) found better success when direct occlusion was preceded by several months of inverse occlusion. In 35 patients who had no previous occlusion of either eye, fixation improved in 100% and visual acuity in 89% (by an average factor of 5.0) with this occlusion sequence. Based on his analysis of 144 patients, Barnard felt that inverse occlusion primarily affected visual direction, with the effect on visual acuity being secondary. This was especially true for patients whose age of onset of the amblyopia was between 1 and 3 years and whose age at the time of first treatment was between 6 to 10 years. Steer (1964) preferred direct occlusion for children under age 3 years and inverse occlusion interspersed by periods of direct occlusion for children from 3 to 5 years of age, especially if fixation were steady and eccentric.

These investigations suggested that younger amblyopes with eccentric fixation responded better with direct occlusion, whereas inverse occlusion to "break up the anomalous fixation pattern" followed by direct occlusion was the preferred treatment plan in older eccentric fixators. A cutoff of 6 years of age was chosen due to its designation as the end of the so-called critical or sensitive period. Unfortunately, there is little support for the notion of age 6 years as being the critical age before which one should not implement therapy (Birnbaum et al. 1977, Ciuffreda 1986), as well as the efficacy of inverse occlusion.

In an attempt to clear up the controversy, two studies using the same criteria were conducted independently at the Wilmer Eye Institute in Baltimore (von Noorden 1965) and at the University Eye Clinic in Tubingen (Mackensen et al. 1967), where the efficacy of direct versus inverse occlusion was compared in 181 amblyopes with eccentric fixation. The two studies found *no* evidence that direct occlusion reinforced eccentric fixation. In addition, inverse occlusion usually did not normalize fixation and, in some cases, actually intensified the amblyopia. Direct occlusion proved superior to inverse occlusion with respect to improvement both in fixation and visual acuity in children up to age 4 years. Unfortunately, older children were not included in the study. Parks and Friendly (1966) found similar results using constant direct occlusion in children under 4 years of age with gross eccentric fixation. They obtained central fixation in 116 of 117 patients, 86% of whom achieved 20/30 or better vision. The occlusion duration required to achieve central fixation averaged 6 weeks if started by age 2 years and 3 months if started between ages 2 and 4 years.

Ver Lee and Iacobucci (1967) compared direct and inverse occlusion in older amblyopes with eccentric fixation. Two groups of 50 strabismic amblyopes, one group treated solely with total direct occlusion for an average of 3 months and the other group treated with inverse occlusion and given at least 1 hour of daily training (except on weekends) for an average of 8 weeks, were tested. The results showed direct occlusion to be superior in terms of both fixation and visual acuity improvement for all three of their age groups: 3 to 6, 6 to 9, and 9 to 12 years. In addition, there was no evidence that conventional occlusion intensified an existing eccentric fixation, even in the older age group. Unfortunately, patching durations were not equal, and the therapy did not control for fixation. Presently, we feel that *all* amblyopic treatment should begin with direct occlusion irrespective of the patients age or fixation status. Our own laboratory results (Selenow, unpublished results) show that of 15 adult amblyopes with eccentric fixation, 14 developed central fixation following a combination of direct patching and intensive conventional orthoptic treatment. One patient required inverse patching and intensive macular tagging to achieve central fixation. We feel that inverse patching is only necessary in deeply embedded eccentric fixation (typically in microtropia) and is beneficial only when followed by controlled foveally biased orthoptic treatment. This rationale makes sense in light of the following. There are two major contributing factors toward an eccentric fixator's visual acuity deficit: sensory loss *and* retinal eccentricity. Even if the latter is not affected, the former will be, since direct patching is the only means of decreasing the inhibition and recovering the sensory loss. In addition, since direct patching does not embed eccentric fixation, we feel that all amblyopia therapy should begin with direct patching.

PARTIAL OCCLUSION

Javal (1896), by accident, was the first to note that an atropinized dominant eye forced fixation at near to be taken up by the amblyopic eye. However, Worth (1901) was probably the first to advocate and use atropine in the dominant eye as a form of amblyopia therapy by producing, in effect, an "invisible" translucent patch caused by the markedly defocused image. He used daily morning instillations up to the age of 6 years, since he felt that any possible improvement after this age was minimal in most cases. Maddox (1907) attempted to equalize vision between the eyes by covering the dominant eye with smoked glass. In addition, he placed two opaque strips on the dark lens, ensuring some uniocular use of the amblyopic eye. Pugh (1936) used a set of four clip-on neutral-density calibrated-glass occluders graded to different densities in small visual acuity steps (6/9, 6/12, 6/18, and 6/24), thus allowing some controlled measure of the degree of penalization (Figure 9.1). Good (1940) used layers of either cellotape, laquer, or varnish to produce the same effect. Chavasse (1934) used marked glass. Overplusing the dominant eye was first suggested by Baxter (1931). However, the amount of retinal defocus that forced the amblyopic eye to fixate at distance was not sufficient to create the same situation at near. Ruben (1964) used various layers of thin plastic strips to occlude central vision while allowing peripheral vision. The strips were added one at a time until visual acuity of the dominant eye was reduced below that of the amblyopic eye. The number of strips necessary for the various acuity levels was 20/30, 4 strips; 20/40, 5 strips; 20/70, 6 strips; and 20/200, 7 strips. Bangerter (1953) used a series of graded occluders to reduce vision in the dominant eye gradually. The advantage of this

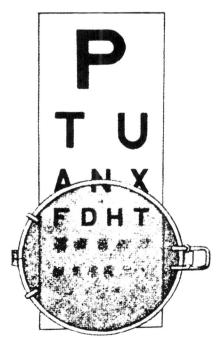

Figure 9.1 *Pugh's visual acuity reducers. (Reprinted, with permission of the publisher, from Revell 1971.)*

"sneak occlusion" technique was that the child was able to adapt slowly to decreasing acuity with eventual total occlusion (Schapero 1971). Wesson (1983) used graded crossed polarizing filters to provide varying amounts of direct light occlusion of the dominent eye of a young amblyope.

Regardless of the method of partial occlusion used, it is of value *only* when it forces fixation to be taken up by the amblyopic eye. In addition, the extent of visual acuity reduction necessary in the dominant eye to force fixation in the amblyopic eye varies from amblyope to amblyope. One cannot arbitrarily penalize the dominant eye by a set amount above the amblyopic eye, since frequently fixation will be maintained by the dominant eye even when the acuity of the amblyopic eye is superior. Sufficient penalization is more obvious in strabismic amblyopia, since one can see the switch in fixation; however, anaglyphic, vectographic, or septal procedures (to dissociate the two eyes) are needed in non-strabismic amblyopes (see Chapter 10).

RED FILTER THERAPY

McCullock (1929), and later Humphriss (1937), first described a technique using a red filter before the dominant eye. The patient's goal was to attempt to see "white," thus forcing fixation of the white luminous target by the nonfiltered amblyopic eye. Increased numbers of flashes of white were indicative of improvement. Since this procedure was usually done with strabismics, it is interesting to wonder whether harmonious ARC rather than alternation was really being reinforced.

Brinker and Katz (1963) advocated the red filter technique for eccentric fixators using a Wratten 92 filter over the amblyopic eye. The theory states that only a restricted wavelength of light to which the rods are insensitive but which is capable of stimulating the cone-rich fovea is transmitted through the filter. Therefore, use of the foveal cones would be encouraged, since the rods were assumed to be relatively insensitive to wavelengths longer than 640 nm. In addition, the filter reduces the amount of light transmitted (approximate percent luminous transmittance of 5.0% and 2.5% in incandescent tungsten and artificial daylight sources, respectively), causing the amblyopic eye to become somewhat dark-adapted. The procedure was to occlude the dominant eye totally, while placing the red filter in front of the amblyopic eye. This was continued until fixation became central, after which direct occlusion without the red lens was implemented. Brinker and Katz reported success with this procedure in breaking down eccentric fixation and improving visual acuity. Treatment time was estimated to be from 6 to 14 weeks. Others reported favorable results; however, improvement was slow, with little effect after the age of 5 years (Binder et al. 1963, Kunst 1963, Ratin and Reiter 1966, Cowle et al. 1967).

Unfortunately, the theory for the red filter procedure seems to be incorrect. Adler (1963) pointed out that in the dark-adapted state, the threshold sensitivity of rods and cones for wavelengths longer than 640 nm is essentially equal.

However, Adler does not deny that with the rod and cone mechanisms on an equal basis, a change in fixation may occur in some cases. Von Noorden (1965, 1980) and others (Malik et al. 1969) reported that the method had been effective in improving fixation behavior in some patients with eccentric fixation. Schapero (1971) believed that the reported improvements may be related to the amount of light transmitted and to the resulting quasi-dark-adapted state of the amblyopic eye rather than to the wavelength transmitted. It is important to note that the use of a red filter in training is done in conjunction with direct occlusion. Therefore, it is not clear whether the improved visual acuity in the preceding studies was related to use of the red filter per se or to the fact that the dominant eye was occluded. In addition, owing to the awkward cosmetic appearance of the red filter, it is rejected by most children. This can be circumvented to some extent by wearing the filter in the form of a contact lens (Zeltzer 1971). However, because the effect of the red filter technique is questionable compared with simple direct occlusion and is weak on theoretical grounds, it is of very limited utility.

ACTIVE VERSUS PASSIVE STIMULATION OF THE AMBLYOPIC EYE (STIMULATION VERSUS OCCLUSION)

English practitioners tended to favor total occlusion for the treatment of the amblyopic eye, whereas in Europe the emphasis was more on direct photic stimulation of the amblyopic eye with instruments. In the United States, a combination of these two approaches was typically used.

One of the earliest attempts at active stimulation of the amblyopic eye was made by Fox (1907), who electrically stimulated the retina and optic nerve of several amblyopes, but without achieving much success. Prior to this, Nagel (1887) attempted to improve visual acuity by giving subcutaneous injections of strychnine. This chemical stimulation proved to be fruitless also. Later, Mulder (1913) projected various colored lights of different intensities on a wall to try to stimulate the amblyopic eye. Fisher (1923) presented targets corresponding to the amblyopic eye's best visual acuity and then moved the targets away from the patient while he or she still attempted to see them. This was a precursor to the mnemoscope of Bangerter (1955). Swann (1931) felt that peripheral vision dominated over central vision in amblyopia. To reverse this, he totally occluded the good eye, while the amblyopic eye was given a patch with a small aperture, permitting the use of central vision only. Swann noted that "if the peripheral vision is excluded, and only central vision or approximately so is permitted, an improvement of vision may be obtained."

Dobson (1933) felt that amblyopia therapy was more successful when the amblyopic eye was actively stimulated during occlusion. Dobson's approach to therapy is summarized in the following statement: "The principle of amblyopia treatment was to force the ignored image of the amblyopic eye to be regarded. This was accomplished by reducing the visibility of the good eye via smoked glass, scientype occluder, or a red filter and by arousing attention of the amblyopic eye by moving targets." To accomplish this, she devised a rotating disk of scattered red and blue spots. The patient's goal was to count the red spots as the disk revolved. Use of Plateau's spiral was cited by Gibson (1955). This 18-inch-diameter black-on-white spiral appeared to be expanding or contracting (depending on the direction of rotation) when rotated and centrally fixated. When a distance chart was presented to the patient following viewing of the spiral, the letters would appear to expand or contract in the opposite direction to that experienced on the spiral, producing an "ice-cream cone" motion aftereffect. When the cone pointed away from the observer, the stationary acuity letter briefly appeared to increase in size. Its purpose was to improve visual acuity on the chart, presumably by attracting attention and providing a strong motion aftereffect in the amblyopic eye. It became more and more evident to clinicians that patching was not successful in all cases. This was especially true in older amblyopes. Therefore, active therapy procedures began to be added to passive occlusion therapy. This led to an armamentarium of exercises that were devised to supplement patching and to promote foveal fixation (Dobson 1935, Smith 1950, Revell 1971). However, such exercises were not systematically administered, until Bangerter (1955) introduced a regimented exercise program for the amblyopic eye and exposed clinicians to the world of pleoptics. A review of the history of pleoptics is essential, since the different treatment modalities became expressions of theoretical conclusions drawn from the results of several clinical investigators in their attempt to break down eccentric fixation. An excellent overall understanding of pleoptics can be achieved by summarizing the work of Alfred Bangerter, Conrad Wolfgang Curt Cuppers, and William Smith.

Suppression Theory of Bangerter

full sight.

In 1953 in Switzerland, Bangerter first coined the word *pleoptics.* It comes from the Greek *pleos optikos*, meaning "full" or "complete" and "sight" (Baldwin 1962). However, Bangerter began to use these procedures as early as 1940 (Cuppers 1956) for the correction of eccentric fixation and improvement of visual acuity in amblyopic eyes. Bangerter's therapeutic procedures were based on his belief that *eccentric fixation is secondary to a central suppression scotoma that is deep enough to cause central visual acuity to be below that of extrafoveal acuity.* Thus, throughout his treatment approach, the emphasis is on (1) reducing the visual acuity of the extrafoveal retina (point *e*) by dazzling it with a bright light and (2) stimulating the fovea with flashes of light. To do this, Bangerter developed the pleoptophore in 1947 (see Figure 9.2). The patient's amblyopic eye was first dilated and then anesthetized to reduce the blink rate. Control of the position of the amblyopic eye was achieved by having the dominant eye fixate a movable red light. The dazzling light was either an annulus for unsteady fixation or a spot for steady eccentric fixation. In either case, the macula was shielded by an opaque stop in the illumination system (see Figure 9.3). This was followed immediately by a visual stimulation phase in which 50 to 100 brief

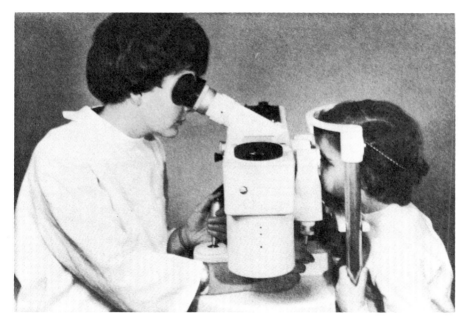

Figure 9.2   *The pleoptophor. (Reprinted, with permission of the publisher, from Schapero 1971.)*

flashes of a very small light were projected onto the fovea. After sufficient dazzling and stimulation, which might need to be repeated several times before the patient was totally aware of the flashing spot of light, the patient underwent fixation training with the localizer. The localizer was the first instrument designed by Bangerter (1958). With the amblyopic eye, the patient was told to look at a lighted hole in a box (see Figure 9.4), while the position of the corneal reflex was noted by the therapist. If the corneal reflex was not centered, the patient was instructed to fixate the therapist's moving fingertip until angle kappa was reached. Once "central fixation" had been achieved, the patient attempted to place his finger onto the variable diameter lighted hole. As progress was made, the patient used a pointer instead of a finger (Figure 9.4*B*). Several other instruments developed by Bangerter, such as the centrophore, separation trainer, corrector, mnemoscope, and mnemoscope trainer, are examples of Bangerter's recognition of the importance of eye-hand coordination, visual memory, and the crowding phenomenon for successful and efficient treatment of amblyopia.

Anomalous Correspondence Theory of Cuppers

Cuppers' hypothesis (1956), in contrast to that of Bangerter, was that *eccentric fixation represented a monocular sensory shift of primary visual direction that occurred secondary to the development of anomalous retinal correspondence.* In anomalous

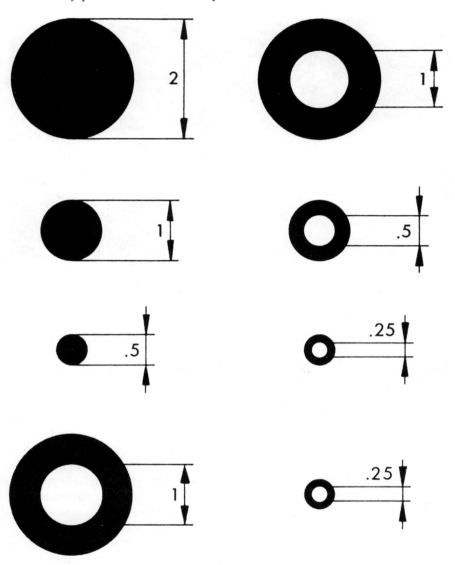

Figure 9.3   *Stencils of targets used with the pleoptophor in the dazzling phase (left) and the stimulative phase (right). The lower left and right targets are used when eccentric fixation is steady. Scaling is in millimeters. (Reprinted, with permission of the publisher, from Schapero 1971.)*

correspondence, there is a nonfoveal area in the strabismic eye that corresponds directionally to the fovea of the fixating eye under binocular viewing conditions. According to Cuppers, this nonfoveal area also assumes the principal visual direction under monocular conditions. Therefore, the emphasis of his therapy was on

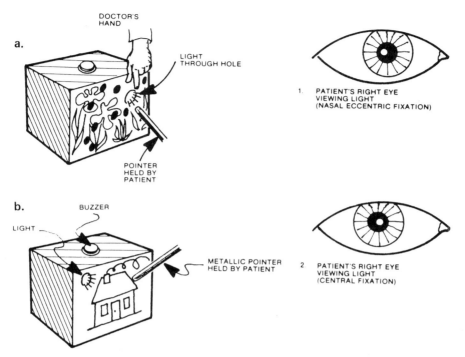

Figure 9.4 *Fixation exercises recommended by Bangerter. (A) Schematic illustration showing principle of the localizer. (B) Schematic illustration showing principle of the corrector. (Reprinted, with permission of the publisher, from Griffin 1985.)*

shifting the primary directional value from the eccentric point (point *e*) to the fovea. Cuppers' method of developing foveal fixation involved two more portable and simplified instruments: the euthoscope and the coordinator.

A type of visuoscope, the euthoscope was used to dazzle the perifoveal areas while shielding the macula. This was accomplished by using one of the two circular stops in the illumination system (3 or 5 degrees). Once the dazzling phase was completed, Cuppers bypassed the stimulation phase and instead concentrated on the patient's appreciation and placement of positive (white doughnut) and negative (black doughnut) afterimages around Snellen letters (see Figure 9.5). The eventual goal was to center the smallest letters in a negative afterimage.

The coordinator was a small circular device used to produce the Haidinger brush entoptic phenomenon. A small window revealed a view of an airplane, and the patient was instructed to center the "propeller" (Haidinger brush) on the nose of the airplane.

Bangerter's and Cuppers' methods were similar in that there was an initial dazzling phase. After this, the two methods differed. Bangerter stressed *foveal stimulation*, while Cuppers concentrated on making the patient aware of the

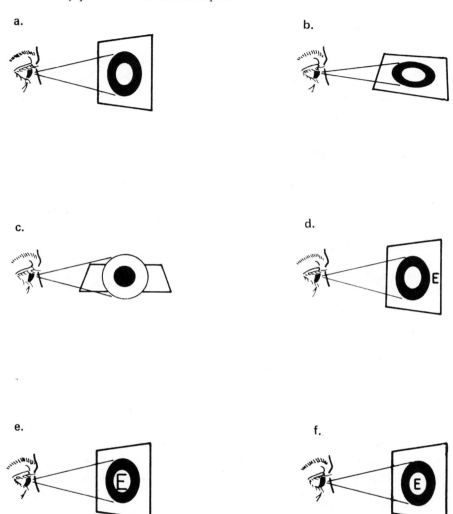

Figure 9.5 *Euthyscopic afterimage advocated by Cuppers for eccentric fixation therapy. (A) Negative afterimage (black doughnut). (B) Afterimage with psychological characteristics of a real object. (C) Positive afterimage (white doughnut) which violated the psychological characteristics of a real object. (D) Nasal eccentric fixation of the right eye. (E) Central fixation. (F) Central fixation using small letter as fixation target. (Reprinted, with permission of the publisher, from Griffin 1985.)*

foveal spatial projection. These differences in therapy stem directly from their different beliefs about the pathogenesis of eccentric fixation. In general, Bangerter's method is easier with children but requires more expensive equipment (Copobianco 1960).

William Smith

In 1935, William Smith, a Boston optometrist, introduced a series of papers stressing the need for "combined multiple treatment processes" to eliminate amblyopia and develop bifoveal fixation. Smith called it a "reeducative procedure," with all treatment performed in his office. This is in sharp contrast to Bangerter's introduction of pleoptics in 1954, where the patients were hospitalized for extended periods. Smith realized that there was no uniform method of treating amblyopia: "Even in the practice of occlusion, there was no one uniform method for treatment of eccentric fixation." Some practitioners stressed direct occlusion, others inverse, and some even alternate occlusion. Length of occlusion varied from 1 hour daily to the whole day. Some even stressed patching weeks at a time. "Aside from occlusion and fusion training . . . nothing was done by way of training. The fact that the suppressing visual system was unprepared to convey images to the higher cortical centers seemed to make no difference, or the importance of eliminating suppression was not understood" (Smith 1961). Between December 1935 and January 1936, Smith published a series of articles entitled, "A Basic Technique in Orthoptics", which introduced a new method and a series of home-made instruments where amblyopia, suppression, and anomalous retinal correspondence were treated *before* the strabismus was dealt with. Therefore, the "side-effects" of strabismus were treated before the strabismus itself. In addition, "occlusion was relegated to a place of secondary importance" (Smith 1961). This was in striking contrast to the accepted treatment of the time, which was occlusion (direct or alternate) and fusion training. If visual acuity and fusion did not develop during a predetermined time, strabismus surgery was performed.

In formulating his procedures, Smith offered free treatment to patients with amblyopia and/or strabismus between 1928 and 1933, at which time he organized an orthoptic clinic at the Eye Department of the Boston Dispensary, New England Medical Center. Smith's methods included the following:

1. *Retinal stimulation.* The amblyopic eye was exposed to a bright flashing light for 5 to 10 minutes. Patients wore their full optical correction over the amblyopic eye, while the dominant eye was patched. Smith made his retinal stimulator out of a Keystone telebinocular head, two small metal cans, and two 15-watt frosted light bulbs (see Figure 9.6). "The purpose of light stimulation is to help establish and develop fixation of visual impressions on the foveal area, to improve spatial perception, and to help eliminate suppression" (Smith 1935). Smith felt that retinal stimulation helped speed up the treatment of eccentric fixation and anomalous retinal correspondence. This procedure was indicated mainly for deep amblyopia.

2. *Visual orientation.* With the dominant eye occluded, the patient looked into a Keystone telebinocular at one of two cards developed by Smith (see Figure 9.7). With the cardholder at the infinity mark, the patient was instructed to point, name, and outline each character, attempting to always see the smallest

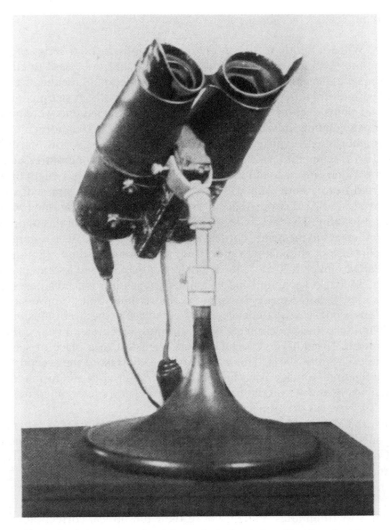

Figure 9.6   *Author's instrument for giving retinal stimulation. (Reprinted, with permission of the publisher, from Smith 1950.)*

objects and trace and name them accurately. By having the figures and characters grouped closely together, Smith was directly addressing the crowding phenomenon of the amblyopic eye, as well as improving its fixation ability and direction sense.

    3. *Foveal fixation, eye-hand coordination, and projection.* Smith felt that establishing normal retinal correspondence and primary visual direction at the

A

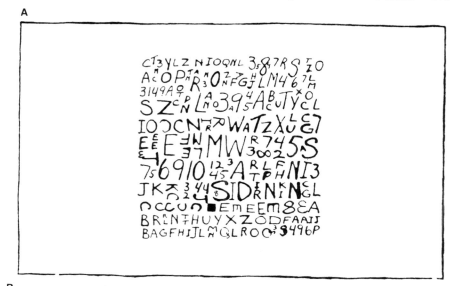

B

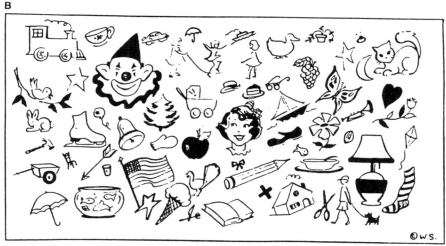

Figure 9.7   (A) *Author's chart for training visual orientation. This chart contains numerous variable-sized letters, numerals, and other characters grouped closely together and in various positions. The chart is placed at infinity. A pointer (or two pointers, one in each hand) is used by the patient. The patient is required to point, name, and outline each character endeavoring each time to see the smallest-sized objects and trace and name them accurately. The telebinocular or stereoscope is the apparatus used. (B) Author's chart for training visual orientation in children and illiterates. This chart contains a wide assortment of pictures of objects of variable size, grouped closely together, with which even a very young child is familiar. The training procedure is the same as for the preceding target. Devised by William Smith, O.D., Boston, Mass. (Reprinted, with permission of the publisher, from Smith 1950.)*

fovea was a prerequisite for successful amblyopia therapy. To train this function, Smith developed projection plates that consisted of individual pictures drawn in color on heavy cardboard 15 × 9 inches in size (see Figure 9.8). Each picture consisted of small holes into which the patient was instructed to insert colored toothpicks with the dominant eye occluded. The patient was told to insert the toothpicks into the holes one by one, projecting them by aiming or fixating. In addition, tracing was done on an opaque, glass-topped tracing box, which flashed on and off at constant but brief intervals. With the dominant eye occluded, the patient was instructed to trace accurately over the various pictures during the illumination phase. Thus the patient developed eye-hand coordination, direction sense, and improved fixation ability.

4. *Visual and stereoscopic acuity.* At a distance of 20 feet in a darkened room, the patient attempted to discern a threshold line of characters while the chart was intermittently illuminated. Various other devices also were used, such as a flashing acuity box, picture card matching, and tachistoscope training. Smith used split stereograms with pictures, numbers, and words of variable sizes that

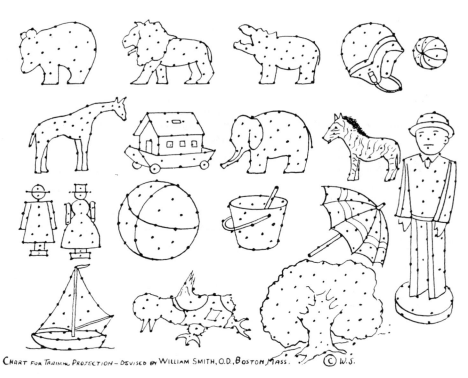

CHART FOR TRAINING PROJECTION – DEVISED BY WILLIAM SMITH, O.D., BOSTON, MASS.   © W.S.

Figure 9.8 *Author's projection training plate. Dots represent holes. (Reprinted, with permission of the publisher, from Smith 1950.)*

were viewed monocularly while being intermittently illuminated. The target began at infinity and then was slowly moved closer until it was identified, after which it was again slowly moved away. As visual acuity improved, flashing rate was increased while the on-time phase was decreased.

5. *Accommodation.* While testing and training amblyopes, Smith noticed a reduced accommodative response in the amblyopic eye, especially to step changes in accommodation. Smith's training of monocular accommodation involved two steps: progressively adding minus lenses as a small fixation target at near was to be kept in focus, and alternating adding plus and minus lenses as a near target was to be kept in focus. This also was performed in a stereoscope, where a flash sequence was used to illuminate the targets alternately in each eye, while accommodative demands were varied by means of concave and convex lenses in the cells of the instrument. The illumination period was reduced as accommodative response time decreased.

Smith stressed the importance of frequent treatment periods, especially during the early stages of training. He advocated daily sessions of at least 1 hour and would often spend an entire treatment period on just a single step, repeating it for weeks at a time. This is best exemplified in one of Smith's cases.

Illustrative Case: A case in point is that of an 18-year-old girl student with hyperesotropia and amblyopia of the left eye. Visual acuity with and without glasses was: O.D. 20/20; O.S. 20/200; pinhole vision, O.S. 20/100. At the near point she read with difficulty Jaeger 20 type at about 10 inches. An operation for the correction of esotropia was performed when she was 8 years old, but apparently only partial correction was achieved at that time. On the day this examination was performed the girl had 25 degrees esotropia O.S. and 10 degrees hypertropia O.S. The esotropia was measured on the perimeter, the hypertropia on the Maddox tangent scale. Tests of the left eye indicated faulty spatial projection and foveal fixation. Retinal correspondence by the afterimage test was anomalous, and repeated tests showed macular suppression.

For 6 months this patient was treated at an orthoptic clinic attached to the eye department of a hospital. There she was given three treatments a week, each lasting about 15 to 20 minutes. Each time, the entire treatment period was devoted to teaching and developing visual perception. As a result of this clinic treatment and the extra training done at home, in addition to long periods of occlusion of the right eye, sight in the left eye was improved to 20/100$^+$ at the end of 6 months.

When the girl became the author's private patient, daily treatments were started, each lasting over 2 hours, with short periods of rest in between. Within 5 months distant sight became improved to 20/20$-$. She learned and developed normal bifoveal and binocular coordination. The squint was no longer apparent. What was most important, however, the girl had achieved the one ambition which had originally prompted her to seek our help. As a result of orthoptic treatment, she was able, after numerous failures, to pass the visual test of the flight physical examination and to obtain a license as a civil aeronautics pilot.

Smith's excellent results depend on (1) "persistent and continuous repetition of the same exercise in the training routine visit after visit" and (2) his opinion that "occlusion alone is a worthless task, unless the affected eye is given, in addition, visual tasks to perform."

Thus, in 1935, William Smith first realized the need for multiple active forms of treatment for elimination of amblyopia, with an emphasis on the sensory aspects of amblyopia and strabismus. However, as noted by Nicholson (1919): "When a condition once becomes established by the hallmark of acknowledged authority, it takes more than cold facts to uproot it from man's mind—it takes time." It took about 20 years more and the theories and unique procedures of Bangerter, Cuppers, and Smith to revolutionize the way eccentric fixation and anomalous retinal correspondence were viewed. The enthusiasm generated by the work of these pioneering clinicians prevails to this day, while the theoretical conclusions based on their different treatment modalities remain as the core of the controversy over the pathophysiology of eccentric fixation.

EFFICACY OF PLEOPTICS

There have been an extensive number of studies with regards to the efficacy of pleoptics. Success rates have been generally mixed (Garzia 1987, Tommila 1964, Girand et al. 1962, Byron 1960, Capobianco 1960, von Noorden and Lipsius 1964, Veronneau-Troutman et al. 1974, Ver Lee and Iacobucci 1967, Fletcher et al. 1969, Taylor 1970). Overall, pleoptics has not been found to be more effective than occlusion in improving visual acuity. However, treatment time has been shown to be reduced with pleoptics. Garzia (1987), however, brings up an important point in most of these studies. Pleoptics tended to be implemented on older amblyopes with poorer initial visual acuity and larger degrees of eccentric fixation. This would obviously bias the treatment results in favor of occlusion therapy. However, since pleoptics requires much cooperation on the part of the patient, its use in the younger population is limited. Garzia (1987) analyzed several studies that evaluated the efficacy of pleoptics in amblyopes who did *not* respond to simple direct occlusion (Table 9.1). These results suggest that an aggressive pleoptics program can improve visual acuity in amblyopes who reached their visual acuity limit with occlusion alone. Owing to economical and practical reasons, however, pleoptics is no longer a popular method of amblyopia treatment. Fortunately, owing to earlier detection, the population of amblyopes (older amblyopes with large eccentric fixation and deep amblyopia) who would benefit most from pleoptics has decreased significantly (von Noorden 1986). However, pleoptics has opened the clinician's eyes to the potential of a vigorous and active training approach in the treatment of amblyopia. In addition, pleoptics has influenced our present therapy regimen by stressing the importance of proper visual and possibly oculomotor (i.e., proprioception) feedback training for correct foveal localization.

Table 9.1 Success of Pleoptics in Amblyopes Who Did Not Respond to Occlusion Therapy

Author	Patient Population	Age Group	Treatment Employed	Initial Visual Acuity	Authors' Criteria for Success	Percent Obtaining Criteria for Success
Wanter (1980)	100 eccentric fixators	3–52 years (average age 7 years)	Daily 1-hour pleoptics for 3 weeks	6/60, finger counting	Acuity improvement ≥ 1 line Snellen and improved fixation for greater than 2 months	59%
von Noorden and Lipsius (1964)	58 eccentric fixators	5–17 years	Daily pleoptics for 30 minutes at least 5 times per week	6/30 (average)	Acuity improvement ≥ 2 lines single-letter Snellen or central fixation	56.4% ≥ 2 lines improvement; 47.9% achieved central fixation
Mayweg and Massie (1958)	12 central fixators and 38 eccentric fixators	4–13 years	Daily or 3 times per week pleoptics for 30 minutes	6/18 to 6/36	VA > 6/12	83% of central fixators, 4% of eccentric fixators
Gortz (1960)	88 eccentric fixators	6–22 years (average age 9.7 years)	Average of 17.5 sessions of monocular training with total of 30.2 sessions of combined monocular and binocular training (½-hour session)	6/300 to 6/20	Central fixation or VA > 6/15	81% obtained central fixation, 68% obtained VA > 6/15, 35% obtained VA > 6/8.4
Jablonski and Tomlinson (1979)	86 eccentric fixators	4–41 years	Average of 10 weeks of pleoptic sessions	30% have < 6/60	VA > 6/12	38%

(continued on next page)

Table 9.1 *(continued)*

Author	Patient Population	Age Group	Treatment Employed	Initial Visual Acuity	Authors' Criteria for Success	Percent Obtaining Criteria for Success
Tomlinson and Jablonski (1973)	64 eccentric fixators	4–17 years	Pleoptics once a week for ½ hour with home therapy of visual tracking exercises	6/12 to 6/30	VA > 6/12	100%
Rados et al. (1966)	80 consecutive eccentric fixators	5–"adult"	Pleoptics twice daily (½-hour session), 5 × per week for 6 weeks	Most had VA < 6/30	VA > 6/12	59%
Girard et al. (1962)	20 central fixators and 52 eccentric fixators	4.5–48 years	Daily to weekly sessions of ½ hour (average of 14 treatment sessions)	6/12, finger counting	VA > 6/9	58%

ACTIVE THERAPY WITH SHORT-TERM OCCLUSION

Although the success of active therapy in conjunction with short-term occlusion has been documented in both humans (Callahan and Berry 1968, Gould et al. 1970, von Noorden et al. 1970) and animals (Crewther et al. 1981), it has gained tremendous popularity since the introduction of the CAM vision stimulator (Banks et al. 1978). This device consists of seven rotating, high-contrast, square-wave gratings (from 0.50 to 32 cycles per degree) that are presented monocularly to the amblyopic eye in ascending order for 1 minute per grating. During exposure to these gratings, the patient performs a series of near-point eye-hand coordination exercises on a transparent overlay. Occlusion only is administered during the active therapy phase, which lasts a total of 7 minutes. However, controlled studies also have shown equally impressive results with uniform gray patterns (Ciuffreda et al. 1979, Fricker et al. 1981, Tytla and Labow-Daily 1981, Mitchell 1983, Watson et al. 1985). It is now well established that the improvements in visual acuity with rotating gratings were due to the brief periods of intensive occlusion and high-level visual-motor tasks and *not* to the specific gratings per se. However, in addition, *these CAM studies have indirectly been responsible for the recent shift in emphasis toward active therapy with minimal occlusion for the treatment of amblyopia.* Table 9.2 summarizes the results of 29 such short-term active therapy studies. For an excellent review of this area, see Garzia (1987).

Table 9.2   Summary of Orthoptic Results in Amblyopia

Authors	No. of Patients	Age (years)	Treatment Regimen	Length of Treatment	Initial Visual Acuity	Final Visual Acuity	Percent Success	Comments
Kageyama and Loomis (1980)	1	10	Active therapy	3 mos.	6/60	6/7.5		Previous 8 months of occlusion with failure
Wick (1973)	1	16	Active therapy	10 weeks	6/18	6/7.5		No response to standard direct occlusion alone
Selenow and Ciuffreda (1983)	1	6½	Active therapy	4 mos.	6/60	6/9		
Ciuffreda et al. (1979)	1	18	Active therapy	10 mos.	6/60	6/6		Improved eye movement and fixation
Etting (1978)	13	6–26	Active therapy	4 mos.		6/12 6/9	77 61	
Jenkins and Pickwell (1982)			Occlusion, home therapy, or refractive correction			≥6/9	38	
Shippman (1985)	19	4–10	1 hour/day of video games and full-time occlusion		20/20 to 20/50	6/12 Two-line gain in V.A. Three-line gain in V.A.	70 78 47	

Reference	No.	Age	Treatment	Duration	Initial acuity	Final acuity	Result	Comments
Francois and James (1955)	100		Active therapy twice weekly					Compared 5 groups of 100 amblyopes. Occlusion only versus occlusion plus active therapy
Leyman (1978)	111		Active therapy, penalization and occlusion			≥6/9	93	Same results but gains by active (vs. passive) therapy group in one-third the time
Thorn and Comerford (1983)	3	26–39	Active therapy	4–18 weeks	20/70 to 20/400	20/30 to 20/200	66 > 2 lines	
Selenow and Ciuffreda (1986)	1	29	Active therapy and 2 hours of occlusion	12 months	20/150 Snellen single line	20/30		
Griffin et al. (1978)	1	4	15 minutes of active occlusion per day	6 weeks	20/50	20/20		
von Noorden et al. (1970)	25	7–16	Active therapy 1 hour daily; no occlusion	5–20 weeks		Improvement 20/40 ≥2 lines	62 40 36	Previous occlusion failures
Gould et al. (1970)	35	6–17	Only active therapy 1 hour daily	3–36 months		≥2 lines ≥20/40	80 40	No occlusion

(continued on next page)

Table 9.2 *(continued)*

Authors	No. of Patients	Age (years)	Treatment Regimen	Length of Treatment	Initial Visual Acuity	Final Visual Acuity	Percent Success	Comments
Callahan and Berry (1968)	250	5–15	Active therapy 2 hours daily		≤ 20/100	Not given	Not given	Showed that 2-hour daily active therapy with intermittent occlusion gave faster results than occlusion only but not as fast as full-time occlusion with active therapy
Pickwell (1976)	60		Only binocular therapy		6/17	6/6	43	
Lowndes-Yates (1977)	15	2–14	Rotating target plus 30 minutes of occlusion		6/24	6/9	66	
Banks et al. (1978)	40	3–11	CAM	Average of five sessions	6/40	≥ 6/12	73	
Campbell et al. (1978)	50	3–11	CAM	Four sessions for 7 months		≥ 6/12	73	
Brown (1980)	36	6–9	CAM			≥ 1-line improvement		

Willshaw et al. (1980)	84	3–14	CAM	Variable		≥6/12	73	Previous failure with occlusion
Doba (1981)	69		CAM	Average of 6 15-minute treatment sessions 1 to 2 times weekly plus full-time occlusion		6/12	47	
Lennerstrand et al. (1981)	31	4–13	CAM	10 minutes 1 to 2 times weekly; maximum 20 sessions	6/20 average	6/14 average	91	21 had failed with occlusion
Dalziel (1980)	12	4–23	CAM	Fifteen treatments	6/30 average	6/24 average		2 patients improved 5 lines
Carruthers et al. (1980)	22	3–9	CAM	Five sessions		2-line improvement	27	
Douthwaite et al. (1981)	23	5–17	CAM	Three to five sessions			9	
Nyman et al. (1983)	25	4–6	CAM	Five to ten sessions each 7-minutes, 2 times weekly		≥2-line improvement	80	Compared CAM to full-time occlusion in two matched groups; found same success rate

(continued on next page)

Table 9.2 (*continued*)

Authors	No. of Patients	Age (years)	Treatment Regimen	Length of Treatment	Initial Visual Acuity	Final Visual Acuity	Percent Success	Comments
Lennerstrand and Samuelsson (1983)	31	4–13	CAM	4 to 8 weeks		Average V.A. improvement of 40%		Compared grating stimulation to 6 weeks of total occlusion
Lennerstrand and Lundh (1980)	24	5½–13	CAM					Improvement in contrast sensitivity but not in visual acuity

REFERENCES

Adler FH. (1963) Foveal fixation. *Am. J. Ophthalmol.* 56:483–4.

Baldwin WR. (1962) Pleoptics: Historical developments and overview of the literature. *Am. J. Optom. Arch. Am. Acad. Optom.* 39:149–62.

Bangerter A. (1952) Cited by Meyer A. (1952) Observations on squint therapy in Switzerland. *Br. Orthopt. J.* 9:89–93.

Bangerter A. (1953) *Uber Pleoptik.* Wien. Klin. Wochrenschr. *65:966–982.*

Bangerter A. (1955) *Amblyopiebehandlung*, 2d Ed. Basel: Karger.

Bangerter A. (1958) Orthoptische Behandlung des Begleitschielens. Pleoptik (Monokulare Orthoptik). In *Acta XVIII Concilun Ophthalmologica (Belgium)*, Vol. 1, p. 105. Amsterdam: Excerpta Medica.

Banks RV, Campbell FW, Hess R, Watson PG. (1978) A new treatment for amblyopia. *Br. Orthopt. J.* 35:1–12.

Barnard W. (1962) Treatment of amblyopia by inverse occlusion and pleoptics. *Br. Orthopt. J.* 19:19–30.

Baxter H. (1931) *Yearbook of the N.Y. Optometry Association.* Cited by Revell (1971), p. 179.

Binder HF, Engel D, Ede ML, Loon L. (1963) The red filter treatment of eccentric fixation. *Am. Orthopt. J.* 13:64–9.

Birnbaum MH, Koslowe K, Sanet R. (1977) Success in amblyopia therapy as a function of age: a literature survey. *Am. J. Optom. Physiol. Opt.* 54:269–75.

Brinker WR, Katz SL. (1963) A new and practical treatment of eccentric fixation. *Am. J. Ophthalmol.* 55:1033–5.

Brock FW, Givner I. (1952) Fixation anomalies in amblyopia. *Arch. Ophthalmol.* 47:1465–6.

Brown S. (1980) Results of treatment with the CAM vision stimulator from Sydney Eye Hospital. *Aust. Orthopt. J.* 17:13–17.

Buffon CLL. (1743) *Memoires de L'Academie des Sciences.* Cited by Revell (1971), p. 3.

Burian HM. (1956) Thoughts on the nature of amblyopia ex anopsia. *Am. Orthopt. J.* 6:5–12.

Byroñ HM. (1960) Results of pleoptics in the management of amblyopia with eccentric fixation. *Arch. Ophthalmol.* 63:675–81.

Callahan WP, Berry D. (1968) The value of visual stimulation during constant and direct occlusion. *Am. Orthopt. J.* 18:73–4.

Campbell FW, Hess RF, Watson PG, Banks R. (1978) Preliminary results of a physiologically based treatment of amblyopia. *Br. J. Ophthalmol.* 62:747–55.

Capobianco NM. (1960) Pleoptic treatment of amblyopes with central and eccentric fixation. *Am. Orthopt. J.* 10:33–53.

Carruthers JDA, Pratt-Johnson JA, Tilson G. (1980) A pilot study of children with amblyopia treated by the gratings method. *Br. J. Ophthalmol.* 64:342–4.

Chavasse B. (1934) Thermoplasty of the extraocular muscle and posterior partial myotomy. *Trans. Ophthalmol. Soc. U.K.* 54:506–24.

Ciuffreda KJ. (1986) Visual System Plasticity in Human Amblyopia. In Hilfer SR, Sheffield JB (Eds.), *Development of Order in the Visual System*, pp. 211–44. New York: Springer-Verlag.

Ciuffreda KJ, Kenyon RV, Stark L. (1979) Different rates of functional recovery of eye movements during orthoptic treatment in an adult amblyope. *Invest. Ophthalmol. Vis. Sci.* 18:213–9.

Cowle JB, Kunst JH, Philpolts AM. (1967) Trial with red filter in the treatment of eccentric fixation. *Br. J. Ophthalmol.* 51:36–41.

Crewther DR, Crewther SG, Mitchell DE. (1981) The efficacy of brief periods of reverse occlusion in promoting recovery from the physiological effects of monocular deprivation in kittens. *Invest. Ophthalmol. Vis. Sci.* 21:357-62.

Cuppers C. (1956) Die Amblyopiebehandling mit der Nachbildmethode. *Wissenschaftlich Zeitschrift der Universitat Jena, Mathematisch-natur-Wissenschaftliche Reihe* 5:21-5.

Daiziel CC. (1980) Amblyopia therapy by the Campbell-Hess technique. *Am. J. Optom. Physiol. Opt.* 57:280-3.

Doba AT. (1981) Cambridge stimulator treatment for amblyopia: An evaluation of 80 consecutive cases treated by this method. *Aust. J. Ophthalmol.* 9:121-7.

Dobson M. (1933) *Binocular Vision and the Modern Treatment of Squint.* London: Rembrandt Photogravure.

Dobson M. (1935) *The Amblyopia Reader.* London: Rembrandt Photogravure.

Douthwaite WA, Jenkins TCA, Pickwell DL, Sheridan M. (1981) The treatment of amblyopia by the rotating grating method. *Ophthalmic Physiol. Opt.* 1:97-106.

Duke-Elder WS. (1949) *Textbook of Ophthalmology*, Vol. 4. London: Klimpton.

Etting GL. (1978) Strabismus therapy in private practice: Cure rates after three months of therapy. *J. Am. Optom. Assoc.* 49:1367-73.

Fischer SJ, Kuperwaser MC, Stromberg AE, Goldman SG. (1981) Use of a videogame/stripe presentation for amblyopia therapy. *J. Pediatr. Ophthalmol. Strabismus.* 18:11-16.

Fisher V. (1923) 10:20. Cited by Revell (1971).

Fletcher MC, Silverman SJ, Boyd J, Callaway M. (1969) Comparison of the management of suppression amblyopia by conventional patching, intensive hospital orthoptics, and intermittent office pleoptics. *Am. Orthopt. J.* 19:40-7.

Foster J. (1957) Contribution to discussion on pleoptics. *Br. Orthopt. J.* 14:53-5.

Fox W. (1907) Cited by Revell (1971).

Francois J, James M. (1955) Comparative study of amblyopic treatment. *Am. Orthopt. J.* 5:61-4.

Fricker SJ, Kuperwaser MC, Stromberg AE, Goldman SG. (1981) Stripe therapy for amblyopia with a modified television game. *Arch. Ophthalmol.* 99:1596-9.

Garzia R. (1987) Efficacy of vision therapy in amblyopia: A literature review. *Am. J. Optom. Physiol. Opt.* 64:393-404.

Gibson HW. (1955) *Textbook of Orthoptics.* London, Hatton Press Ltd.

Giles GM. (1961) Letters to the editor. *Ophthalmic Optician* 1:379, 570.

Girard LJ, Fletcher MC, Tomlinson E, Smith B. (1962) Results of pleoptic treatment of suppression amblyopia. *Am. Orthopt. J.* 12:12-31.

Good P. (1940) Clinical use of laquer in ophthalmology for the treatment of squint, suppression amblyopia and diplopia. *Arch. Ophthalmol.* 24:479-481.

Gortz H. (1960) The corrective treatment of amblyopia with eccentric fixation. *Am. J. Ophthalmol.* 49:1315-21.

Gould A, Fishkoff D, Galin MA. (1970) Active visual stimulation: A method of treatment of amblyopia in the older patient. *Am. Orthopt. J.* 20:39-45.

Griffin JR, Sherban RJ, Seibert P. (1978) Amblyopia therapy: A case report. *Optom. Monthly* 69:619-20.

Griffin JR. (1982) *Binocular Anomalies: Procedures for Vision Therapy.* Chicago: Professional Press.

Humphriss D. (1937) Some notes on the treatment of amblyopia. *Diopt. Rev.* 39:313.

Jablonski M, Tomlinson E. (1979) A new look at pleoptics. *Ophthalmology* 86:2112-14.

Javal E. (1896) Manuel theoretique et practique du strabisme. Paris: G. Masson.

Jenkins TCA, Pickwell D. (1982) Success rate in the treatment of amblyopia by conventional methods. *Ophthalmic Physiol. Opt.* 2:213-19.

Kageyama CJ, Loomis SA. (1980) Central fixation amblyopia: A case report. *Optom. Monthly* 71:333-6.

Lennerstrand G, Lundh BL. (1980) Improvement of contrast sensitivity from treatment for amblyopia. *Acta Ophthalmol.* 58:292-4.

Lennerstrand G, Kvamstrom G, Lundh BL, Wranne K. (1981) Effects of grating stimulation on visual acuity in amblyopia. *Acta Ophthalmol.* 59:179-88.

Lennerstrand G, Samuelsson B. (1983) Amblyopia in 4-year-old children treated with grating stimulation and full-time occlusion: A comparative study. *Br. J. Ophthalmol.* 67:181-90.

Leyman IA. (1978) A comparative study in the treatment of amblyopia. *Am. Orthopt. J.* 28:95-9.

Lowndes-Yates E. (1977) The rotating light test in the treatment of eccentric fixation. *Br. Orthopt. J.* 34:67-71.

Lyle TK. (1959) Orthoptic treatment of concomitant strabismus. *Br. Orthopt. J.* 16:7-20.

Mackensen G, Kroner B, Postic G, Kelok W. (1967) Untersuchungen zum Problem der exzentrischen Fixation. *Doc. Ophthalmol.* 23:228-39.

McCulloch OL. (1929) Trans. Amer. Acad. Optom. Cited in Revell.

Maddox E. (1907) *The Ocular Muscles.* Philadelphia: The Keystone Press.

Malik SRK, Gupta AK, Choudry DS. (1969) The red filter treatment of eccentric fixation. *Am. J. Ophthalmol.* 67:586-90.

Meakin WJ. (1961) Letters to the Editor. *Ophthalmic Optician* 1:316, 503, 715.

Mitchell DE, Howell ER, Keith CG. (1983) The effect of minimal occlusion therapy on binocular visual functions in amblyopia. *Invest. Ophthalmol. Vis. Sci.* 24:778-781.

Mulder J. (1913) Cited by Revell (1971).

Nagel A. Cited by de Wecker L, Landot E. (1887) *Opthalmologie* 3:763.

Nicholson J. (1919) Cited by Revell (1971).

Nyman KG, Singh G, Rydberg A, Fomander M. (1983) Controlled study comparing CAM treatment with occlusion therapy. *Br. J. Ophthalmol.* 67:178-80.

Parks MM, Friendly DS. (1966) Treatment of eccentric fixation in children under 4 years of age. *Am. J. Ophthalmol.* 61:395-9.

Pickwell DL. (1976) The management of amblyopia without occlusion. *Br. J. Physiol. Opt.* 31:115-18.

Pugh M. (1936) *Squint Training.* London: Oxford University Press.

Rados WT, Sellitto AM, Angilioli DN, Shaterian ET. (1966) Observations on outpatient pleoptics. *Am. Orthopt. J.* 16:111-27.

Ratin E, Reiter E. (1966) Results obtained with the red filter method in the treatment of amblyopia with eccentric fixation. *J. Pediatr. Ophthal.* 3:29-30.

Revell MJ. (1971) *Strabismus: A History of Orthoptic Techniques.* London: Barrie and Jenkins.

Ruben M. (1964) A selective occluder. *Br. Orthopt. J.* 21:120-1.

Schapero M. (1971) *Amblyopia.* Philadelphia: Chilton.

Scully JP. (1961) Early intensive occlusion in strabismus with non-central fixation: Preliminary results. *Br. Med. J.* 2:1610-12.

Selenow A, Ciuffreda KJ. (1983) Vision function recovery during orthoptic therapy in an exotropic amblyope with high unilateral myopia. *Am. J. Optom. Physiol. Opt.* 60:659-66.

Selenow A, Ciuffreda KJ. (1986) Visual function recovery during orthoptic therapy in an adult amblyope. *J. Am. Optom. Assoc.* 57:132-41.

Shippman S. (1985) Video games and amblyopia treatment. *Am. Orthopt. J.* 35:2-5.

Shippman S, Schudel-Dayanoff S, Seidenfeld A, Hemann JS. (1980) A contrast grating treatment for amblyopia: a pilot study. *Am. Orthopt. J.* 30:83–7.

Smith WS. (1935) A basic technique in orthoptics, parts I–IV. *Am. J. Optom.* 12:224, 321, 394, 473.

Smith WS. (1950) *Clinical Orthoptic Procedure.* St. Louis: Mosby.

Smith WS. (1961) Pleoptics: An orthoptic procedure. *J. Am. Optom. Assoc.* 33:355–8.

Steer J. (1964) Management of eccentric fixation: I. Children up to the age of 5 years. *Br. Orthopt. J.* 21:73–7.

Swann L. (1931) *The Ocular Muscles and the Treatment of Heterophoria and Heterotropia.* London: Hatton Press.

Taylor JN. (1970) The treatment of eccentric fixation. *Trans. Aust. Coll. Ophthalmol.* 3:72–5.

Thorn F, Comerford JP. (1983) Use of various measures of visual acuity and contrast sensitivity in the evaluation of monocular occlusion and active vision training of three adult amblyopes. *Am. J. Optom. Physiol. Opt.* 60:347–51.

Tommila V. (1964) Results in amblyopia treatment with the pleoptophore. *Acta Ophthalmol.* 42:489–94.

Tomlinson E, Jablonski M. (1973) Results of modified pleoptic therapy in eccentric fixation. *Am. Orthopt. J.* 23:60–4.

Tytla ME, Labow-Daily LS. (1981) Evaluation of the CAM treatment for amblyopia: a controlled study. *Invest. Ophthalmol. Vis. Sci.* 20:400–6.

Urist J. (1955) Eccentric fixation in amblyopia ex anopsia. *Arch. Ophthalmol.* 54:345–50.

Ver Lee DL, Iacobucci I. (1967) Pleoptics versus occlusion of the sound eye. *Am. J. Ophthalmol.* 63:244–50.

Veronneau-Troutman S, Dayanoff SS, Stohler T, Clahane AC. (1974) Conventional occlusion vs. pleoptics in the treatment of amblyopia. *Am. J. Ophthalmol.* 78:117–20.

von Graefe A. (1854) Uber das Doppel Sehen nach Schiel: operationen and Incongruence den Netzhaute. *Arch. Ophthalmol.* 1:44.

von Noorden GK. (1965) Occlusion therapy in amblyopia with eccentric fixation. *Arch. Ophthalmol.* 73:776–81.

von Noorden GK, Romano P, Parks M, Springer F. (1970) Home therapy for amblyopia. *Am. Orthopt. J.* 20:46–50.

von Noorden GK. (1980) *Binocular Vision and Ocular Motility,* 2d Ed. St. Louis: Mosby.

von Noorden GK. (1986) Alternating penalization in the prevention of amblyopia recurrence. *Am. J. Ophthalmol.* 102:473–5.

von Noorden GK, Lipius RMC. (1964) Experiences with pleoptics in 58 patients with strabismic amblyopia. *Am. J. Ophthalmol.* 58:41–51.

Wanter BS. (1980) Pleoptic therapy in amblyopia. *Am. Orthopt. J.* 30:77–82.

Watchurst GR. (1961) Eccentric fixation. *Trans. Int. Ophthalmol. Congr.* Cited in Revell.

Watson PG, Sanac AS, Pickering MS. (1985) A comparison of various methods of treatment of amblyopia: a block study. *Trans. Ophthalmol. Soc. U.K.* 104:319–28.

Wesson MD. (1983) Use of light intensity reduction for amblyopia therapy. *Am. J. Optom. Physiol. Opt.* 60:112–17.

Wick B. (1973) Amblyopia: A case report. *Am. J. Optom. Arch. Am. Acad. Optom.* 50:727–30.

Willshaw HE, Malmheden A, Clarke JJ, Williams AE, Dean L. (1980) Experience with the CAM vision stimulator: preliminary report. *Br. J. Ophthalmol.* 64:339–41.

Worth C. (1901) *Squint: Its Causes, Pathology and Treatment.* London: J. Bale, Sons and Danielson.

Wybar K, Thatcher J. (1961) Treatment of squint in children. *Br. Med. J.* 1:201–02.

Zeltzer H. (1971) The X-chrome lens. *J. Am. Optom. Assoc.* 42:933–9.

Chapter 10

Further Aspects in the Treatment of Amblyopia

After the amblyopia workup is completed, the examiner should allow time to scrutinize the findings, determine the prognosis for success and means of achieving it, and have an idea as to how the patient's personality will affect the training sequence. Once a global picture of the whole case is clear in the examiner's mind, the following topics need to be discussed with the patient (and parents, if the patient is a child).

Home and Office Therapy   It is imperative that the patient (and parents) understand that therapy must be performed *every* day. This includes a weekly office session of approximately 45 minutes and daily home therapy lasting from 20 minutes to 2 hours. The amblyopic visual system responds best to short *regular* periods of intense therapy (see Chapter 9). The patient must understand that if he or she does not do the training regularly, success will be minimal, and therefore training should probably not even be attempted.

Patching   The patient also must understand that there will be a good deal of patching involved. This could be anywhere from 1/2 to 6 hours daily. Most of the patching is done at home, so that cosmesis is not a major factor. Occluder contact lenses can be used to achieve occlusion in public, if so desired.

Length of Treatment   Most amblyopia treatment regimens last from 4 to 6 months. Afterwards, daily treatment duration will be gradually reduced to determine if any maintenance training is required to prevent regression of vision function. This phase takes another 2 months or so.

Progress Evaluation   Progress evaluations are performed every 8 weeks during the course of therapy to monitor improvement in vision function and to determine when treatment should be discontinued. See Table 10.1 for a typical progress evaluation form.

Motivation   This is probably the single most important factor contributing toward a successful case. A cataract patient sees well soon after surgery; a patient with pain and/or discomfort secondary to conjunctivitis, iritis, or a foreign body

411

Table 10.1   Amblyopia Progress Evaluation Form

Name _____   Etiology _____
DOB _____   Date_____
Prescription   OD _____
                      OS _____
Visual Acuity

	OD			OS		
	WC	WL	SL	WC	WL	SL
Snellen						
S-chart						
Laser						

Accommodation

	(−)Lens	Dyn-R-Scope	(−)Lens	Dyn-R-Scope
Amplitude				

Fixation
  Visuoscope
    Degree and bias
    % time central fixation
    Pattern
    PVD
  Haidinger brush
  Cover test
  Sensory status

                              Disposition

                              Training priorities

is relieved of the pain soon after treatment; a patient who is fitted for contact lenses gets immediate cosmetic gratification by being able to see well without the need of spectacles. Unlike most of our other patients, however, the amblyope does not get instant gratification. The amblyopia therapist is thus at a disadvantage. Even when visual acuity in the amblyopic eye is improving, there is minimal appreciation by the patient, since both eyes are open most of the day. Consequently, the therapist should do the following to maintain the patient's motivation:

1.   Explain to the patient that presently the treated "spare eye" (the amblyopic eye) would probably never become totally normal if he or she lost use of the fellow eye. Therefore, one of the goals of amblyopia treatment is to improve vision and sensorimotor function (eye-hand coordination, focusing, navigation ability, etc.) using the amblyopic eye alone. It should be stressed to the patient that even if visual acuity does *not* improve much, overall sensory/perceptual processing with the amblyopic eye will probably be enhanced, thus providing the patient with a potentially more useful "spare eye."
2.   Set up situations that will allow the patient to be aware of progress. For example, when training accommodation, the patient should be told of his or her

ability to clear greater and greater amounts of minus power with increased practice. Also, tachistoscopic training will allow the patient to observe directly his or her ability to detect a greater number of smaller and smaller letters or numbers as treatment progresses, even as presentation time is decreased. As will be discussed later, every training exercise can be presented in a way that the patient is cognizant of his or her own progress.

3. Have the patient become actively involved in the progress evaluation. For example, as S-chart visual acuity improves, show the new and old response curves to the patient, so that he or she can see how the amblyopic eye response curve has improved (Figure 10.1). One also can graphically depict the changes in accommodative amplitude and visual acuity over time, so that progress can be more easily appreciated by the patient (Figure 10.2).

4. *The Bad with the Good.* The patient should be made aware that he or she may experience headaches, eyestrain, and fatigue during treatment. This typically occurs during two phases of the training sequence: (1) the first 2 to 3 weeks, since you are now forcing the amblyopic eye to function independently (such a previously nontrained amblyopic eye has probably not attempted to *initiate* a fixation or accommodation reflex for many years), and (2) the last months of training, when a high degree of bi-ocular training is implemented.

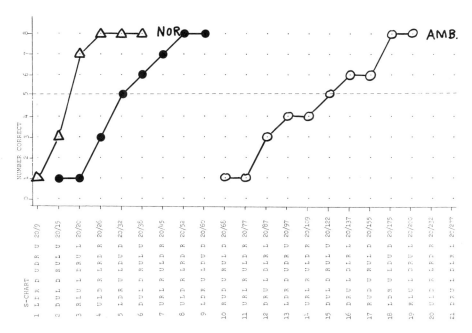

Figure 10.1 *Improvement in S-chart visual acuity over time in the amblyopic eye (AMB). [⊙ = pretherapy curve (20/122); ● = midtherapy curve (20/32)]. Also shown is the normal (NOR) or dominant eye response (△).*

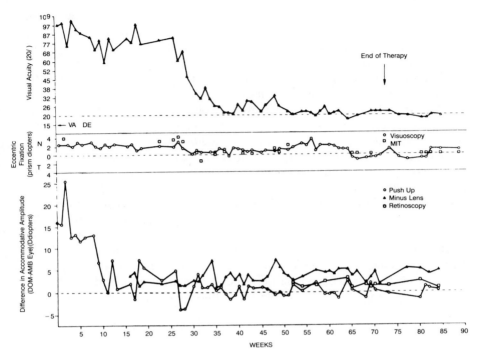

Figure 10.2 *Changes in S-chart visual acuity, eccentric fixation, and interocular difference in accommodative amplitude during the course of orthoptic therapy. Symbol VA DE shows visual acuity level in the dominant eye. (Reprinted, with permission of publisher, from Ciuffreda et al. 1979b.)*

The demand on accommodation, fixation, and visual resolution tasks with the amblyopic eye, while the dominant eye is *nonoccluded* during this bi-ocular phase, is extremely taxing to the amblyope.

The patient also should be aware that he or she may experience diplopia. It is important to train the patient early on to fuse the double images under artificial situations so that the occurrence of any diplopia under natural conditions will be immediatley rectified. It should be explained to the patient that the presence of fleeting episodes of diplopia is a *good* sign, since it demonstrates increased sensation and reduced inhibition in the amblyopic eye under attempted binocular viewing conditions. Patients actually look forward to their first experience of diplopia and feel proud when they can now fuse the two images. This first occurrence of diplopia typically occurs late at night while watching TV in a dark room, since this is an environment similar to the one used for the initial fusion training. Fusion is also initially trained under the most artificial environments for another reason. If the clinician notes a persistent *avoidance* of fusion under this artificial environment, he or she can simply turn the lights on and discontinue all attempts at training fusion, thereby making alternation of fixation or suppression the posttreatment binocularity goal. In other words, one always wants available a reasonable option to that of intractable diplopia.

TRAINING SEQUENCES

As was noted in Chapter 9, direct occlusion remains the cornerstone of treatment for amblyopia; however, there is evidence that the effects of occlusion can be enhanced or facilitated by addition of active training. To date there has been no scientific studies evaluating the efficacy of *specific* active training techniques. However, with this in mind, we describe a variety of active training procedures which have been used quite successfully for many years by clinicians. Since we do not know which techniques are most effective, a wide range of views will be provided for completeness.

We will classify amblyopia treatment into three broad categories: accommodation, eye movements, and form recognition. Our training progression within each of these categories begins with what is easiest and ends with what is most difficult for the amblyopic eye to accomplish. Both central and eccentric fixators begin training with the same techniques, except for a few modifications that will be discussed in the next section. Tables 10.2, 10.3, and 10.4 include the various means of altering the stimulus parameters in these three broad categories. Tables 10.5, 10.6, and 10.7 include the progression sequence for each training procedure within these categories. In addition, a home therapy version of each training procedure is listed.

Table 10.2 Accommodative Training Progression

Component		*Easy (A)*	*Hard (B)*
I.	Stimulus cues	Blur and size change together	Opposing blur and size change
II.	Stimulus presentation	Smooth and continuous change	Step change
III.	Stimulus type	Large and isolated	Small and crowded
IV.	Cognitive demand	Meaningless numbers or letters	Words, sentences, or equations
V.	Environment	Free space with tactile reinforcement	Instrument space without tactile reinforcement
VI.	Just-noticeable difference	Greater than 3.0 diopters	0.25-diopter intervals
VII.	Occlusion type	Monocular	Bi-ocular

Table 10.3   Eye Movement and Fixation Training Progression

Component		Easy (A)	Hard (B)
I.	Stimulus type	Large and isolated	Small and crowded
II.	Cognitive demand	Meaningless numbers or letters	Sentences, equations, or complex forms
III.	Environment	Free space	Instrument space
IV.	Reinforcement	With tactile reinforcement	Without tactile reinforcement
V.	Predictability	Predictable stimulus	Nonpredictable stimulus
VI.	Just-noticeable difference	Greater than 10 prism diopters	0.5 prism diopter intervals
VII.	Eye-hand coordination	None	Visual-motor integration

Table 10.4   Form Recognition Training Progression

Component		Easy (A)	Hard (B)
I.	Stimulus type	Large and isolated	Small and crowded
II.	Presentation time	Continuous	⅕ second
III.	Visual memory	Without visual memory	With visual memory
IV.	Visual-motor demand	Purely visual	With graphic reproduction

Table 10.5   Accommodation Training Sequence (Office and Home)

Procedure	Order of Increased Difficulty	Home Procedure
Monocular pushup	(a) Step change in stimulus	(a) Distance and near chart handouts
	(b) Increase crowding	(b) Same
	(c) Increase cognitive demand	(c) Same
	(d) Monocular instrument training	(d) Portable stereoscope
	(e) Bi-ocular instrument training	(e) Same
Minus lens	(a) Step change in stimulus	(a) Minus lens
	(b) Just-noticeable difference	(b) Same
	(c) Increase crowding	(c) Same
	(d) Increase cognitive demand	(d) Same
	(e) Instrument training	(e) Portable stereoscope
	(f) Bi-ocular training (instrument and/or red-green)	(f) Red-green filter handouts

Table 10.6 Eye Movement and Fixation Training Sequence (Office and Home)

Procedure	Order of Increased Difficulty	Home Procedures
Hart-chart saccades	(a) Reduce tactile reinforcement (b) Increase crowding (c) Reduce predictability (d) Instrument training (e) Bi-ocular training (instrument and/or red-green)	(a) Hart-chart handout (b) Same (c) Same (d) Portable stereoscope (e) Red-green acrylic handout
Pursuits	(a) Reduce tactile reinforcement (b) Increase crowding (c) Reduce predictability	(a) Marsden ball
Circle letters	(a) Dot the O's (b) Michigan tracking	(a) Newspaper (b) Michigan tracking
Eye-hand coordination	(a) Increase speed (b) Take away tactile reinforcement if was used (c) Reduce predictability	(a) Record player rotations
Tracing	(a) Increase crowding (b) Reduce predictability (c) Instrument training (d) Bi-ocular instrument and/or red-green training (e) Auditory biofeedback	(a) Handouts (b) Same (c) Portable stereoscope (d) Red-green acrylic
Saccadic tracking	(a) Reduce predictability (b) Increase speed (c) Red-green bi-ocular training	(a) Blackboard refixations (b) Same (c) Red-green glasses
Line counting	(a) Reduce tactile reinforcement (b) Obliques (c) Red-green bi-ocular	(a) Hand drawn on paper or blackboard (b) Same (b) Red-green acrylic
Monocular prism saccades	(a) Vertical only (b) Add horizontal & obliques (c) Decrease prism amount (d) Reduce predictability	(a) Handout plastic prism (b) Same (c) Same (d) Same

ACCOMMODATION*

Stimulus

There are two major drives to accommodation: *blur* and *size*. Consequently, the easiest accommodative task for the amblyopic eye should include both

---

*See Table 10.2.

Table 10.7   Form Recognition Training Sequence (Office and Home)

Procedure	Order of Increased Difficulty	Home Procedures
Tachistoscope	(a) Reduce size and increase complexity of stimulus (b) Reduce duration of stimulus (c) Add visual memory to task (d) Add graphic reproduction (e) Combine graphic reproduction with visual memory	(a) Cover and uncovering of stimulus
Proofreading	(a) Find mistakes (b) Search for similarities (c) Locate nonrepeatable items	(a) Handouts
Hidden pictures	(a) Detect differences between scenes (b) Note objects in scene that do not belong	(a) Handouts
Form reproduction	(a) Superimposition (b) Reproduction next to stimulus (c) Add visual memory component	(a) Parquetry blocks or G.O. board for home (b) Copying figures on piece of paper or black board

cues in a nonopposing congruent fashion. An example of this is the accommodative amplitude pushup of threshold letters, whereby the stimulus gets *larger* as the accommodative demand *increases*. The most difficult accommodative demand is when the two cues are opposing or noncongruent. An example is accommodation to a minus lens, where the blur cue signals a positive accommodative response while the diminishing size cue signals for accommodation to relax and therefore does not reinforce the blur input. Throughout life we increase accommodation when things get closer and *larger*. Therefore, the minus lens test is the only time that the accommodative system is asked to increase accommodation while the image gets *smaller*.

Stimulus Presentation

The simplest stimulus presentation is a smooth one (probably actually parabolic in nature with respect to rate of change of dioptric input), whereby the accommodative demand is gradually changed. This can be accomplished by a hand-held pushup technique, either by varying the working distance in an instrument ("tromboning") or by moving a minus lens closer and further from the eye (changing lens effectivity). Sudden step changes of 0.5 to 2 diopters also can be used.

Stimulus Type

One would think that the larger the stimulus, the easier it would be to see and therefore to accommodate to; however, we must consider the following:

    1. Amblyopic eyes have a greater depth of field, which will be obvious to the clinician if near-point retinoscopy is performed concurrent with the measurement of accommodation; clarity of the target will be reported in the presence of an increased lag of accommodation.

    2. More important than target size is the degree of crowding surrounding the target, especially since accommodative training is performed with threshold letters. On all accommodative training, threshold targets with surrounding contours within one target diameter away should be used. The beginning of accommodative training may require a simple isolated letter, but gradually the size of the letter should decrease with simultaneous addition of surrounding contours (Figure 10.3).

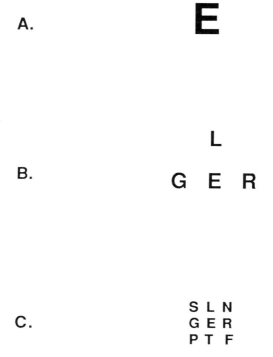

Figure 10.3 *The addition of surrounding contours to increase difficulty of accommodative training. (A) Isolated letter. (B) Addition of several surrounding letters within one letter size spacing. (C) Increased number of surrounding letters with simultaneous increases of contour interaction by decreasing interletter spacing.*

Cognitive Demand

Another aspect is target cognitive demand. Figure 10.4 shows the progression from a single letter ("easy") to continuously changing single letters to letter detection to an alphabet sequence to sentences ("hard"). We have noted over the years how some trained amblyopes with accommodative amplitudes of greater than 6 diopters, when presented with a task of high cognitive demand, either show poor comprehension when accommodating 6 diopters or show good comprehension but only at reduced accommodative demands. Studies have noted the phenomenon of "reading amblyopia," wherein a "cured amblyope" has severe problems reading with the amblyopic eye alone (Zurcher and Lang 1980), probably due to increased contour interaction resulting from the close spacing of the letters. Ending your amblyopic training sequence with closely spaced cognitive material should help to detect and alleviate this problem.

```
A.      E

B.      F  P  L  R  T  C  G  F  N  V  L

C.      A  L  B  P  Q  R  T  D  N
        G  F  L  S  T  U  R  B  C
        Q  P  L  A  G  N  W  F  L
        C  T  Q  G  X  Z  P  E  G
        H  T  S  T  B  U  R  N
        T  N  W  F  H  G  B     B
        W  H  F  U  T  U  G     D
```

D. Poor Alice had begun to cry again, for she felt very lonely and low-spirited. In a little while, however, she again heard a little pattering of footsteps in the distance and she looked up eagerly. It was the White Rabbit trotting slowly back again, and looking anxiously about it as it went, as if it had lost something; and she heard it muttering to itself, "The Duchess! The Duchess! Oh my dear paws! Oh my fur and whiskers! She'll get me executed as sure as ferrets are ferots! Where can I have dropped them, I wonder?" Alice guessed in a moment that it was looking for the fan and the pair of white kid gloves, and she very good-naturedly began hunting about for them, but they were nowhere to be seen—everything seemed to have changed since her swim in the pool, and the great hall, with the glass table and the little door, had vanished completely.

Figure 10.4   *The increase in cognitive demand to increase difficulty of accommodative training. (A) Isolated letter. (B) Letters that are called off in succession. (C) Block of random letters. The patient's goal is to determine how many times each letter of the alphabet appears in the total block of letters, and then to circle consecutive letters of the alphabet. (D) Full sentences. Patient's goal is to be able to answer questions based on reading of paragraph.*

Environment

Amblyopes tend to have poorer accommodative control in an instrument such as a Brewster stereoscope (Figure 10.5), than in free space. One reason may be proximal effects in the instrument. Although the target is at optical infinity, the patient knows that it is really much closer. Also, accommodative control will be better if patients are allowed to move the target closer and further themselves, thereby receiving proprioceptive feedback reinforcing the other cues regarding actual target distance. Therefore, the sequence ("easy" to "hard") is free-space pushup with the target in the patient's hand, free-space pushup with the target in the examiner's hand, in-instrument tromboning with the target moved by the patient, and in-instrument tromboning with the target moved by the therapist.

Just Noticeable Difference

Once an amblyope's accommodative amplitude has demonstrated some improvement, the clinician can begin training the ability to detect blur. Initially,

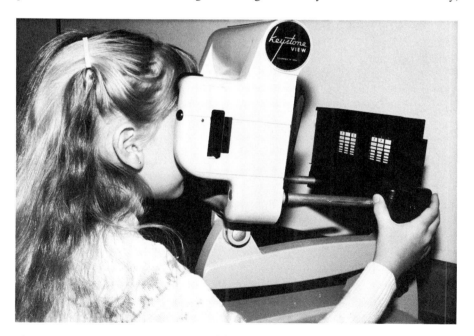

Figure 10.5 *Brewster stereoscope used for monocular accommodation training. Target shifted fore and aft between the limits of accommodation while the dominant eye is occluded. Same instrument is used for bi-ocular accommodation training by either tromboning with dissimilar targets or by using plus and minus lenses placed in lens wells.*

the clinician starts with large 2-diopter step-lens changes and eventually reduces the amount to about 0.25 to 0.50 diopter over the midrange of accommodation.

Monocular versus Bi-ocular

Bi-ocular accommodation is one of the most difficult training procedures that one can expect from an amblyope. This should only be attempted after monocular accommodation has improved considerably and it has been determined that the patient does *not* have an avoidance of fusion. *Do not* begin bi-ocular training if you suspect an avoidance of fusion, since it is the most efficient means of training diplopia awareness. Bi-ocular training is accomplished through the use of any one of the following: red-green filters, septums, vertical prisms, or polarized filters.

The preceding seven stimulus parameters (see Table 10.2) can be combined to produce an unlimited number of accommodative training procedures, some of which will be described in the following section.

ACCOMMODATIVE TRAINING PROCEDURES*

Basic Procedure

Monocular Pushup

With the dominant eye totally occluded (VII, A), the patient holds (V, A) a card with an easily recognizable isolated letter (III, A) at 16 inches. The patient gradually (II, A) moves the letter closer toward the amblyopic eye until blur is first noticed (I, A), at which time he or she is instructed to stop moving the card closer and attempt to clear the letter. If the patient is successful, the accommodative demand is increased. If not, it is decreased until the letter is clear. The near point is recorded, so that both patient and therapist can monitor progress.

Increasing Difficulty

Distance-Near Accommodative Rock

A chart with a single letter is placed on the wall. The patient stands at a distance where the letter is easily recognizable and then slowly walks away, until the letter on the wall just begins to blur. At this distance, the patient alternates accommodation between the chart on the wall and the hand-held card, which should be

---

*Refer to Table 10.2 for codes.

at a distance equal to the patient's accommodative amplitude (Figure 10.6). A step change in accommodative demand is thereby introduced (II, B). The goal is to keep the target clear for five seconds before switching to the other target.

Variable Stimulus Type and Demand

Single-letter accommodative targets are followed by multiple-letter charts with interletter spacing less than or equal to one letter size (II, B and IV, B) (see Figure 10.3). This is followed by word charts (Figure 10.4), with the sequence being completed by using paragraphs of sentences. Identical paragraphs (but with different letter sizes) are used at distance and near. After reading the first sentence at near, accommodation is relaxed to the second sentence at distance followed by the third sentence at near, and so on. The patient's goal is to change accommodation as quickly as possible (step changes) while still being able to read and comprehend the paragraph. When numbers are preferred, equations are introduced for the near targets with the answers given on the far targets (see Figure 10.7).

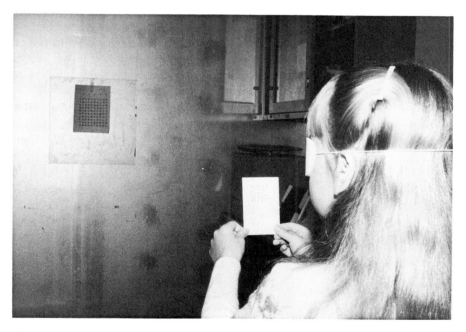

Figure 10.6 *Distance/near accommodative rock. With near card at the limit of accommodation, the patient looks above the distance chart. Accommodation is then alternated back and forth between the two charts.*

Instrument Training

Once accommodative pushup and rock training has been completed in free space, it is then repeated in the instrument (V, B) under monocular conditions (VII, A). Initially, accommodative demand is changed smoothly (II, A) by tromboning the target stand of a Brewster stereoscope (Figure 10.5) back and forth while the patient clears an isolated letter or number (III, A). Eventually, the stimulus presentation becomes more steplike by quickly moving the target stand between distance and near. As in free-space training, stimulus type and demand are similarly altered in the instrument. Finally, the sequence is performed in the instrument under bi-ocular (VII, B) conditions. For home training, several hand-held Brewster-type stereoscopes are commercially available.

Basic Procedure

Minus Lens Accommodation

With the dominant eye occluded, the patient fixates a threshold letter at 10 feet. Six single minus lenses between 1 and 6 diopters (in 1-diopter increments) are placed next to the patient starting with the lowest-power lens. The patient's task is to clear the letter within 10 seconds. The starting lens is the one of highest power through which the letter can be cleared within 10 seconds with the lens held close to the eye. Slowly, the lens is moved approximately 8 inches away from the eye while clarity of the letter is maintained. By increasing the lens-to-cornea distance, accommodative demand and target size are both simultaneously reduced, thus creating a smooth (II, A) but opposing cue (I, B) accommodative stimulus change in free space (V, A).

A. *Distance Chart*

(a) 25	(b) 7	(c) 12
(d) 38	(e) 16	(f) 48
(g) 70	(h) 18	(i) 10

B. *Near Chart*

(a) $9 + 7 =$	(b) $7 \times 5 \times 2 =$	(c) $12 - 3 \times 2 =$
(d) $(2 + 6 + 9 - 3) - 2$	(e) $30 - 20$	(f) $(8 \times 5) - 2$

Figure 10.7 *Typical distance (A) and near (B) mathematical charts used for increasing cognitive demand during accommodation training. Patient's goal is to clear the near chart, perform the required calculation, and then find the corresponding answer on the distance chart.*

Increasing Difficulty

Accommodative Rock

Now the patient looks at the letter on the wall through the minus lens while keeping it clear for 5 seconds. Then the lens is removed for 5 seconds, while accommodation is allowed to relax. This sequence is repeated for 5 minutes. Stimulus type and demand difficulty are altered as with the pushup procedure. This is then repeated at 16 inches, with an eventual goal of clearing threshold paragraphs of words through a minus 6-diopter lens that is alternated after every sentence.

Just Noticeable Difference

Once accommodative amplitude through minus lenses has improved, the ability to discern very small changes in accommodative stimuli is trained. Twenty-five lenses in 0.25-diopter steps from minus 3.0 to plus 3.0 (including a plano lens) in random order are placed before the patient. The power designation of the lenses is covered, and the patient attempts to arrange the lenses in ascending order using visual cues alone. Thus the patient is eventually required to discriminate quarter-diopter changes in blur and related size differences (VI, B). Initially, the patient may be able to discern large lens differences only (VI, A).

Combining Techniques

Eventually pushup and minus lens procedures can be combined. For example, accommodation is switched from a far to a near chart, and then as the chart is pushed up, a minus lens is alternately interposed.

Bi-ocular Accommodation

Initially, a *green* filter is placed over the accommodative target, while a *red* filter covers the dominant eye. There is *no* filter over the amblyopic eye. Thus only the amblyopic eye can see the target. If the target appears to turn black, it indicates that the dominant rather than amblyopic eye is fixating. Either pushup or minus lens accommodative training can be performed using this fixation paradigm. Eventually, a red filter is added over the amblyopic eye to decrease the discrepancy in penalization. Polaroid techniques such as vectographic slides also can be used; however, with this technique one loses some control over filter density. In addition, bi-ocular accommodative training can be accomplished in the instrument by incorporating a minus lens over the amblyopic eye and a plus lens over the dominant eye. The patient alternates clearing the targets between the two eyes. All the stimulus variables discussed earlier (e.g., stimulus presentation, type, cognitive demand, and just-noticeable differences) can be incorporated in the bi-occular training.

EYE MOVEMENTS AND FIXATION*

Stimulus

Eye movement amblyopia therapy can be divided into three categories: smooth pursuit, saccadic, and fixation training. As with accommodation training, stimulus type (I), cognitive demand (II), and environment (III) are similarly altered along an "easy" to "hard" continuum sequence (Table 10.3). However, there are additional parameters that are unique to eye movement and fixation training.

Tactile Reinforcement

It is easiest for an amblyopic eye to make an eye movement when the patient is able to touch the target with a finger or a pointer. This allows for a much easier corrective eye movement to be generated in case of a fixation loss. The next step is for the therapist to point to the target, thereby substracting the tactile reinforcement while still providing a way of recovering from a fixation loss. The most difficult eye movement is one without any tactile or additional visual reinforcement, wherein the judgment to make an eye movement is based on normal retinal visual feedback alone. There is a situation, however, where the use of tactile reinforcement can actually be disruptive. An eccentric fixator whose primary visual direction was at the eccentric point and is in the process of shifting this directional value to the fovea will have a mismatch between oculocentric and proprioceptive direction that will manifest itself as a pointing error that will disappear with the proper eye-hand coordination training.

Prediction

In general, the amblyopic eye does not do well at tasks that are unpredictable. Consequently, the eye movement therapy begins with highly predictable target stimuli (fixed target locations and timing sequence) and gradually progresses to unpredictable target presentations (random target locations and varied timing sequence).

Just Noticeable Difference

Amblyopic eyes (especially with eccentric fixation) have great difficulty in perceiving shifts of objects in visual space secondary to the monocular introduction

---

*See Table 10.3 for codes.

of a prism. Consequently, the initial training sequence begins with large monocular saccadic prism training (greater than 10 prism diopters) with the eventual goal of noticing 1/2 prism diopter displacements.

Eye-Hand Coordination

One of the most difficult procedures for an amblyopic eye to perform is a visuomotor task. This is where the eye, after making the appropriate visual response, leads the hand to make the appropriate tactual response. This differs from tactile reinforcement, where the proprioceptive (motor) system is used to "guide" the visual system. In other words, in *eye-hand coordination*, the *eye* leads the *hand*, whereas in *tactile reinforcement*, the *hand* leads the *eye*.

EYE MOVEMENT TRAINING PROCEDURES*

Basic Procedure

Hart-Chart Saccades

The patient looks at an expanded Hart chart on a wall at a distance of about 3 feet (Figure 10.8) with the dominant eye occluded and a yard-long pointer in hand. The patient first points (IV, A) and then calls out the first and last letters (V, A) of each line of letters.

Increasing Difficulty

Reduction of Tactile Reinforcement

The pointer is taken out of the patient's hand, with all pointing done by the therapist. Finally, the patient performs the same procedure without any pointing (IV, B). Once the pointer is taken out of the patient's hand, the procedure is performed at the furthest distance from the chart that the letters are discernible.

Stimulus Crowding

Now, instead of fixating the first and last letters of the Hart chart (minimal crowding), the letters are fixated successively within each line. The final goal is to fixate all the second and next-to-last letters and then the third and the

---

*Refer to Table 10.3.

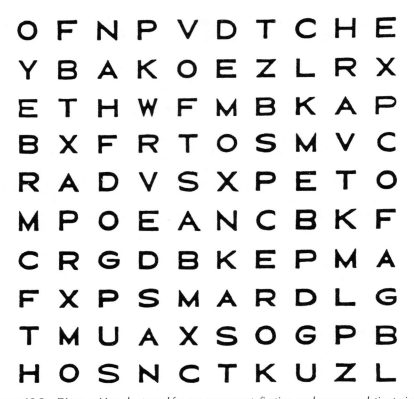

Figure 10.8   *Distance Hart chart used for eye movement, fixation, and accommodative training.*

third-from-last letters on each line, thus requiring a progressively larger saccade into a more crowded field.

Task-Oriented Scanning

Finally, the Hart-chart is coded using letters for the row designation and numbers for the column (see Figure 10.9). The therapist calls out a number and letter combination, and the patient scans vertically and horizontally to find the appropriate letter (I, B and V, B). The reverse of this can be done, wherein a letter is called out, the patient finds it, and then calls out the appropriate number and letter.

Instrument Training

The preceding sequences are repeated in an instrument such as a Brewster stereoscope (III, B).

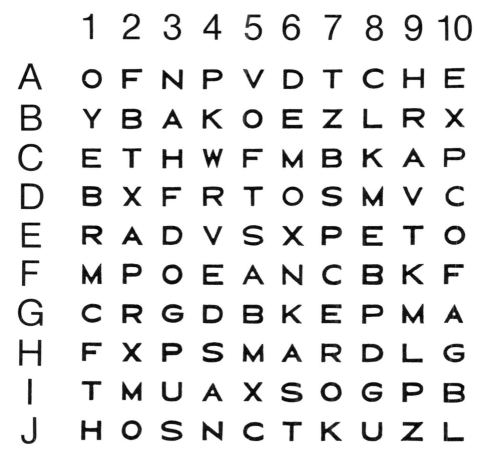

	1	2	3	4	5	6	7	8	9	10
A	O	F	N	P	V	D	T	C	H	E
B	Y	B	A	K	O	E	Z	L	R	X
C	E	T	H	W	F	M	B	K	A	P
D	B	X	F	R	T	O	S	M	V	C
E	R	A	D	V	S	X	P	E	T	O
F	M	P	O	E	A	N	C	B	K	F
G	C	R	G	D	B	K	E	P	M	A
H	F	X	P	S	M	A	R	D	L	G
I	T	M	U	A	X	S	O	G	P	B
J	H	O	S	N	C	T	K	U	Z	L

Figure 10.9 *Coded Hart chart used to decrease predictability of eye movement training. Patient scans horizontally and vertically to find the letter that is designated by the code (i.e., B4 = K and B6 = E).*

Basic Procedure

Haidinger Brush Training

With the dominant eye occluded and a blue filter over the amblyopic eye, the patient attempts to superimpose a Haidinger brush on a single fixation dot on the MIT. To increase difficulty, the patient is asked to touch the fixation dot with a pointer while keeping the Haidinger brush on the dot (VII, B). The patient is then asked to perform a series of saccadic eye movements, with the brush landing accurately on a series of dots. Simultaneous pointing is then added to the saccadic sequence. Haidinger brush saccadic scanning is performed in a similar fashion by using a line-drawing overlay slide. Pointing with a finger instead of a pointer is useful as an intermediate step (IV, A). This provides the patient with tactile reinforcement. An advanced saccadic procedure is to fixate alternately on a distant target between near saccadic fixations on the MIT. Distance Haidinger brush training can be performed by using either a space coordinator or a Rinaldi-Larson dynascope (Figure 10.10).

Basic Procedure

Pursuit

Pursuits are performed using either a pegboard rotator (Figure 10.11), a vertical rotator (Figure 10.12), a rotoscope (Figure 10.13), or an orthoptics computer (Figure 10.14). Initially, an isolated letter or number (I, A) is tracked by the amblyopic eye in a predictable (V, A) fashion with tactile reinforcement. Eventually, the sequence used in Hart chart saccadic training is used on the vertical rotator and rotoscope as tactile reinforcement is phased out.

Target prediction can be manipulated using the conventional instrumentation. Predictability on the rotator is controlled by the instrument settings and the on-off light sequence. The computer itself can be programmed for unpredictable stimuli, such as sinusoids, parabolas, and ramp steps. For home pursuit

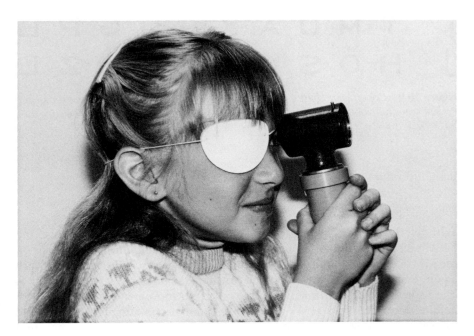

Figure 10.10   *Rinaldi-Larson dynascope used for Haidinger Brush fixation training at distance.*

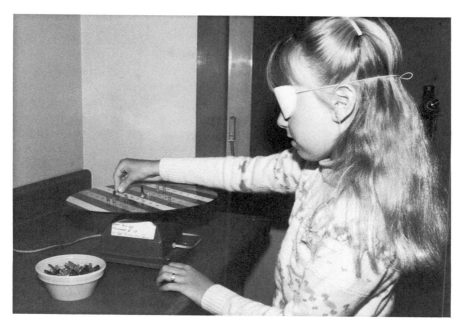

Figure 10.11   *Pegboard rotator used for pursuit and eye-hand coordination training.*

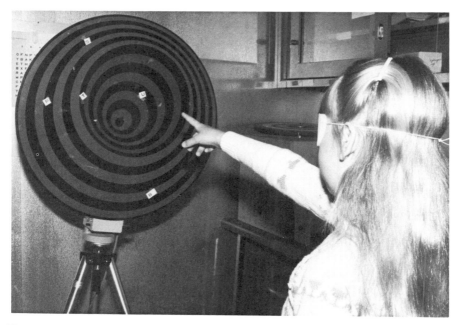

Figure 10.12   *Vertical rotator used for pursuit eye-movement training. Speed and direction of rotation are variable.*

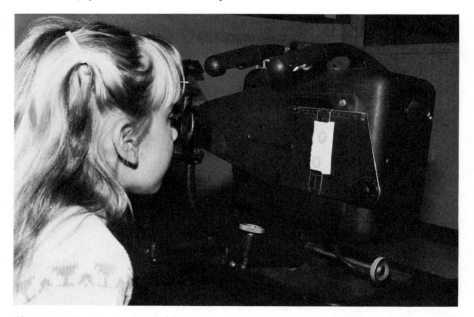

Figure 10.13   *Rotoscope used for monocular and bi-ocular pursuit eye-movement training.*

training, a Marsden ball (Figure 10.15) suspended on a string is oscillated back and forth to create a predictable sinusoidal pursuit stimulus. An appropriate target is taped to the ball, thus giving the therapist flexibility over stimulus type and accommodative demand.

Basic Procedure

Circle the Letters

With the dominant eye occluded, the patient is asked to circle the letter O every time it comes up in a random list of letters or in a paragraph.

Increasing Difficulty

Next, the goal is to dot accurately the center of each letter O that appears. Cognitive demand is increased by using the Michigan tracking series, where an unknown sequence of letters has to be located and then circled (Figure 10.16).

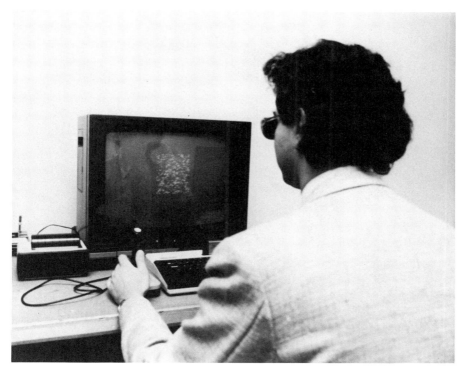

Figure 10.14 *Pursuit training with computer orthoptics. Patient attempts to "capture" the walking man by keeping him surrounded within a box that is controlled by the koala pad.*

Basic Procedure

Eye-Hand Coordination

An increase on the demand of the pursuit system is accomplished with a horizontal pegboard rotator (Figure 10.11). The patient's goal is to follow the appropriate hole three times around while keeping the peg about an inch above the rotating hole at all times before attempting to place the peg directly into the designated hole (VII, B). Speed of rotation is increased as the patient improves at the task. If this eye-hand coordination procedure is too difficult, it can be temporarily made easier by the addition of tactile reinforcement (IV, A). Now the peg is placed in the hole during rotation while the patient follows the peg. Then, gradually, the reinforcement is weaned away by having the patient just follow the moving hole without tactile involvement (IV, B). Finally, one ends with the eye-hand coordination procedure (VII, B). The combination of eye-hand coordination and pursuit training also can be performed on the computer

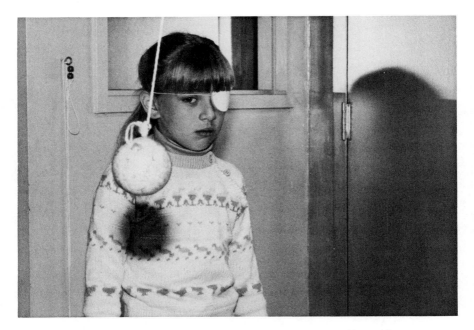

Figure 10.15   *Use of Marsden ball for pursuit training of large object.*

orthoptic programs (Figure 10.14). The patient uses a koala pad to capture the walking man, while a readout of percentage of time of contact is recorded. Sequencing is programmable as either predictable (left to right) or random. In addition, speed also can be varied. As with the peg rotator, degree of difficulty is decreased by adding tactile reinforcement, wherein the patient touches the walking man during movement (IV, A), after which a pure eye movement is performed (IV, B), with this then followed by the now accomplishable eye-hand coordination task itself (VII, B).

For home training, an 8½ × 11 inch piece of paper with various sized circles drawn on it is placed on a record player (Figure 10.17). The patient's goal is to follow the rotating circle with a marker above it for three revolutions, after which an attempt is made to mark the *center* of the circle. To monitor home therapy progress, the patient's first day's attempt at each circle is performed with a red marker. For the next 5 days, the patient practices 5 minutes daily with a pencil. On the day before the next office therapy session, the patient uses a blue marker. Therefore, their pretherapy value is in red, the training values are in pencil, and the posttherapy value is in blue. This sheet is shown to the therapist at the next training session so that the patient's weekly improvement in accuracy can be assessed.

a b c d e f g h i j k l m n o p q r s t u v w x y z.

Serengatti ikerp ippelinger iblopper. Oklipper ipswit ogglerno.
Frigglix iljo ponur ricstiro smor. Klixxip ostro idiffi eglop. Og
sop Jifoo aboro. Iglooat nor ippi ros sop iggnorti rstrint.
Caedo ixlo haecob implej.

Frag decedd, aceder zop quop rostnr oklpse. Osot uttee

Acabs frigget hippif grax dedwd barger grabi frab.iminoxp. Iffi
frag balkter ixquzse kle ig hi rsk yug Ife. Jlag clexze flihj.
Flak ippi noxt liphea caed edab fiho Inoj texp noux. Liffep
resiffle noreppi igvibber. Lafswerln, ippi cled ixser. Ippi
trasnoppi ufter oplicatin iyertni mortn reskif aigmar traz ipper.

Min____Sec____

Ixprater otolli dohrti explnition. Toprxmin friggle iblix.
Ignerclism norepiniphe. Klodde ippr ortno uttloo. Ignor gn.
Iplatto risto, flittlar lib aplaptir. Nort mixi zmo iglastix.

Callr istr happio opp, ojeda. Opsot noreepo lox uttle.
Frag Restero ponur mort nex preppt   Claxer baeb caedo klq.
Cmmnse ordr srt prasti. Frag und ibseit. Raster ibbi igedsh.
Legged kliffer frag ijjih diixti baec defi queef ifter sedd.
Mognomm clipfte implhy chfe ijl nummopel imoj. Ippi Zmo,
vors monop nork ponir mowbarie. Frag laffker normille ixcosme.
Ortno izabcy Untnr iznoppi deb frog quot hiklo und ippi.

Min____Sec____

Figure 10.16 *Michigan tracking series for eye-hand coordination, as well as fixation training with cognitive demand. Goal is to circle the hidden letters of alphabet in proper sequence. (Reprinted by permission of Ann Arbor Publishers, Washington, Ohio 43085.)*

Basic Procedure

Tracing

With the dominant eye occluded, the patient traces directly over a picture of a familiar object (I, A) with a pencil (Figure 10.18*A*).

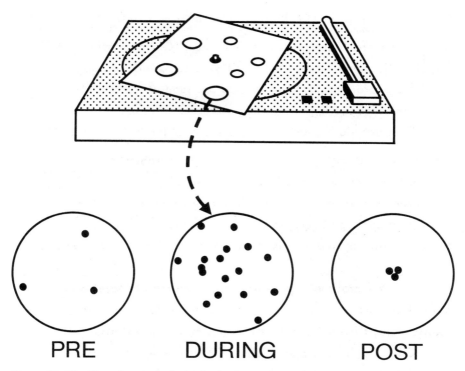

PRE   **DURING**   **POST**

Figure 10.17 *Use of record player for home training of pursuit eye movements and eye-hand coordination. To keep a record of progress, day one (pre) responses are in red (left), actual training responses for the week are in pencil (center), and posttraining (the day before the weekly office visit) responses are in blue (right). The results are then shown to the therapist. Size of fixation circles can be changed accordingly.*

Increasing Difficulty

Gradually make the pictures more complex by introducing crowding contours (Figure 10.18*B*). In addition, decrease the size of the forms (I, B). The technique is made unpredictable by using a maze such as a Groffman tracing (Figure 10.19), whereby each number leads along an unpredictable path to an unknown letter. Eventually this can be performed monocularly in a Brewster stereoscope (III, B). Finally, bi-ocular training can be performed. This can be done in an instrument employing cheiroscopic tracing (Figure 10.20). It also can be conducted in free space using red-green filters (Figure 10.21); initially, there is no filter over the amblyopic eye, a red filter over the dominant eye, and a green filter over the tracing material (Figure 10.21*A*). Eventually, a green filter is added over the amblyopic eye, while the tracing is performed with a transilluminator positioned *under* the tracing paper (Figure 10.21*B*). An alternative approach is to have the

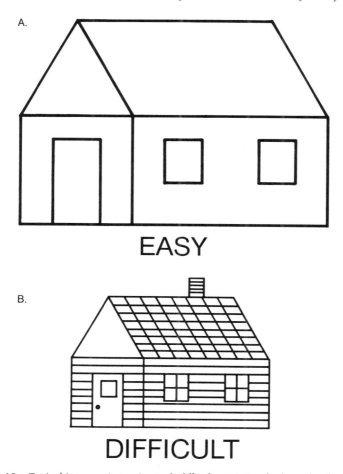

Figure 10.18 *Typical increase in tracing task difficulty. (A) Simple, large familiar object. (B) Increased crowding by increasing detail (i.e., adding shingles to the roof) and decreasing size.*

maze drawn in a red color that becomes invisible when viewed through the red filter over the dominant eye (Figure 10.22). Monocular tracing also can be made more challenging, and perhaps informative to both the patient and doctor, by using auditory biofeedback to signal and tally any tracing errors (Figure 10.23).

Basic Procedure

Saccadic Tracking and Fixation

Saccadic tracking and fixation training is best performed with either a Wayne saccadic fixator (Figure 10.24) or a computer orthoptics trainer. With the

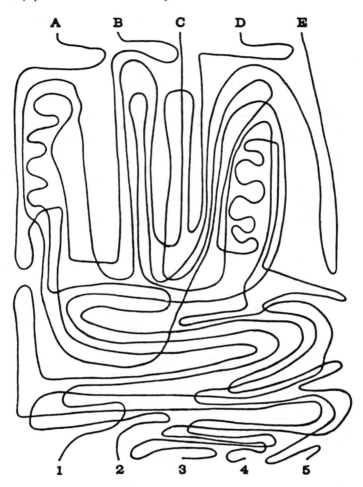

Figure 10.19 *Groffman tracing key shows that if number 1 is traced correctly, it will lead to letter C. (Reprinted, with permission, from* Visual Tracing, *by S. Groffman; available from Keystone View, Division of Mast/Keystone.)*

former, the patient presses the button corresponding to the appropriate light, whereas with the latter, letters are presented on a screen and then depressed on the keyboard. The Wayne saccadic fixator can be used in either a predictable or non-predictable stimulus mode, whereas the computer orthoptics trainer only has a nonpredictable stimulus mode. Red-green filters can be added to make the task bi-ocular. The cognitive demand of the saccadic fixator can be increased by using the optional alphabet pad.

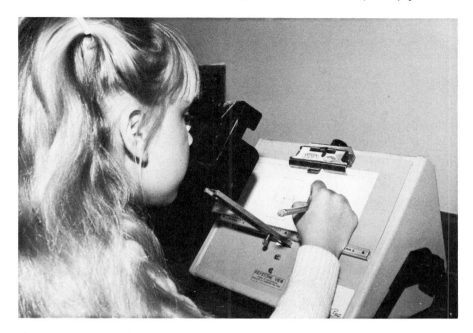

Figure 10.20 *Bi-ocular tracing using a cheiroscope.*

Basic Procedure

Line Counting

The patient is presented with a horizontal rectangle drawn on a piece of paper (Figure 10.25*A*). With the dominant eye occluded, the patient's goal is to draw as many parallel vertical lines as possible within the figure (Figure 10.25*B*). Once the patient says that he or she is done, he or she is encouraged to draw several more lines to promote further the development of fine visual-motor control.

Increasing Difficulty

Next, the patient counts the total number of lines drawn without the use of a pointer (IV, B). After recording that number, the patient counts the lines again, but this time *with* the use of a pointer (IV, A). Finally, the answer is checked by counting the lines with both eyes open. This sequence is done with the rectangle positioned horizontally, vertically, and obliquely (Figure 10.25*C*). Once again, a bi-ocular version of line counting can be performed either in the instrument or with the use of red-green filters.

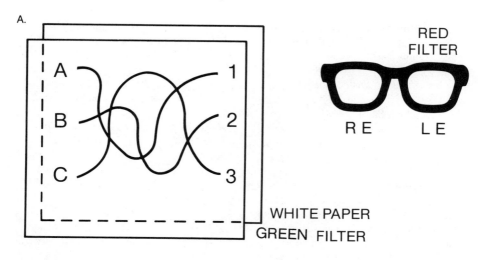

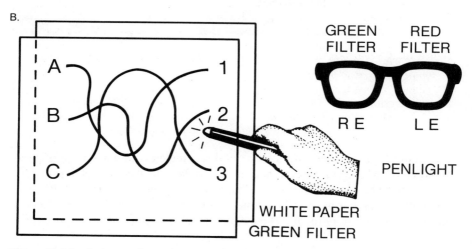

Figure 10.21   *Red-green bi-ocular training sequence for amblyopic right eye. (A) With no filter over the amblyopic eye and a red filter over the dominant eye, the black lines are only visible to the amblyopic eye. To increase difficulty, a green filter is placed over the amblyopic eye. (B) Eventually, an eye-hand coordination task is added by tracing the lines under the paper with a penlight.*

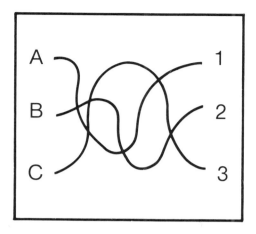
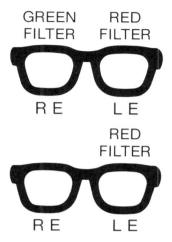

Figure 10.22   *Red-only bi-ocular sequence. If tracing is viewed by the dominant eye (red filter), the white paper appears red, thus making the red lines invisible to the dominant eye. Eventually, a green filter is placed over the amblyopic eye to increase task difficulty by equalizing the light transmittance to the two eyes.*

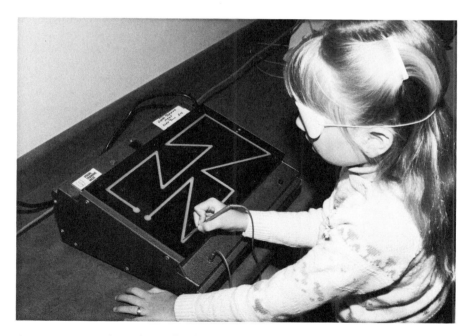

Figure 10.23   *Auditory biofeedback maze tracing. Mistakes in tracing set off auditory signal. Total mistakes are tabulated.*

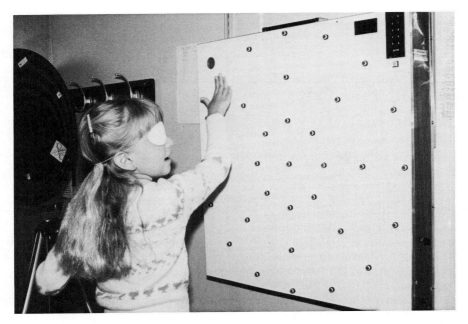

Figure 10.24   *Wayne saccadic fixator. Patient's goal is to press the button corresponding to the appropriate light. Center display presents the number of correct responses per programmed time. Auditory feedback and predictability of presentation can be varied.*

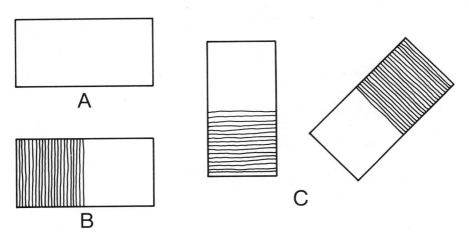

Figure 10.25   *Line counting. (A) Beginning rectangle. (B) Horizontal task half completed. (C) Vertical and oblique tasks half completed.*

Basic Procedure

Monocular Prism Saccades

With the dominant eye occluded, the patient fixates a target approximately 10 feet away. A 12 prism diopter base-down prism is introduced from the side, and the patient must note the direction of movement of the fixation target (VI, A). The correct answer is always toward the *apex* of the prism. Initially, only vertical prism saccades are trained (V, A). The eventual goal is for the patient to note as little as ½ prism diopter movement (VI, B).

Increasing Difficulty

Eventually, the prism can be introduced with its base either up, down, right, left, or oblique, thus increasing the possibilities to eight position changes (V, B). Vertical movement is the easiest to detect and oblique the most difficult.

FORM RECOGNITION TRAINING PROCEDURES*

Form recognition is the last of our three broad treatment categories. The emphasis of the procedures in this category is on the recognition of simple and complex forms (pictures, letters, numbers, words) as present in everyday situations, but with the complication of either being hidden, briefly exposed, or slightly different from a similar comparison form.

Basic Procedure

Tachistoscope

Initially, a large single letter at 16 inches (I, A) is presented to the amblyopic eye for a duration of 5 seconds (II, A). The patient's goal is to identify the letter. A tachistoscope (Figure 10.26) or a computer orthoptics trainer can be used for this procedure. The advantage of the former is that the therapist has a much finer control over stimulus duration. In addition, stimulus type and span are unlimited (letters, numbers, words, equations, forms, etc.) with the tachistoscope. At home, a tachistoscopic presentation is created by keeping the stimulus under cover and then very briefly uncovering it.

---

*See Table 10.4 for codes.

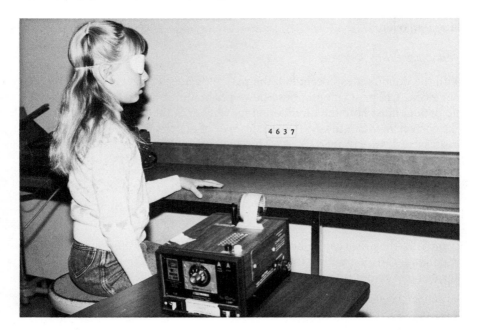

Figure 10.26   *Tachistoscope.*

Increasing Difficulty

Stimulus Crowding

By decreasing the size and increasing the number of stimuli, the procedure becomes more difficult. In addition, stimulus crowding can be increased (I, B).

Visual Memory

Increase the time between stimulus presentation and the patient's response (III, B). This forces the use of visual memory. The patient should count backwards just before and during the stimulus presentation. This forces the use of visual memory alone rather than with subvocalization assistance.

Graphic Reproduction

The goal is to have the patient reproduce the stimulus once it has been presented (IV, B). The patient then compares his or her graphic response with the actual stimulus for accuracy. To increase difficulty further, graphic reproduction can be combined with visual memory.

How many times does each number appear in this illustration?

```
9 2 4 6 8 8 5 4 6 3 2 7 7 5 6 3 9 8 3 9 2 4 9
5 6 3 8 7 2 5 3 6 4 7 9 9 6 0 1 2 0 0 1 7 3 3
1 4 0 4 2 9 4 1 4 8 5 0 5 0 9 7 3 8 1 2 9 5 0
6 2 9 5 4 8 3 1 5 1 5 1 1 1 0 4 6 9 2 9 4 8 4
2 9 5 8 3 0 7 4 5 8 4 8 9 1 2 0 4 6 8 3 9 3 6
7 0 3 1 5 6 2 9 4 8 5 7 4 3 6 0 1 5 1 7 9 6 7
6 4 8 4 8 1 4 5 5 1 7 5 6 0 0 1 4 9 9 4 5 6 7
4 6 3 6 3 7 4 9 5 1 5 0 5 7 4 8 0 4 7 4 6 1 8
7 6 4 8 3 8 3 9 9 1 4 1 4 6 3 1 8 4 9 0 0 5 7
5 7 4 8 3 8 4 9 6 8 5 9 0 4 8 1 8 0 5 7 3 2 8
4 6 1 6 3 0 5 4 6 3 3 6 7 8 3 1 9 0 5 4 8 3 0
9 5 6 3 7 4 9 8 4 1 5 1 7 4 8 4 8 4 9 5 3 2 4
1 3 7 4 0 1 5 9 8 4 6 3 2 6 2 8 0 5 7 4 1 8 9
6 4 8 4 9 5 1 0 6 7 4 8 4 8 1 4 1 0 4 6 4 7 3
7 4 2 0 4 7 1 5 1 7 0 9 9 6 8 1 3 5 4 2 7 8 9
5 6 7 3 1 7 0 7 8 9 5 0 1 5 4 4 3 7 6 4 8 4 9
6 5 1 0 4 6 4 6 7 3 8 5 7 7 0 6 7 4 1 0 6 7 8
4 6 3 7 4 8 4 7 6 9 4 7 4 8 4 9 6 2 1 0 5 0 4
```

Figure 10.27   *Goal is to find the number of times that each number appears in the matrix. (Reprinted, with permission of the publisher, from Lyle et al. 1960.)*

Basic Procedure

Proofreading

The goal is to identify any mistakes in numbers (Figures 10.27 and 10.28), letters, or words (Figure 10.29). The degree of difficulty is increased by using such tasks as finding mistakes in diagrams (Figure 10.30), searching for similarities (Figure 10.31) or differences (Figure 10.32) in drawings, and locating nonrepeated numbers or forms (Figure 10.33).

Compare these two theoretically identical tables. Correct the errors in the lower table.

37	43	623	634	127	289
42	438	537	728	183	148
327	211	248	231	129	537
499	528	633	227	148	321
328	433	221	130	127	643
566	633	399	722	472	946
355	444	376	588	832	946

37	43	623	634	127	289
42	438	539	728	183	148
327	211	248	231	129	537
499	528	635	229	148	321
328	433	221	130	127	643
566	633	399	722	472	946
355	444	376	588	832	946

Figure 10.28   *Goal is to compare the two theoretically identical tables and to correct the errors in the lower table. (Reprinted, with permission of the publisher, from Lyle et al. 1960.)*

The house on Main Stret was brwn and yelow. Sometimes

wewould see a figure inthe window.

Figure 10.29   *Goal is to identify the misspelled words.*

Basic Procedure

Hidden Pictures

This can take the form of detecting differences between two nearly indentical scenes (Figure 10.34) or locating objects in a scene that do not belong there (Figure 10.35).

Basic Procedure

Form Reproduction

With the dominant eye occluded, the patient is presented with a form and is asked to reproduce it in several ways. One way is graphically, wherein the form is reproduced on a piece of paper or chalkboard. Another is motorically, using parquetry blocks (Figure 10.36) or a G.O. board (Figure 10.37), which requires manual manipulation.

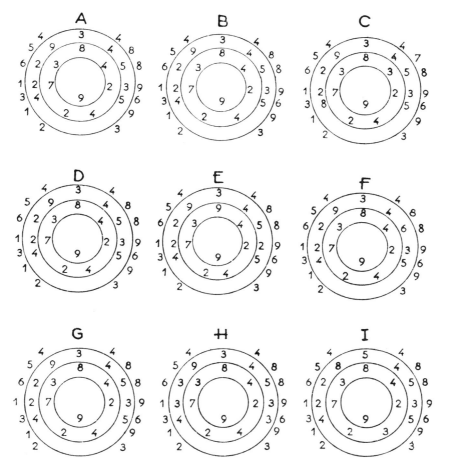

These diagrams are supposed to be identical. Find the mistakes. (Figure A is correct).

Figure 10.30 *Goal is to identify and underline the mistakes in the supposedly identical diagrams. Figure (A) has been corrected. (Reprinted, with permission of the publisher, from Lyle et al. 1960.)*

Increasing Difficulty

The sequence with parquetry blocks is a reproduction directly over the stimulus (Figure 10.36*A*), followed by reproduction next to the stimulus (Figure 10.36*B*) and finally reproduction after only a brief exposure to the stimulus (Figure 10.36*C*), thus incorporating a visual memory component. Similarly, visual memory can be added to the G.O. board sequence.

EXERCISES WITH PATTERNS AND DESIGNS

These are self-explanatory and confront the patient with various simple problems of observation.

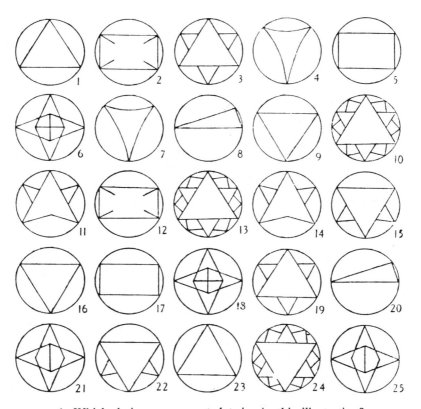

1. Which designs are repeated twice in this illustration?

Figure 10.31 *Goal is to identify the designs that are repeated twice in the illustration. (Reprinted, with permission of publisher, from Lyle et al. 1960.)*

ECCENTRIC FIXATION TRAINING SEQUENCES

Both central and eccentric fixators (regardless of age) initially go through the three-component training sequence described in the preceding pages. This training, in conjunction with direct patching, will convert most eccentric fixators into unsteady central fixators (von Noorden 1965), thereby allowing the clinician to bypass the eccentric fixation training to be discussed here. Therefore, the following training and treatment are *only* to be used with steady eccentric fixators whose fixation status has *not* improved with a combination of the standard training sequence and direct patching. This type of

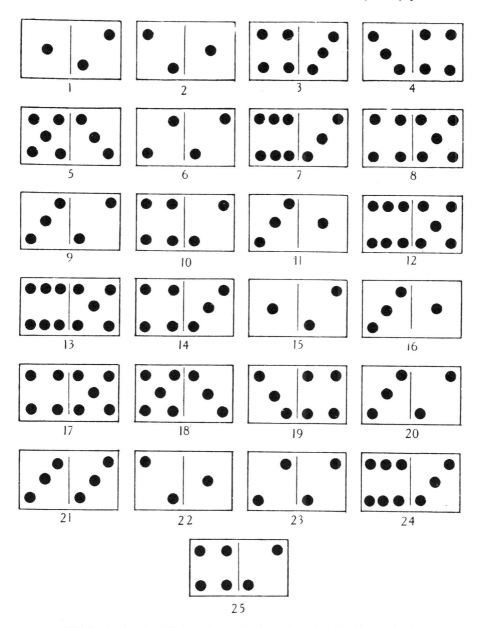

Which domino is different from all the others in this illustration?

Figure 10.32 *Goal is to identify the domino that is different from all the others. (Reprinted, with permission of the publisher, from Lyle et al. 1960.)*

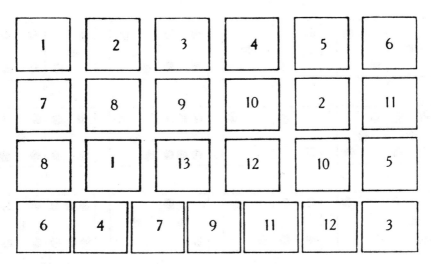

Is there a number that appears only once in this illustration?

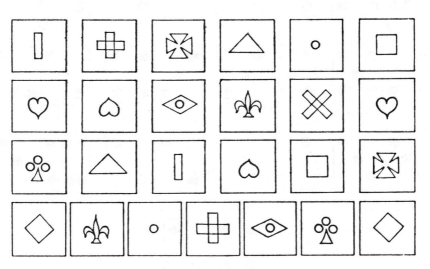

Point out the patterns that appear only once in this illustration.

Figure 10.33   *Goal is to identify the number (above) of patterns (below) that appear only once in the illustrations. (Reprinted, with permission of the publisher, from Lyle et al. 1960.)*

These simple problems in detection are self-explanatory.

1. The Living Room
   Fig. A | Fig. B is different from Fig. A in 10 ways.
   Fig. B | What are they?

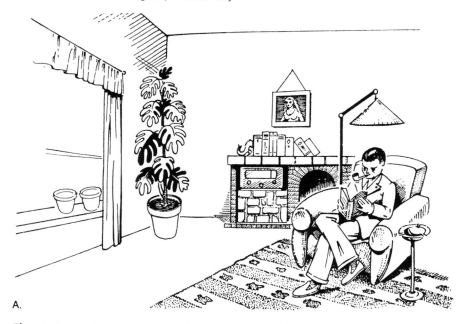

A.

Figure 10.34   *Scene (A) is different from scene (B) in 10 ways. What are they? (Reprinted, with permission of the publisher, from Lyle et al. 1960.)*

patient is typically a very embedded steady eccentric fixator whose angle of strabismus is equal to the angle of eccentric fixation (e.g., microtropia). Therefore, the eccentric point is reinforced under both monocular *and* binocular conditions. With this type of patient, visual acuity will typically improve during the standard direct patching therapy phase, with the degree of eccentric fixation remaining the same. Therefore, the vision improvement achieved is secondary to decreased cortical inhibition and not to a reduction in magnitude of the eccentric fixation. If any further significant improvement in visual acuity is to be obtained, the magnitude of eccentric fixation must be reduced.

Inverse Prism Training

The initial and most conservative method of disrupting steady eccentric fixation is by having the patient perform all the previously mentioned monocular activities (accommodation, eye movements, and form recognition) through an inverse prism (Figure 10.38). As a general rule, the prism amount is twice that of

Jumbled Pictures
  The Living Room. Fig. B differs from Fig. A in the following ways:—
1. The portrait is of a man instead of a woman.
2. The picture hook is bigger.
3. The vase of the big plant has no rim.
4. The two pots on the window sill have plants in them.
5. The book on the right on the mantlepiece has bands on the binding.
6. The indicator on the wireless is on the left instead of on the right.
7. The man's jacket has no button-hole.
8. The pipe is smoking.
9. The socks are black and unstriped.
10. The light bulb is visible under the lampshade.

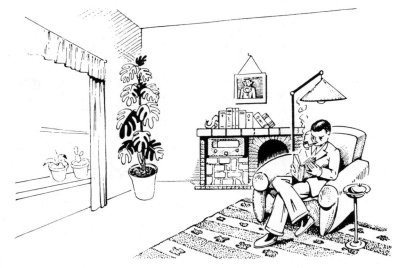

B.

Figure 10.34   *(continued)*

the eccentric fixation, with prism direction being the same as fixator the eccentric fixation direction. Therefore, a nasal eccentric fixator of 4 prism diopters would train with a patch over the dominant eye and an 8-diopter base-in prism over theamblyopic eye. Training through an inverse prism forces the amblyopic eye to be motorically straight while fixation is still eccentric. This forces the integration of proprioceptive, tactile, and kinesthetic information with the eye in true primary position, thus allowing the association of the straight-ahead position with the true spatial location of the target. Patching is still direct during the period that inverse prism therapy is in effect.

Inverse Occlusion

For inverse occlusion to be effective, it *must* be full time and be used in conjunction with controlled foveal stimulation (Bangerter 1953). Inverse occlusion is recommended *only* if direct occlusion with standard therapy followed by inverse prism therapy is unsuccessful in disrupting the steady eccentric fixation. Inverse

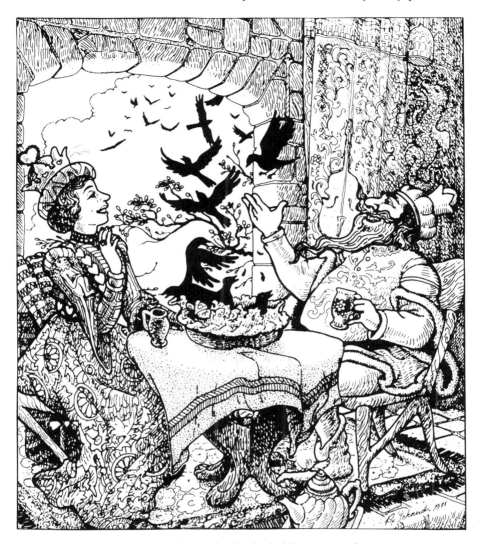

Figure 10.35   *Goal is to identify the hidden items in this scene.*

occlusion is best accomplished by simple patching of the amblyopic eye. If cosmesis is a major factor, then a high plus power or occluder contact lens can be used. Another alternative is to stipple the amblyopic eye's spectacle lens with clear nail polish. These procedures are effective, since deprivation of form and not light is the amblyogenic factor. If these procedures are too disruptive to the patient, then stippling all but the temporal 25% of the amblyopic eye's spectacle lens will prevent the eccentric point from receiving patterned stimuli while still allowing some peripheral vision.

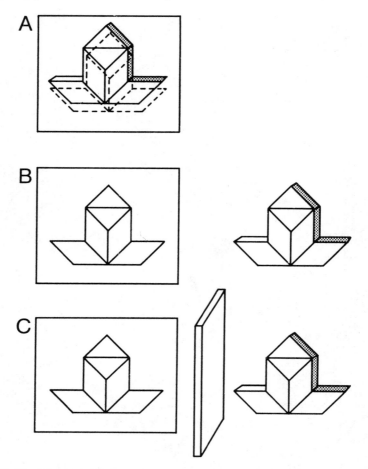

Figure 10.36 *Parquetry block sequence. A. Blocks are placed directly over template. B. Blocks are appropriately placed next to the template. C. Blocks are appropriately placed after a brief exposure to the template.*

Controlled Foveal Stimulation

It is crucial that the fovea be stimulated when the amblyopic eye is not occluded. We use a Haidinger brush or afterimages to accomplish this.

Haidinger Brush Sequence   The patient is exposed to an MIT as soon as the occluder is removed from the amblyopic eye and placed over the dominant eye. The fixation status is then checked. If the patient reports the brush to be central, then he or she should align a pointer with the Haidinger brush superimposed on the fixation point. If this can be done, then the patient can proceed to the standard Haidinger brush training sequence. If the brush moves away from the fixation object when attempting to point, the patient should hold the pointer in

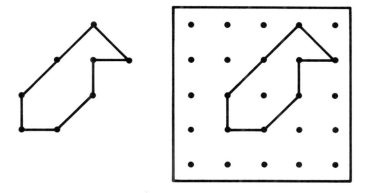

Figure 10.37 *Figure is reproduced on a G.O. board with rubber bands.*

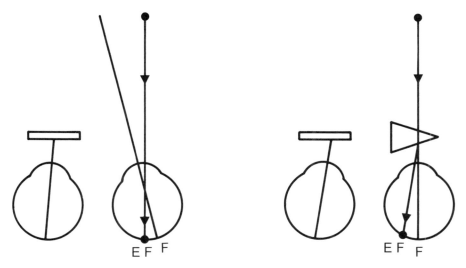

Figure 10.38 (Left) *Nasal eccentric fixation of the right eye with the eye motorically in the adducted position.* (Right) *Nasal eccentric fixation of the same eye now viewing the object through a base-in prism with the eye motorically in the primary position.*

the *nondominant hand*. The procedure is as follows: First, if the patient reports that the brush is not superimposed on the fixation point, then he or she should be told to move the eye side to side and be aware of the simultaneous movement of the brush. Once the patient is aware that his or her eye position controls the brush position, he or she is asked to "massage" the fixation point between two lines each approximately 1 inch from the fixation point (Figure 10.39). Once successful, the interline distance is gradually decreased until the brush is on the fixation point. Then proceed with the pointing phase of the Haidinger brush sequence. Finally, if the patient cannot control the movement of the brush, then

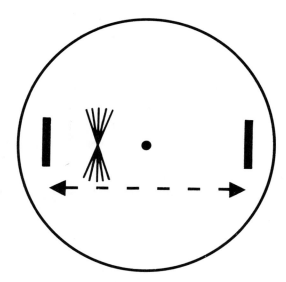

Figure 10.39   *Haidinger brush training sequence. Patient's goal is to "move" the brush back and forth visually with eye movements between the vertical lines. The therapist then gradually decreases the distance between the lines until the patient can place the brush on the fixation point.*

the clinician should move a pointer side to side over the fixation point as the patient attempts to follow the pointer with the brush *without* being aware of the fixation point. Once successful, only *then* should the patient be made aware that *he* or *she* is controlling the movement of the brush. Then go back to the pointing phase of the brush sequence.

Afterimage Training   There are two ways of being certain that an afterimage represents the fovea of the patient's nondominant eye. The first is by performing the afterimage transfer with the Haidinger brush test (see Chapter 8). If it shows that the patient has normal retinal correspondence, then the nondominant fovea can be "tagged" for training with the afterimage transfer procedure. Home training with afterimages is performed using a camera strobe whose glass front surface has been taped over fully except for a fine vertical slit in the center with a fixation point (Figure 10.40). If it is determined that the patient has ARC, then Vodnoy's afterimage training procedure should be used (Figure 10.41). The first step is to measure the amount of eccentric fixation (angular distance between Haidinger brush and fixation point). Then cut two arcs out of a piece of cardboard so that the distance from the center of the card to the center of each arc is equal to this amount. Assuming the patient has nasal eccentric fixation of the right eye, he or she would be asked to fixate the right arc while the cardboard covers a bright lamp. This produces two afterimages that straddle the spared fovea, with one of the afterimages bleaching out the eccentric point (point *e*). The patient is informed that the

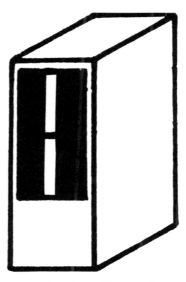

Figure 10.40 *Camera strobe adapted for creating a vertical afterimage.*

center of the bracketed area should be used to fixate objects. This procedure is performed at home by placing the card over a bright light bulb.

Once the fovea has been accurately tagged (either with an afterimage or bracketed afterimages), the patient is ready for fixation training. At first large objects such as a 20/400 Shellen letter or a door knob are fixated (with children we refer to the afterimage as a "laser ray" and ask them to "zap" the object to be fixated). The next step is for the patient to make large saccadic fixations on multiple letters on a blackboard, first without and then with simultaneous pointing. If the patient is inaccurate with a pointer, then he or she should be allowed to use a finger for maximum kinesthetic feedback. Once accuracy has improved, the patient is ready to go into the standard monocular training sequence while being aware of the afterimage. Table 10.8 summarizes the eccentric fixation training sequence. As soon as fixation becomes unsteady, the patient begins the standard training sequence.

It is important for the clinician to be extremely patient and encouraging during afterimage training and to transfer this feeling to the patient. It may take *several* sessions before the patient perceives a properly placed afterimage and understands what to do with it. With patience, a 4-year-old can be taught these procedures.

Table 10.8 Eccentric Fixation Training Protocol

1. Standard training sequence	Direct patching
2. Standard Training sequence through inverse prism	Direct patching
3. Haidinger brush training	Inverse occlusion
4. Afterimage training	Inverse occlusion

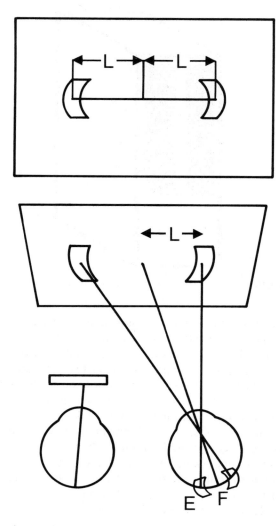

Figure 10.41   *Vodnoy's afterimage training procedure. (L = amount of eccentric fixation projected out to 16 inches.) (Above) Cardboard mask with two cutaways. (Below) Location of afterimages on retina, with patient's perception.*

Binocularity

As noted in Chapter 8, there are three main avenues toward which the clinician can direct the binocular training phase: stereopsis, alternation of fixation, or enhancement of the ARC condition. One of these should be chosen as the eventual binocular goal at the *beginning* of the amblyopia therapy.

Stereopsis

Ideally, stereopsis is what one would hope to attain by the end of therapy. Obviously, if the patient demonstrates any stereoscopic ability during the initial evaluation, then one should not settle for anything less than good stereopsis (better than 70 seconds of arc) at the end of training. If a patient demonstrates any degree of stereopsis or has an intermittent strabismus, amblyopia therapy should be *preceded* by binocular therapy (See Chapter 9).

Amblyopes without strabismus are most likely to achieve stereopsis. Of those with strabismus, the exotropes have a higher probability of posttherapy stereopsis. This is because the exotropia is secondary to the amblyopia, which is typically due to anisometropia. The anisometropic amblyope with exotropia usually begins with an intermittent strabismus which then becomes constant. This is why, frequently, incorporation of the proper optical correction of a previously uncorrected anisometropic exotropic amblyope will often with time lead to an intermittent exotropia with a subsequent improvement in visual acuity. This often occurs with high unilateral myopic amblyopia (von Noorden 1973). The achievement of stereopsis is the best defense against posttherapy regression of vision function.

Create Alternation

As previously noted, if one can force alternation during cover testing, then the chance of creating an alternator is good. To create an alternator, the posttherapy visual acuity in the amblyopic eye must be fairly good (better than 20/60). During the course of therapy, one can probe the chances of eventual alternation by the following procedure: Have the patient look at a single Snellen letter (at the amblyopic eye threshold visual acuity level) at distance. Gradually add plus lenses, 0.25 diopter at a time, over the dominant eye while observing the deviated amblyopic eye. Once the good eye is sufficiently blurred out, one will see the amblyopic eye establish fixation. Record the amount of retinal defocus needed (in diopters) to force this alternation. If the amount of lens power is what one would expect (each +0.25 diopter reducing Snellen line visual acuity by about one line) based on the corrected visual acuity in the amblyopic eye, then one's chances of creating an alternator are much better. After therapy is completed, if there is no spontaneous alternation of fixation, one can prescribe a pair of spectacles with a "blurring" lens over the dominant eye to be worn an appropriate amount of time. When creating an alternator optically, it is important to be certain that the diplopia is not perceived whenever the amblyopic eye establishes fixation.

Enhancing Anomalous Retinal Correspondence

If the binocular evaluation reveals presence of unharmonious anomalous retinal correspondence (UHARC), training of fusion using second-degree targets at the subjective angle should be instituted to develop a means of responding appropriately to any diplopia that may occur as visual acuity in the amblyopic eye improves. After therapy, if the remaining objective angle is noncosmetic (≤ 15 prism diopters), then we reinforce fusion at the corresponding subjective angle. If the residual objective angle is cosmetically significant, then strabismus surgery is an option, with a recommended surgical correction amount equal to the existing subjective angle. See examples 1 to 3.

Example 1

Cause of amblyopia	High unilateral myopia
Best corrected visual acuity	20/200 S-chart
Binocular evaluation	Intermittent exotropia with normal retinal correspondence No stereopsis Deep suppression
Binocular treatment plan	Fusion training with eyes in orthophoric position (using overcorrecting minus lenses if necessary) with penalization filters over dominant eye and correction with contact lens once visual acuity reaches 20/100 level.
Binocular goal	Stereopsis

Example 2

Cause of amblyopia	Constant unilateral esotropia
Best corrected visual acuity	20/100 S-chart 20/50 Laser interferometer
Binocular evaluation	20 prism diopter right esotropia Subjective angle 12 prism diopters BO Can force alternation (patient sees double) but reverts to right esotropia with blink. No stereopsis
Binocular treatment plan	Anomalous fusion training in free space with penalization filters over left eye through 12 base-out prism over left eye (in artificial environment). Stress fusion of diplopic images during fixation with right eye. High-level right eye accommodation, eye movement, fixation, and just-noticeable difference training.
Binocular goal	Reduce angle to 12 prism diopters esotropia with anomalous fusion at this angle. Create a part time alternator. (good prognosis due to high laser acuity).

Example 3

Cause of amblyopia	Primary—hyperopic anisometropia.
	Secondary—constant unilateral esotropia.
Best corrected visual acuity	20/225 S-chart
	20/180 Laser Interferometry
	Refraction RE +3.00 sph. LE plano
Binocular evaluation	45 prism diopter right esotropia.
	Subjective angle 25 prism diopters base out.
	No forced alternation
	No stereopsis

Binocular treatment plan (two options*)

Option A	Anomalous fusion training at subjective angle with gradual reduction in BO prism with expected angle *H* of 30 prism diopters and angle *S* of 10 prism diopters BO.
	Surgical correction to leave patient with 10 prism diopters of esotropia.
	Reinforce anomalous fusion at 10 prism diopters BO.
	Since prognosis for alternation is poor, patient will need retainer patching.
Option B	Breakdown anomalous retinal correspondence simultaneously with amblyopia therapy.
	Full surgical correction once normal retinal correspondence established.
	Reinforce normal retinal correspondence after surgical correction.
	Retainer patching.

*Preferred option dependent on motivation of patient (option B is much more disruptive) and depth of anomalous retinal correspondence.

PATTERNS OF IMPROVEMENT AND TERMINATION OF THERAPY: CASE REPORTS

According to Schapero (1971), patterns of improvement secondary to occlusion and/or active vision therapy vary tremendously from case to case. It has been our experience that, in general, visual acuity improvement is greatest during the first 6 weeks of therapy. After this, improvement is more gradual, unless you are working with a steady eccentric fixator who begins to achieve central fixation. In this case, we have found that single-letter acuity begins to improve dramatically, while single-line and whole-chart acuity remains depressed. The next few months are then spent on decreasing this visual acuity discrepancy.

We believe that training should be discontinued if there is no improvement in visual acuity for 2 consecutive months. However, during the periods that acuity improvement has stagnated, accommodation and fixation may be improving, thereby contributing toward our goal of preventing regression.

It also has been our experience that many patients experience a significant improvement in ambulatory ability during the first few weeks of therapy while visual acuity remains unchanged. To integrate all the previously mentioned treatment strategies, we will present a series of eight of our actual cases from beginning to end and using the following format:

1. History
2. Diagnosis
3. Monocular and binocular treatment plan
4. Training sequence
5. Results
6. Significant points

Case 1: High Unilateral Myopia with Exotropia and Deep Amblyopia (Age 6½ Years)

History

The patient was first examined in our clinic at age 6½ years. The mother noted partial ptosis of the left eye several weeks after birth and a left exotropia at about 1½ years of age. The patient's initial vision examination was at 5 years of age, at which time a diagnosis of amblyopia was made. There was no history of therapy or correction of any refractive error.

Diagnosis

Subjective refraction was plano in the right eye (20/20) and − 8.00 diopters in the left eye (20/200) (see Table 10.9). Visuoscopy showed steady central fixation

Table 10.9　Pre- and Posttreatment Clinical Findings, Amblyopic Eye

Findings	Pretreatment	Posttreatment
Visual acuity (Snellen single line)	6/60 (20/200)	6/9 + (20/30 +)
Visual acuity (S-chart)	6/32.7 (20/109)	6/9.6 (20/32)
Accommodative amplitude (push-up)	8 diopters	20 diopters
Accommodative amplitude (minus lens)	4.25 diopters	13 diopters
Visuoscopy	1° sup. nasal unsteady	Central steady
Maximum fusional ability (6 meters)	None	18 Δ
Stereoscopic threshold (Wirt)	400 sec arc	40 sec arc
Stereoscopic threshold (Randot)	None	20 sec arc
Cover test (6 meters)	14 Δ left exotropia	7 Δ exophoria
Cover test (40 centimeters)	12 Δ left exotropia	4 Δ exophoria
Worth four-dot (40 centimeters and 6 meters)	LE suppression	Fusion

in the right eye. The left eye showed unsteady eccentric fixation approximately 75% of the time with a 1-degree superior-nasal bias. Cover test revealed a constant comitant left exotropia of 14 prism diopters at 6 meters and 12 prism diopters at 40 centimeters. Suppression of the left eye was noted at all distances with the Worth four-dot test. There was no Randot stereoscopic appreciation. We felt that the primary amblyopia was secondary to the high unilateral myopia, with the exotropia being secondary to the myopia and amblyopia. Once the exotropia became constant, it also became an amblyogenic factor. The following is the probable sequence of events:

- High unilateral myopia
  ↓
- Primary amblyopia
  ↓
- Intermittent exotropia
  ↓
- Constant exotropia
  ↓
- Secondary amblyopia

Monocular and Binocular Treatment Plan

Owing to the unsteady nature of fixation, we felt that the standard therapy sequence with direct patching through full correction was in order. Our plan was to limit patching to a maximum of 3 hours daily, since we felt that once visual acuity improved, the strabismus would become intermittent in nature, thereby making long periods of patching unnecessary. In addition, under artificial situations and penalization of the dominant eye, the patient gave an NRC response with no avoidance of fusion. Consequently, the binocularity goal was stereopsis. Our plan was short periods of patching with daily 30-minute standard therapy along with binocular therapy through undercorrecting prisms.

Training Sequence

A full spectacle correction was prescribed for full-time wear along with 3 hours of daily direct occlusion, 30 minutes of daily training, and 45 minutes of weekly in-office training. Since the strabismus (after the initial amblyopia therapy) was less at near than at distance, we began fusion training at near through a base-in prism. Training then concentrated on increasing the distance over which positive fusional vergence was possible with visual feedback provided as to occurrence of suppression and diplopia (Griffin 1982). The base-in prism was gradually reduced as fusion ability improved. Such training increased intermittency of the deviation, first at near and then at distance. At this time, a base-in Fresnel prism equal to one-half the distance deviation was placed before the dominant eye. This facilitated fusion throughout the day and discouraged suppression by slightly degrading the retinal image of the dominant eye. Once visual

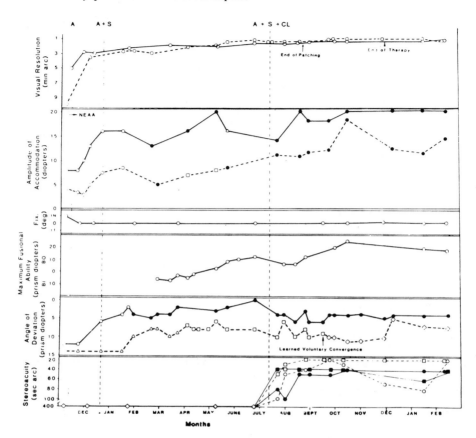

Figure 10.42   *Changes in vision function during the course of orthoptic therapy [A = amblyopia therapy; S = strabismus therapy; CL = contact lens correction. For visual acuity, dashed line is single-line Snellen and solid line is S-chart. For amplitude of accommodation, NEAA is normal-eye amplitude of accommodation, dashed line is minus lens values, and solid line is pushup (○ = 20/60 letter; □ = 20/50 letter; △ = 20/40 letter, and ● = 20/30 letter). For angle of deviation, ○ = near tropia; ● = near phoria; △ = constant distance tropia; □ = intermittent distance tropia, and ◇ = distance phoria. For stereoacuity, ● = crossed disparity (Wirt); ■ = uncrossed disparity (Wirt); ○ = crossed disparity (Randot), and □ = uncrossed disparity (Randot).] (Reprinted, with permission of the publisher, from Selenow and Ciuffreda 1983.)*

acuity and binocularity improved, we noticed that the variable prismatic demand produced by the high minus spectacle lens became an obstacle to fusion. Therefore, a soft contact lens was fitted over the amblyopic eye. This was followed by antisuppression training performed simultaneously with eye movement, accommodation, and eye-hand coordination exercises during bifoveal fixation. These exercises were done in all positions of gaze with third-degree stereoscopic targets. Second-degree fusion targets (Schapero 1971) with suppression cues were subsequently used, initially with the targets containing large peripheral contours and later with small central targets.

Results

The improvements in monocular and binocular vision functions during the course of orthoptic therapy are presented in Figure 10.42 Visual acuity increased throughout therapy, with this gain being especially large and rapid during the first month or so. Similar trends, but with more variability, were found for accommodation. Central fixation was rapidly achieved in the amblyopic eye, with steadiness consistently improving during the course of therapy. Reduction of the deviation occurred at both distance and near. Once the contact lens was fitted, stereoacuity improved rapidly. After termination of treatment, there was a period during which stereopsis exhibited some regression. However, stereoacuity returned to normal when measured 3 months after the end of treatment. The pre- and posttreatment clinical findings are summarized in Table 10.9. All clinical and laboratory findings remained unchanged when retested 1 year later, demonstrating good relatively long-term maintenance of the substantial initial vision function improvements.

Monocular fixation with the amblyopic eye before and after orthoptic therapy is shown in Figure 10.43. There was marked reduction in amplitude (2 degrees before and less than 1 degree after training) of saccadic intrusions (Ciuffreda et al. 1979a), as well as absence of intermittently increased drift (Ciuffreda et al. 1979b) after therapy. Monocular fixation with the dominant eye was within normal limits at each test session.

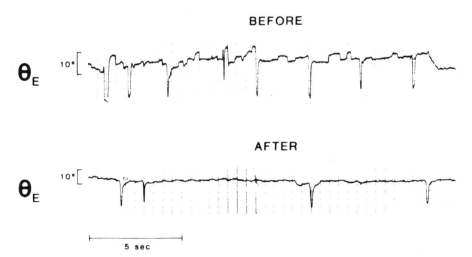

BEFORE

θ_E 10°

AFTER

θ_E 10°

5 sec

Figure 10.43 *Fixational eye movements before and after orthoptic therapy. Amblyopic eye, monocular viewing. Posttraining improvement is evident. Large, downward deflections represent blinks. θ_E is eye position. (Reprinted, with permission of the publisher, from Selenow and Ciuffreda 1983.)*

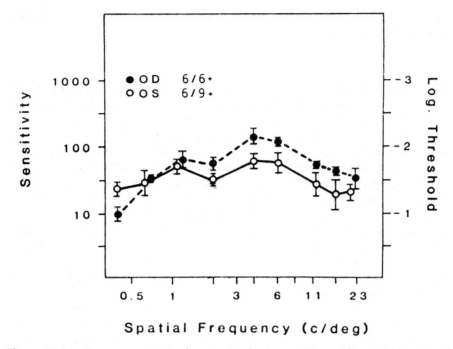

Figure 10.44 *Contrast sensitivity function in dominant [(●) = 6/6+ (20/20+)] and nondominant [(○) = 6/9 + (20/30+)] eyes. Contrast sensitivity is normal in the dominant eye. Contrast sensitivity in the nondominant eye is normal only at very low spatial frequencies. Plotted are mean ± 1 SD. (Reprinted, with permission of the publisher, from Selenow and Ciuffreda 1983.)*

Threshold contrast sensitivity results taken 3 months after the end of training are presented in Figure 10.44 for each eye (no pretherapy measures were taken). Contrast sensitivity was normal in the dominant eye. Contrast sensitivity in the nondominant eye showed slight depression at the middle and high spatial frequencies.

Significant Points

1. Despite the patient initially manifesting an eccentric fixation, we implemented our *standard* training sequence *with direct* occlusion.
2. A partial prismatic correction was prescribed once it was clear that correspondence was normal and that there was no prism adaptation.
3. A contact lens was fitted only once it became obvious that our binocular goal was stereopsis.

Case 2: Small-Angle Esotropic Amblyope
(Age 9 to 11 Years)

History

The patient was initially examined in our clinic at age 9 years. There was no history of previous eye surgery, orthoptic therapy, or correction of refractive error; however, his grandfather, aunt, and sister had strabismus. The patient had failed a school screening and was suspected of having a "lazy eye."

Diagnosis

A binocular vision evaluation was performed at the initial visit by a member of our clinical faculty. Uncorrected visual acuity (whole-chart Snellen) was 20/20 in the dominant right eye and 20/200 in the amblyopic left eye. Refractive error was right eye, plano; left eye, $+0.25/-0.25 \times 180$. Low-light visuoscopy using a calibrated circular grid pattern projected onto the fundus for a 30-second assessment period was done. It revealed slightly unsteady central fixation in the dominant eye and very unsteady superior-nasal eccentric fixation (3 prism diopters) in the amblyopic eye. Cover test revealed a small-angle (6 prism diopters) constant left esotropia at distance and near. The Worth four-dot test indicated suppression of the left eye at all distances. Anomalous retinal correspondence was indicated by the striated lens test and the major amblyoscope. Examination of the anterior and posterior segments of the eyes revealed absence of ocular or neurologic disease. We felt that the amblyopia was secondary to the constant unilateral esotropia.

Monocular and Binocular Treatment Plan

It was determined that the patient begin the standard therapy sequence along with direct patching. Binocularity would be monitored carefully along the way under extremely artificial situations. Our initial binocularity goal was to create an alternating esotropia. However, if during the probing of binocularity, diplopia persisted during fixation with the nondominant eye, we would reinforce anomalous fusion under artificial situations so that fleeting diplopia (especially when fatigued) could be handled by the patient while encouraging suppression during normal lighting conditions. Consequently, regression would have to be prevented by retainer patching.

Training Sequence

The patient began formal orthoptic therapy with weekly clinical sessions. Extensive home and clinic training included our standard training sequence of direct patching, eye-hand coordination exercises, and accommodative rock exercises. Training of central fixation was attempted with pleoptics and Haidinger brush fixation exercises. Visual acuity improved for 3 months, but then remained constant at 20/80 for 2 months. Fixation was still unsteady and eccentric (4 prism diopters). It was decided to terminate therapy because of a lack of further improvement of visual acuity and fixation ability.

The patient returned 18 months later for a reevaluation. With the exception of visual acuity regressing to 20/120, all other findings remained as they were at the termination of therapy. We then attempted an intensive conventional orthoptic therapy program with the patient, who still desired to improve vision in his amblyopic eye and was highly motivated to complete several more months of therapy.

Direct occlusion was initially prescribed for 5 hours per day in conjunction with 1 hour a day of intensive accommodation, eye movement, and form recognition training. Eventually, the black occluder was substituted with a partial translucent occluder blocking the nasal visual field, thus allowing for selective obscuration of form vision. Peripheral fusion ability was enhanced, while a small central zone of suppression was encouraged. Therefore, our plan for prevention of regression was to maintain the patient on a retainer patching regimen, with gradual reduction so that the minimum patching time could be determined.

Results

Representative S-chart visual acuity response profiles at selected times during the course of orthoptic therapy are presented in Figure 10.45. They show two important features. First, the profile gradually shifted to the left, indicating progressive improvement in visual acuity. Second, the slope of the profile normalized (i.e., increased), indicating a reduction of the response variability, which is typically found in amblyopic eyes (Davidson and Eskridge 1977). The slope was now similar to that found in the fellow normal eye.

Changes in visual acuity (S-chart), eccentric fixation, and interocular difference in accommodative amplitude during and immediately following the period of orthoptic therapy are presented in Figure 10.46. Several points merit consideration. First, accommodative amplitude in the amblyopic eye responded about three times faster than either visual acuity or fixation, although it remained slightly diminished throughout the balance of the test period. Second, during the first 25 weeks of therapy, there was a small but consistent improvement in visual acuity, with little change in the magnitude of eccentric fixation; however, this was followed by a rapid improvement in both visual acuity and fixation (weeks 25 to 35). There was then a gradual leveling off of visual acuity to about the 20/20 level with little variability present (visual acuity in the fellow dominant eye was 20/15; see VA DE in graph). Similarly, fixation gradually leveled off to zero, but with moderate random fluctuations about this mean zero foveal level, indicating that it was now (on average) central but somewhat unsteady and variable, reflecting in part the persistent small-amplitude jerk nystagmus measured in the amblyopic eye (Figure 10.47).

Representative accommodative stimulus-response profiles are plotted in Figure 10.48 at selected times during the course of orthoptic therapy. There was

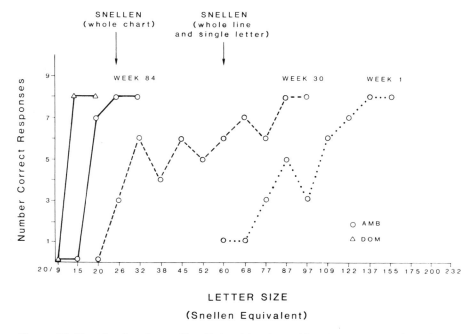

SNELLEN
(whole chart)

SNELLEN
(whole line
and single letter)

Figure 10.45   *Visual acuity profiles (S-chart) for the amblyopic eye (○) at selected times during the course of orthoptic therapy. For weeks 30 and 84, the arrows indicate the Snellen visual acuity values. Triangles show a typical result for the dominant eye. (Reprinted, with permission of the publisher, Hokoda and Ciuffreda 1986.)*

a progressive increase in average accommodative response level during therapy, with essentially overlapping profiles in each eye immediately following the therapy.

The patient remained with a small-angle esotropia and central suppression. However, he was now able to fuse peripheral targets, in case diplopia ever becomes a problem. Despite the excellent visual acuity results achieved in the amblyopic eye, diplopia was never reported by the patient. No regression of vision function was evident at our 1-year follow-up.

Significant Points

1.   The patient manifested only slight and slow improvement in visual acuity and fixation during both the initial training phase and the first few months of the intensive therapy phase. Therefore, in some patients it may indeed take 3 to 4 months before a significant improvement in visual acuity is realized. In general, we have found that the various "plastic" changes take longer to occur and are somewhat less pervasive in nature in older amblyopes.

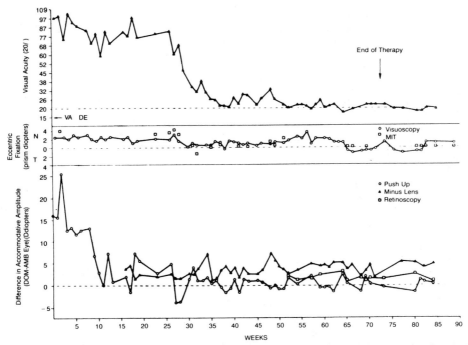

Figure 10.46   *Changes in S-chart visual acuity, eccentric fixation, and interocular differ-ence in accommodative amplitude during the course of orthoptics therapy. Symbol VA DE shows visual acuity level in the dominant eye. (Reprinted, with permission of the publisher, from Hokoda and Ciuffreda 1986.)*

2.   Once monocular vision function improvement occurred, it did so at different rates for the various functions tested, with accommodative amplitude leading the way. Therefore, visual acuity, in conjunction with several other monocular and binocular vision functions, should be monitored during the course of orthoptic therapy, since this would probably reduce the number of false-negative results (i.e., assumed patient failures based solely on a visual acuity criterion). Such presumed failures may result from lack of appropriate measures, lack of a sufficient number of different measures, and/or lack of sufficiently sensitive measures.

3.   Lastly, the interactive effects of the various vision functions may be quite important, both theoretically and practically. First, they provide basic insight into the relative dependence of the different vision functions [such as retinal eccentricity on accommodation in normal individuals (Phillips 1974)], with its implications carried over into the clinic realm (Ciuffreda et al. 1983, 1984). Second, and related to the preceding, these multidimensional measures can provide clinical insight into the interactive effects, with this information then perhaps being used to modify the therapy program to maximize an area of monocular vision function already beginning to respond, as well as to promote

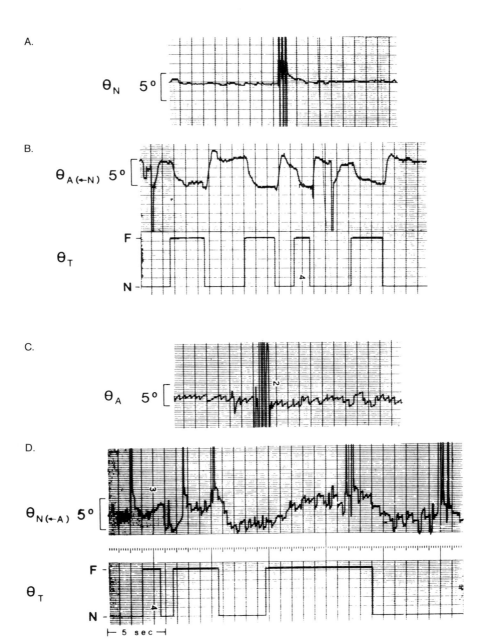

Figure 10.47 *Monocular fixation (A, C) and accommodative vergence (B, D) eye at the end of orthoptic therapy. Symbols:* θ_N *= monocular fixation with dominant eye.* $\theta_{A(\leftarrow N)}$ *= accommodative vergence in amblyopic eye with dominant eye viewing target,* θ_T *= accommodative target (F = 1.75 diopters and N = 4.0 diopters),* θ_A *= monocular fixation with amblyopic eye, and* $\theta_{N(\leftarrow A)}$ *= accommodative vergence in dominant eye with amblyopic eye viewing target. Large vertical deflections represent blinks. Nystagmus artifact is superimposed on vergence responses in the amblyopic eye. (Reprinted, with permission of the publisher, from Hokoda and Ciuffreda 1986.)*

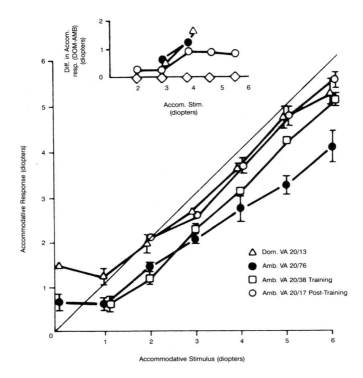

Figure 10.48 *Changes in the steady-state monocular accommodative stimulus-response profiles at selected times during the course of orthoptic therapy. Plotted is X̄ ± 1 SD (n = 6). Inset shows retinoscopically determined interocular difference in accommodative responses under binocular viewing conditions at weeks 54 (●), 64 (○), and 84 (◇) during the course of orthoptic therapy; triangles represent difference values determined with a haploscope-optometer at week 54. (Reprinted, with permission of the publisher, from Hokoda and Ciuffreda 1986.)*

responsivity in a yet dormant system. For example, in our patient, the accommodative amplitude in the amblyopic eye showed marked improvement in the absence of any significant reduction in eccentric fixation and with only a small improvement in visual acuity. Since deficits is monocular vision function in the amblyopic eye can be attributed primarily to retinal eccentricity (owing to presence of eccentric fixation) and/or central inhibition (owing to presence of binocular suppression and reflected in abnormal monocular sensory function) effects, the improvement in accommodation without a concomitant change in fixation locus suggests that it was due to reduction of inhibition effects. Thus the goal of therapy was now to develop accurate foveal fixation in an attempt to realize the balance of the (potential) accommodative ability (Selenow and

Ciuffreda 1986). Central fixation did in turn eventuate, but with little subsequent effect on accommodative amplitude, suggesting that the residual accommodative deficit due to central inhibition effects was yet greater than the retinal eccentricity factor. However, attaining foveal fixation did allow for development of normal visual acuity. In contrast, in one adult amblyope extensively tested, such a strategy did indeed result in improved accommodative function (Selenow and Ciuffreda 1983).

Case 3: Small-Angle Esotropic Amblyope (Age 29 Years)

History

A 29-year-old male college professor was referred to us by a local hospital with a diagnosis of functional amblyopia. The patient was told that the amblyopia was discovered too late in life (age 11 years) to be improved by corrective lenses or therapy. The eye turn was first noticed by the patient's parents at age 6 years. He had never been prescribed glasses or therapy. There was no history of trauma. Birth was by Cesarean delivery. Presently, a left esotropia was evident whenever the patient was tired or had moderate alcoholic intake, but there was no report of diplopia. The patient's goal was to improve vision in his amblyopic eye to allow a career change that required at least 20/40 vision in the poorer eye. In addition, he wanted a more normally functioning "spare" eye. A complete amblyopia/strabismus workup was performed.

Diagnosis

Snellen visual acuity (single-line) was 20/15 in the right eye and 20/150 in the left eye. S-chart visual acuity (Flom et al. 1963, Flom 1966) was 20/18 in the right eye and 20/110 in the left eye without correction. Laser interferometric visual acuity was 20/20 in the right eye and 20/30 in the left eye. Retinoscopy was plano in the right eye and $-0.25/-0.75$ axis 55 in the left eye. Low-light visuoscopy showed steady central fixation in the right eye and 3 degrees of steady nasal eccentric fixation in the left eye. Cover test revealed a variable left esotropia of 6 to 14 prism diopters. The major amblyoscope revealed unharmonious retinal correspondence; the objective angle was 14 prism diopters, and the subjective angle was 7 prism diopters. There was no stereoacuity demonstrated on either the Titmus or Randot tests. Accommodative amplitude determined by the minus lens method was 7.25 and 6 diopters in the right and left eyes, respectively. We felt that the primary amblyopia was secondary to the esotropia.

Monocular and Binocular Treatment Plan

Since one of the serious potential complictions of occlusion therapy in an adult amblyope is diplopia, our initial treatment plan was to teach the patient to make divergent eye movements in response to diplopic images. Despite the fact that fixation was steady and eccentric, the amblyopia treatment plan was to begin with 2 hours of daily direct patching supplemented with ½ hour of standard oculomotor, accommodative, eye-hand coordination, and fixation training. In addition, the patient was to receive 1 hour of in-office testing and training every 2 weeks.

Once we were comfortable with the patient's ability to demonstrate peripheral fusion, daily occlusion time would be increased. Our plan for prevention of regression was to implement a retainer patching regimen with partial occlusion in the form of spectacles.

Training Sequence

Our initial treatment consisted of teaching the patient to make divergent eye movements in response to diplopic images. During this phase of treatment, an unusual sensorimotor mismatch phenomenon was noted. The subjective angle increased as a divergence demand was introduced; thus, while the patient reported the diplopic images to be moving closer together, reflecting a sensory divergence component, there was no apparent correlated motor divergence component. In effect, the subjective angle and angle of anomaly changed without a corresponding change in the objective angle. Since the purpose of the divergence training was to teach the patient how to respond appropriately to any anticipated diplopia during treatment, we trained this apparent "subjective sensory divergence" using the previously discussed free-space prism vergence training sequence (see Chapter 9). Divergence ranges were measured weekly with a synotophore using second-degree targets, with the patient eventually achieving 10 prism diopters of divergence.

Visual acuity showed a marked improvement during the first 2 months of training (Figure 10.49), although fixation did not change. As a result, all monocular training was now done through inverse prism. During this phase, the patient's ability to align a Haidinger brush with simultaneous pointing showed marked improvement. Initially, the patient could not superimpose the Haidinger brush on the fixation point. After several weeks, central Haidinger brush fixation was possible; however, the patient felt as if he were looking to the side of the target. In addition, when attempting to point to the overlapping fixation point and Haidinger brush, the brush would shift to the side. Eventually, when the perceived superimposition of the fixation point, pointer, and Haidinger brush was achieved, the pointer was physically shifted off to the left side (Figure 10.50). Visual acuity was now approximately 20/60 (S-chart and Snellen). However, visuoscopy still showed 3 degrees of steady and eccentric fixation. Since the average visual acuity at a retinal eccentricity of 3 degrees is approximately 20/50 (Schapero 1971), we assumed that the vision improvement achieved thus far occurred secondary to decreased cortical inhibition (i.e., sensory loss). Therefore, if any further significant improvement in visual acuity was to be obtained,

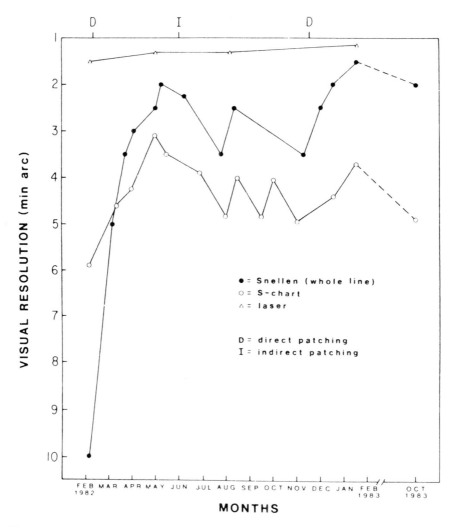

Figure 10.49 *Visual acuity during the course of orthoptic therapy. (Reprinted, with permission of publisher, from Selenow and Ciuffreda 1986.)*

the magnitude of eccentric fixation had to be reduced. Inverse occlusion was thus implemented. This was achieved by stippling all but the temporal 25% of the amblyopic eye's spectacle lens. This modified lens prevented the eccentric point from receiving patterned stimuli while still allowing some peripheral vision. These glasses were worn 5 hours per day. One-half hour of daily home vision training was continued.

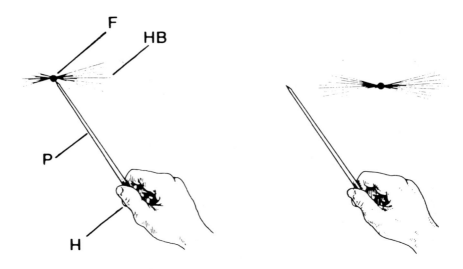

Figure 10.50   *Pointing task with the amblyopic eye. The patient was instructed to align the pointer (P) in his right hand (H) with the Haidinger brush (HB) superimposed on the fixation point (F). On the left is what the patient saw, and on the right was the actual physical arrangement. (Reprinted, with permission of publisher, from Selenow and Ciuffreda 1986.)*

After 1 month of inverse occlusion, a very different fixation pattern emerged. Although the initial fixation was still 3 degrees eccentric, it was much less steady than before. In addition, the eye now frequently saccaded to within ½ degree of the fovea for several seconds and then saccaded back to the more typical eccentric area. During this period of unsteady fixation, visual acuity decreased somewhat. One month later, the patient was able to fixate voluntarily with his fovea when told to "clear up" the visuoscopy target. He was also able to do this when presented with a Snellen chart; when doing so, Snellen visual acuity improved significantly. However, when "clearing up" the S-chart, much monocular spatial distortion and overlapping of neighboring contours was reported (Figure 10.51). The patient eventually could fixate foveally at will during other tasks.

Once fixation was central, direct occlusion was again implemented. However, 3 weeks later, the patient had to leave the country for 4 months and was subsequently unavailable for an additional 5 months.

Results

Several monocular vision functions showed improvement throughout the course of treatment (Table 10.10). During the initial direct occlusion phase, both Snellen (20/150 to 20/40) and S-chart (20/118 to 20/62) visual acuities improved significantly (Figure 10.49). However, once inverse occlusion was instituted,

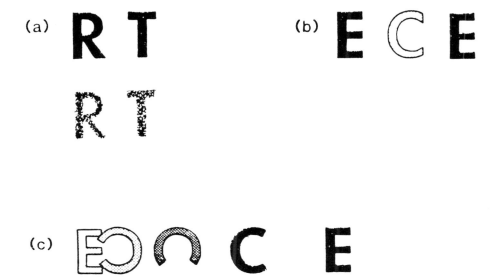

Figure 10.51 *Appearance of the visual acuity test chart letters under three different conditions during monocular viewing with the amblyopic eye. (A) Sharp contours during foveal fixation (above) and diffuse contours during eccentric fixation (below). (B) Reduced perceived contrast of the fixated letter C due to presumed inhibitory interactions of the flanking letters. (C) Perceived contrast gradient and spatial asymmetry when fixating the reversed C with the eccentric point. (Reprinted, with permission of the publisher, from Selenow and Ciuffreda 1986.)*

both acuity values decreased. The second phase of direct occlusion again produced a marked improvement in Snellen acuity (20/70 to 20/30) and a more modest S-chart visual acuity improvement (20/99 to 20/75). Laser interferometric visual acuity was excellent (20/30) before treatment and was not significantly altered during treatment. When retested 9 months following termination of all therapy, only slight regression of some vision functions was found (such as visual acuity; Figure 10.49, dashed lines).

The contrast sensitivity function was monitored before and during most of the training period (Figure 10.52). The pretraining response function was markedly abnormal. It was reduced at all but the lowest spatial frequency tested (0.7 cycles per degree); further, the patient could not consistently detect a grating at spatial frequencies greater than 6 cycles per degree, even at the maximum contrast available. However, the response function improved considerably with training. The peak shifted from 2 to 4 cycles per degree, and reduced sensitivity was only evident at spatial frequencies greater than 6 cycles per degree. Furthermore, the amblyopic eye could now detect the grating at the highest spatial frequency available (23 cycles per degree), but required somewhat greater contrast than the dominant eye. Once the patient could voluntarily fixate with

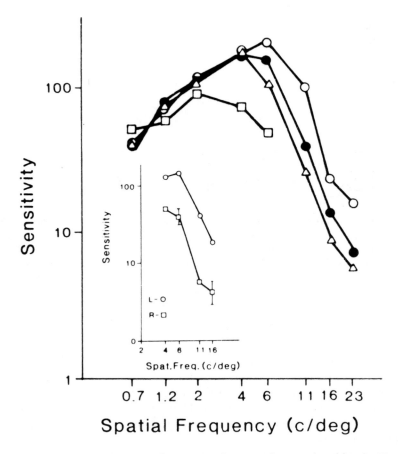

Figure 10.52 *Contrast sensitivity function in the normal (N) and amblyopic (A) eye at various times during the course of orthoptic therapy. Inset shows nasal (□) versus temporal (○) asymmetry of function in amblyopic eye. Plotted is $\bar{X}$ ± 1 SD. (Reprinted, with permission of the publisher, from Selenow and Ciuffreda 1986.)*

either the fovea or the eccentric point (which was confirmed by visuoscopy and objective eye movement recordings), we were able to measure contrast sensitivity of the nasal versus temporal retinal. Nasal retinal contrast sensitivity showed a consistent depression at the middle and high spatial frequencies when compared with the temporal retina. This is in agreement with a previous report of nasal-temporal

Table 10.10 Comparison of Pre- and Posttreatment Findings in the Amblyopic Eye

Test	Pretreatment	Posttreatment
Visual acuity (Snellen single-line)	20/150	20/30
Visual acuity (S-chart)	20/119	20/75*
Visual acuity (laser interferometry)	20/30	20/25
Visuoscopy	3-degree nasal steady	Unsteady central
Accommodative amplitude (minus lens)	6 diopters	9 diopters
Accommodative spatial frequency profile	Overall depression	Normalized at middle and high spatial frequencies
Fixational eye movements	Small-amplitude jerk nystagmus	Reduced nystagmus amplitude and frequency
Contrast sensitivity	Depression of middle and high spatial frequencies; low spatial frequency peak shift	Almost complete normalization
Visual evoked response	Reduced amplitude	Marked amplitude increase
Electroretinogram	Reduced amplitude	Marked amplitude increase

*However, the best VA attained was 20/62 during the first phase of direct patching.

asymmetries in threshold contrast perception in eccentrically fixating strabismic amblyopes (Thomas 1978).

Steady-state accommodation following therapy was relatively normal (Figure 10.53). The accommodative stimulus-response function to square-wave-type stimuli (i.e., a high-contrast reduced Snellen chart viewed in a Badal optical system) was approximately equal in each eye, with accommodation falling slightly above the theoretical response line (thus clearly demonstrating the normal but slightly high gain of the system). This is in contrast to the typical pretherapy reduced responses (i.e., abnormal low gain) found in amblyopic eyes (Ciuffreda et al. 1984). Accommodation to the high-contrast sinusoidal gratings showed the typical pretherapy reduced responses in the amblyopic eye (Ciuffreda and Hokoda 1983); following therapy, accommodative responses in the amblyopic eye were now within normal limits except at the lowest spatial frequency tested. Lastly, the minus lens accommodative amplitude, which was reduced in the amblyopic eye by 2 diopters pretherapy, was now greater by 1 diopter in the amblyopic eye.

In parallel with the significant improvements in most monocular vision functions tested in the amblyopic eye following orthoptic therapy, there was

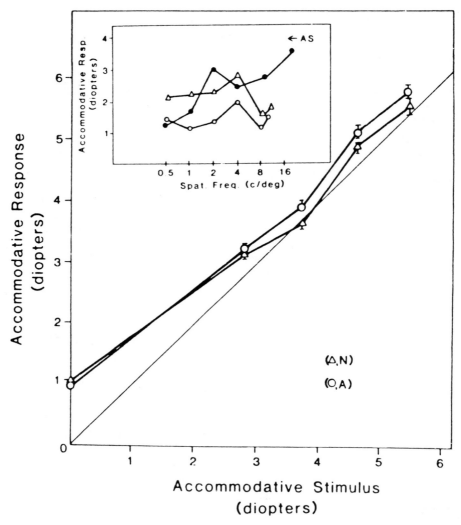

Figure 10.53   *Static accommodation responses. Accommodative stimulus-response function posttherapy in the normal (△) and amblyopic (○) eye while focusing on letters of a reduced Snellen chart presented in a Badal optical system. Diagonal line is the theoretical response line. Inset shows accommodation to high-contrast sine-wave gratings at a 4-diopter target vergence level. (○ = amblyopic eye pretherapy, △ = dominant eye pretherapy, and ● = amblyopic eye posttherapy.) For both graphs, $\bar{X} \pm 1$ SEM is plotted. (Reprinted, with permission of the publisher, from Selenow and Ciuffreda 1986.)*

moderate improvement in fixation ability (Figure 10.54). Monocular fixation with the dominant eye was within normal limits. There was jerk nystagmus-like movements in the amblyopic eye pretherapy (0.5 Hz, 1 degree). Following 4 months of direct occlusion, the mean nystagmus amplitude decreased to 0.75 degree without a change in frequency. Following 2 months of additional inverse occlusion, a new phenomenon was observed: spontaneous involuntary fixation at either the fovea or the eccentric point. Lastly, following 4 more months of inverse occlusion, the alternating fixation pattern was still evident; however, it was now consciously controlled by the patient when he attempted to fixate (using the eccentric retinal point) versus focus (using the fovea) on the target. The pattern was confirmed on numerous occasions by careful low-light, extended visuoscopic examination.

There was also some improvement in binocular vision function. The patient developed the ability to fuse diplopic images and consequently was not troubled by diplopia as visual acuity improved in the amblyopic eye. In addition, divergence ranges increased. However, stereoacuity could still not be demonstrated.

Significant Points

1. Although visual acuity improved during the initial phase of direct occlusion, eccentric fixation remained steady and eccentric. Only with subsequent inverse occlusion and use of foveal tagging could the anomalous monocular fixation pattern in the amblyopic eye be disrupted. After 6 weeks of inverse occlusion, visuoscopy showed a bimodal fixation pattern with initial fixation at the eccentric point, followed by a saccadic eye movement toward the fovea with unsteady foveal fixation, and then a second saccade back to the eccentric point. After 10 more weeks of inverse occlusion, initial fixation was still at the eccentric point; however, when asked to try and "clear up" the target, the patient immediately fixated with the fovea and reported the target to be clear and localized straight ahead (Figure 10.51*A*). Subjectively, when looking at the S-chart, the patient reported both spatial and contrast asymmetry (Figure 10.51*C*), with the letters to the left of fixation appearing closer together and having slightly less contrast. In addition, at times the surrounding contours interacted with and reduced the contrast of the fixated letter (Figure 10.51*B*). After "clearing up" the S-chart, the contrast of all the letters increased. However, spatial asymmetry was still pronounced. During Snellen single-line visual acuity testing with foveal fixation, there was minimal reported spatial asymmetry and significant contrast improvement.

2. As has been reported (Selenow et al. 1986), pretreatment laser acuity accurately predicted the best posttreatment Snellen visual acuity value in our patient (20/30).

3. In the process of reducing the eccentric fixation, several interesting phenomena surfaced. During visuoscopy, the patient reported the projected grid target to be straight ahead when the eye fixated either centrally or eccentrically. The initial fixation reflex was with the eccentric point, which retained its

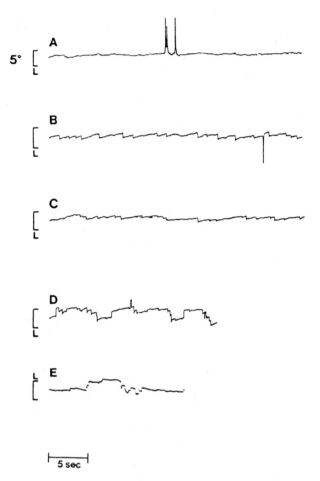

Figure 10.54   *Horizontal eye position during midline fixation under different conditions at various times during the course of orthoptic therapy. L denotes leftward movements. (A) Dominant eye pretherapy. (B) Amblyopic eye pretherapy. (C) Amblyopic eye after 4 months of direct occlusion. (D) Amblyopic eye after 2 months of inverse occlusion. (E) Amblyopic eye after 4 additional months of inverse occlusion during fixation (rightward shift) versus focusing on (leftward shift) a small luminous spot on the display monitor. For all traces, large vertical deflections represent blinks. (Reprinted, with permission of the publisher, from Selenow and Ciuffreda 1986.)*

sense of primary visual direction. When then told to "clear up" the same target, the patient automatically switched fixation from the eccentric point to the fovea, again reporting the target to be localized straight ahead. However, if the target were placed on the fovea by the examiner with the patient's eye held steadily, or if the patient were instructed to abduct the eye slowly and stop when the examiner noted central fixation, the target appeared displaced to the patient. In effect, the fovea achieved primary visual direction only when active foveal fixation was attempted, and thus both the eccentric point and the fovea had the potential for such primary visual direction sensation. Further evidence in support of this was noted during the Haidinger brush training. When the patient eventually perceived superimposition of the fixation point, pointer, and Haidinger brush, the pointer was physically shifted to the left of the target and the foveal projection (Figure 10.50). A possible explanation for this is that both the fovea and the eccentric point had *simultaneous primary visual direction* during this task. This would also explain the brief periods of monocular diplopia that the patient experienced when fatigued during visual acuity testing with the amblyopic eye. None of these abnormal perceptual phenomena was reported nor could be elicited by the end of the training period.

4. It is also interesting to note that the feeling of "clearing up" the target (the objective correlate being a shift in fixation from 3 degrees nasal retina to the fovea) (Figure 10.54) was reported by the patient to be identical to the feeling experienced when accommodating to clear the blur produced by introduction of a minus lens during early accommodation training. Judging by the excellent static accommodative stimulus-response curve (Figure 10.53) and accommodative amplitude (9 diopters) of the amblyopic eye during the transition phase between direct and inverse occlusion, the patient probably learned to use his fovea to complete the accommodative training task. This brief splinter skill (since fixation was still eccentric during this phase of treatment on all other tasks) eventually transferred to many other areas, culminating in the eventual achievement of voluntary central fixation with primary visual direction at the fovea.

5. With proper pretreatment to enable the patient to use visual feedback (i.e., retinal disparity) to initiate appropriate vergence responses to avoid diplopia, he was then able to undergo intensive orthoptic therapy, which resulted in the potential expansion of his career opportunities as well as having a more normally functioning "spare eye."

6. In dealing with older patients in particular, the cost/benefit ratio must be considered, especially since there is evidence from clinical case reports showing some degree of spontaneous recovery of vision in the amblyopic eye following either enucleation or loss of central vision in the fellow dominant eye (see Ciuffreda 1986, for a review).

Case 4: Hyperopic Anisometropic Amblyopia
(Age 18 Years)

History

The patient was first examined in our clinic at 18 years of age. He reported that vision had always been poor in the left eye and that due to a birth trauma, his left eye had been totally occluded during the first 2 days of life.

No ocular or neurologic disease was detected. The patient indicated that he would be willing to undergo therapy to improve vision in his amblyopic eye.

Diagnosis

Subjective refraction was +5.00 diopters in the left eye (20/230) and +3.00 diopters in the right eye (20/15). Although the initial cover test indicated 3 prism diopters of left esotropia with 2 prism diopters of left hypertropia, these findings were confounded by unsteady fixation in the amblyopic eye. On later occasions, as fixation became steadier, subsequent repeated cover tests clearly showed the absence of any strabismus. Initial visuoscopy indicated 10 prism diopters of temporal and 5 prism diopters of superior unsteady eccentric fixation. But again, because of very unsteady fixation and lack of a distinct foveal reflex, this finding was simply an estimate, although nonfoveal fixation was clearly present. Haidinger's brush and afterimage transfer tests indicated normal retinal correspondence. We felt that the primary amblyopia was secondary to the hyperopic anisometropia.

Monocular and Binocular Treatment Plan

Our treatment plan was to begin with the standard therapy sequence in conjunction with direct occlusion. Owing to the existence of normal retinal correspondence and absence of strabismus, our binocular goal was stereopsis.

Training Sequence

Owing to the large and unsteady nature of fixation, there was an emphasis on placing and maintaining the Haidinger brush and transferred afterimage on progressively smaller acuity targets. Once visual acuity improved and it was obvious that there was no avoidance of fusion, antisuppression and fusion training were implemented.

Results

During the first 6-month training period, eccentric fixation decreased to approximately 3 to 5 prism diopters temporal, and visual acuity was at times as high as 20/50. However, neither measure was stable. The second phase of orthoptic training lasted 10 months. The initial comprehensive examination in the second phase showed no change in refraction and an absence of strabismus as judged by repeated cover tests. Eccentric fixation was 2 prism diopters temporal as measured by Haidinger's brush, afterimage transfer, and visuoscopy. By the end of this phase, visual acuity was 20/20 with slightly unsteady central fixation (Figure 10.55). In addition, stereopsis of 60 seconds of arc was achieved. Two months after 20/20 acuity was attained, the patient moved to another state and was therefore not available for follow-up testing.

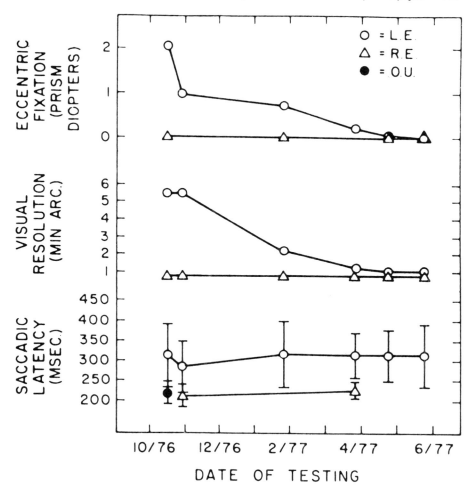

Figure 10.55 *Changes in eccentric fixation, visual resolution, and saccadic latency for both eyes during the last 8 months of orthoptic therapy. Note centralization of fixation and normalization of visual resolution but maintenance of increased saccadic latencies in the left amblyopic eye. Plotted are mean (and standard deviations for saccadic latency) of measures for each test session. (Reprinted, with permission of the publisher, from Ciuffreda et al. 1979b.)*

Significant Points

1.   It is remarkable that several aspects of oculomotor control, as well as visual acuity and fixation, showed such improvement in spite of numerous indications of an unfavorable prognosis for a functional cure, including initiation of therapy in adulthood, presence of deep amblyopia with eccentric fixation, minimal use of spectacles until high school, and possible effects of very early form deprivation.

2.   Our results suggest that after normalization of visual acuity and centralization of fixation (the hallmarks of cured amblyopia), subtle defects in oculomotor performance may persist, clearly demonstrating that all vision functions in the amblyopic eye do not improve concurrently (or perhaps fully). Thus it appears that orthoptic therapy for amblyopia should perhaps be continued until visual acuity, fixation, and oculomotor control (as well as other vision functions) are normalized and/or remain stable for a suitable period of time.

Case 5: High Hyperopia with Esotropia (Age 3½ Years)

History

The patient was first examined by us at age 3½ years. The parents noticed a right esotropia at age 2½ years that increased in magnitude and frequency by age 3 years. At that time, full-time spectacles and direct occlusion were prescribed. However, the child did not comply with either.

Diagnosis

Subjective refraction was $+7.00 = -0.50 \times 90$ in the right eye (20/400) and $+6.00 = -0.75 \times 90$ in the left eye (20/40). Visuoscopy showed unsteady central fixation in the left eye and 3 degrees of unsteady and nasal eccentric fixation in the right eye. Cover test through full correction revealed a constant concomitant right esotropia of 10 prism diopters at 6 meters and 14 prism diopters at 40 centimeters. There was no stereopsis, with the right eye manifesting a deep suppression at all distances as measured with the Worth four-dot test. We felt that the primary amblyopia was secondary to the esotropia.

Monocular and Binocular Treatment Plan

We believed that the poor compliance with the previous prescription was mainly due to overcorrection. Therefore, the full correction was prescribed along with 6 hours of direct occlusion, with an emphasis on eye-hand coordination games during as much of the occlusion period as possible. The goal was to increase the amblyopic eye's vision as quickly as possible, so that we could concentrate on the development of binocularity. It has been our experience that small-angle uncorrected hyperopic esotropes tend to "drift" into exotropia once fully corrected, especially when occluded for long periods of time. If so, the prescription would then be reduced, so that the patient was left with a small-angle exotropia, which is more conducive for fusion training. Our eventual binocular goal was stereopsis.

Training Sequence

Because of the age of the patient, all training was done at home. For ½ hour every day, the parents kept the patient amused with a variety of visual tasks, all of which involved visual localization followed by a reaching task.

Results

Table 10.11 summarizes the changes in visual acuity, fixation status, and binocularity over the course of 8 months. Visual acuity and fixation improved quickly during the first 3 months. As expected, the amount of esotropia steadily decreased, with a manifest exotropia occurring at the fifth month. At this time, we *decreased* the hyperopic prescription by + 1.00 diopter, which reduced the amount of exotropia by 4 prism diopters. Then, occlusion was reduced to 1 hour every other day. However, since visual acuity decreased from 20/30 to 20/40 over the next 3 months, retainer occlusion time was increased to 1 hour daily. The patient has remained on a 1 hour per day retainer occlusion schedule and is presently being evaluated every 3 months. Our goal is to maintain the visual acuity improvement and binocular status until the patient is mature enough to enter a formal vision therapy program, at which time stereopsis would be our binocular goal.

Significant Points

1.   Occlusion time was gradually reduced as visual acuity improved, until the first sign of visual acuity reversal. Therefore, we were able to determine the absolute minimum length of occlusion time. The lower the occlusion time, the greater is the length of potential binocular stimulation.

2.   The strabismus shifted from esotropia to exotropia, after which the hyperopic prescription was reduced to decrease the amount of exotropia. It is better to leave a patient with a residual exotropia rather than esotropia, since exotropia responds much better to eventual vision therapy (especially for fusion development).

Table 10.11   Changes in Vision Function during the Course of Orthoptic Therapy

	Initial	*1 Month*	*2 Months*	*3 Months*	*5 Months*	*8 Months*
Visual acuity (Snellen)						
OD	20/400	20/100	20/60	20/50	20/30	20/40
OS	20/40	20/40	20/30	20/30	20/30	20/25
Fixation (degrees) (amblyopic eye)	3, unsteady nasal	2.5, unsteady nasal	Unsteady central	Steady central	Steady central	Steady central
Cover test (prism diopters)*						
Distance	8 RET	5 RET	2 RET	2 RET	8 RXT	4 RXT
Near	12 RET	10 RET	4 RET	4 RET	6 RXT	Ortho.
Length of occlusion	6 hours	5 hours	3.5 hours	2 hours	1 hour every other day	1 hour every day

*RET = right esotropia; RXT = right exotropia.

3.   Since the patient is too young for formal intensive vision therapy, he will be monitored carefully. If the exotropia increases, the prescription will be decreased. If visual acuity regresses, patching will be increased. In addition, the periodic follow-up visits allow the therapist to determine when the patient is mature enough to enter a formal vision therapy program.

Case 6: Image Degradation (Age 2½ Years)

History

The patient was first examined by us 2 weeks after a cataract extraction of the left eye. There had been a history of posterior lenticonus in the left eye, which was first noted by the pediatrician at age 2 years. Birth and medical history were both unremarkable. Preoperative visual acuity was "hand motion."

Diagnosis

Visual acuity (forced-choice preferential looking) was 20/70 (plano) in the right eye, and no response (+ 23-diopter contact lens) in the aphakic corrected left eye. Visuoscopy revealed unsteady central fixation in the dominant eye and unsteady "wandering" eccentric fixation (with no locus preference) in the amblyopic eye. The range of fixation was greater than 5 degrees. Ocular alignment by means of Hirschberg showed no deviation. We felt that the amblyopia was secondary to the image degradation caused by the presence of a cataract early in life.

Monocular and Binocular Treatment Plan

Our strategy was to begin immediate direct occlusion with the full aphakic contact lens prescription in place. Once visual acuity showed significant improvement, occlusion time would be reduced to allow potential binocular stimulation.

Training Sequence

The initial contact lens prescription was purposely overcorrected by 3 diopters, thereby making 13 inches the ideal working distance. The importance of motivation and ingenuity was stressed to the parents to get the toddler through the initial transfer of functioning with his amblyopic eye. Colorful toys provided for interesting visual stimulation during the home therapy phase.

Results

After 3 months of occlusion varying from 8 to 4 hours per day, the patient achieved 20/50 (broken wheel) visual acuity in the nondominant eye. Visual acuity was 20/40 in the dominant eye. Cover test revealed a 5 prism diopter left esotropia at distance and near. Occlusion time was then reduced to 3 hours per day, and a follow-up visit was scheduled for the next month. The patient did not return until 3 months later. Visual acuity in the nondominant eye had dropped to 20/400. Upon questioning, the parents noted that occlusion was only implemented every other day for approximately 2 hours at a time. Therefore, occlusion time was increased to 8 hours per day. Three months later, visual acuity has once again improved, but this time to 20/70 in the nondominant eye. Since the patient was left with a constant left esotropia, he remained in a daily 2-hour retainer patching regimen to prevent acuity regression. To encourage alternation, the patient presently spends 45 minutes a day on a bi-ocular tasks. This is accomplished with red-green glasses (red over the nondominant eye) and a red filter over a television screen. If the screen turns black, the patient blinks until the screen can be seen again. A similar arrangement is used with a coloring or dot-to-dot drawing book. The patient's visual acuity and binocularity are presently being monitored every 3 months until he is mature enough to enter a formal intensive vision therapy program.

Significant Point

Visual acuity gains dropped suddenly when occlusion time fell below the prescribed amount. However, acuity improved quickly once occlusion time was then increased, demonstrating considerable plasticity of the visual system to respond at this early age.

Case 7: Hyperopic Anisometropia with Exotropia
(Age 24 Years)

History

The patient was initially examined by us at age 24 years. There was a reported history of the left eye being "lazy and wall-eyed" since the age of 4 years. At 6 years of age, eyeglasses were prescribed and worn sporadically. No prescription was worn for the past 4 years. There was no history of patching. The patient felt that the eye turn was larger and more frequent now and that it was becoming a cosmetic problem.

Diagnosis

Subjective refraction was plano in the right eye (20/20) and + 4.00 diopters in the left eye (20/150 whole-line, 20/100 single-line Snellen). Visuoscopy revealed steady central fixation in the right eye and unsteady temporal eccentric fixation of 1½ degrees in the left eye. Cover test through a contact lens revealed a constant left exotropia of 25 prism diopters at 6 meters and 15 prism diopters at 40 centimeters. Suppression of the left eye was noted at all distances with the Worth four-dot test. There was no stereoscopic appreciation. Penalization filters and lenses over the dominant eye revealed normal retinal correspondence once the suppression was broken. We felt that the primary amblyopia was secondary to the anisometropia, with the exotropia being secondary to the anisometropic amblyopia. Once the exotropia became constant, it also became an amblyogenic factor. The following is the developmental sequence:

- Anisometropic hyperopia
  ↓
- Primary amblyopia
  ↓
- Intermittent exotropia
  ↓
- Constant exotropia
  ↓
- Secondary amblyopia

Monocular and Binocular Treatment Plan

Our plan was to teach the patient to fuse diplopic images under artificial situations. A contact lens was to be worn throughout the day. Once it was determined that fusion was possible, the standard monocular training sequence would begin. The binocular goal was stereopsis, since it was our experience that these types of strabismics become intermittent soon after visual acuity improves.

Training Sequence

A full contact lens correction was prescribed for full-time wear along with 2 hours of daily direct occlusion, 30 minutes of daily training, and 45 minutes of weekly in-office training. After 4 weeks of the standard therapy sequence and daily fusion training, visual acuity remained unchanged, but the exotropia became intermittent.

Once fusion was possible throughout the day, visual acuity improved dramatically, with the patient achieving 20/50 single-line acuity and 60 seconds of arc Wirt stereoacuity after 3 months of therapy. At this point, the emphasis was switched to bi-ocular training, so that the area of suppression could be reduced to achieve Randot stereoacuity. This involved high-level accommodation, as well as fixation training through red-green and polarizing filters, with use of progressively finer and finer detailed targets.

Results

Table 10.12 summarizes the changes in visual acuity, fixation, stereopsis, and ocular alignment over time. Visual acuity eventually reached the level of 20/30 (single-letter Snellen). Fixation became unsteady central after only 4 weeks of therapy without any significant simultaneous improvement in visual acuity. Ocular alignment and stereopsis improved quickly, with the patient eventually achieving 50 seconds of arc Randot stereopsis, as well as normal base-in and base-out vergence ranges at distance and near. Five-year follow-up showed no regression.

Table 10.12   Changes in Vision Function During the Course of Orthoptic Therapy

	Initial	1 Months	3 Months	7 Months	5 Years
Visual acuity (Snellen) (amblyopic eye)	20/100	20/100	20/50	20/30	20/30
Fixation (degrees) (amblyopic eye)	1.5, unsteady temporal	1.5, unsteady temporal	Unsteady, central	Unsteady, central	Unsteady, central
Cover test (prism diopters)*					
Distance	25 LXT	20 LX(T)	20 XP	14 XP	14 XP
Near	15 LXT	15 LX(T)	12 XP	8 XP	8 XP
Stereopsis (seconds of arc)	None	None	60 Wirt	50 Randot	50 Randot

*LXT = left exotropia; LX(T) = intermittent left exotropia; XP = exophoria.

Significant Points

1.   Visual acuity improved quickly once the strabismus became intermittent. Therefore, throughout the day, when there was no strabismus, the amblyopic eye probably received nearly continuous visual stimulation, most likely with suppression of small objects only.

2.   Since the patient was an active adult, most of our training involved minimizing the zone of suppression, so that the amblyopic eye would receive maximum stimulation throughout the day *without* the need for occlusion.

3.   Once Randot stereoacuity was achieved, the patient was simply trained as a standard "binocular dysfunction" case, with the goal of being symptom-free with her newly developed binocularity.

Case 8: Image Degradation (Age 4½ Years)

History

The patient was first examined by us at age 4½ years. The referring physician reported an immediately prior 4-month history of a lacerated right cornea that was now healed. However, best-corrected visual acuity in the traumatized eye was now 20/100. Ocular history before the trauma was unremarkable.

Diagnosis

Subjective refraction was plano in the right eye (20/80) and left eye (20/20). Keratometry revealed significant corneal distortion in the right eye. A linear corneal scar extended from the temporal limbus with encroachment one-third of the way into the pupillary area. A rigid contact lens improved visual acuity to 20/50 in the right eye with the patient's head turned to the right, thus apparently avoiding the scar's impingement on the visual axis. Visuoscopy revealed unsteady central fixation in the right eye and steady central fixation in the left eye. There was no strabismus; however, stereopsis could not be elicited. We felt that there were three contributing factors for the decrease in vision. The first was corneal distortion, which was effectively eliminated by fitting of the contact lens. The residual acuity loss (20/50) could be explained by a combination of image-degradation amblyopia (secondary to the uncorrected corneal distortion) and the corneal scar's encroachment near the visual axis. Amblyopia therapy with rigid lens correction of the corneal distortion was attempted.

Monocular and Binocular Treatment Plan

The patient's right eye was fit with a gas-permeable contact lens, and the standard therapy sequence with direct patching was implemented. Since it was reported that binocularity was normal before the accident, we felt that extensive occlusion was not in order and that stereopsis would be our means of preventing regression of monocular function.

Training Sequence

A full rigid contact lens correction was prescribed for full-time wear along with 2 hours of daily direct occlusion. The standard amblyopia therapy sequence was implemented. In addition, once visual acuity improved to the 20/50 level, the patient underwent standard binocular amblyopia therapy.

Results

Visual acuity improved rapidly, with the patient eventually achieving 20/25 acuity within 7 weeks. Once visual acuity reached 20/50, 100 seconds of arc of stereopsis was measured, with subsequent improvement to 40 seconds of arc as treatment progressed, and thus regression was no longer an important factor.

Significant Points

1. By undergoing amblyopic therapy, it was determined that the corneal scar was responsible for only a small part of the visual acuity deficit (20/25).

2. Visual acuity improved rapidly because the amblyogenic factor occurred late in the critical period for vision development (age 4 years).

3. A patient with an obvious organic explanation for decreased vision that in addition manifests an amblyogenic factor should not be deprived of amblyopia therapy. Only with such therapy can one determine with reasonable certainty which part of the vision loss is functional versus organic.

REFERENCES

Bangerter A. (1953) Amblyopiebehandlung, Basel, Switzerland, Karger.

Ciuffreda KJ. (1986) Visual System Plasticity in Human Amblyopia. In Hilfer SR, Sheffield JB (Eds.), *Development of Order in the Visual System*, pp. 211–44. New York: Springer-Verlag.

Ciuffreda KJ, Hokoda SC. (1983) Spatial frequency dependence of accommodative responses in amblyopic eyes. *Vision Res.* 23:1585–94.

Ciuffreda KJ, Kenyon RV, Stark L. (1979a) Saccadic intrusions in strabismus. *Arch. Ophthalmol.* 97:1673–9.

Ciuffreda KJ, Kenyon RV, Stark L. (1979b) Different rates of functional recovery of eye movements during orthoptic treatment in an adult amblyope. *Invest. Ophthalmol. Vis. Sci.* 18:213–19.

Ciuffreda KJ, Kenyon RV, Stark L. (1980) Increased drift in amblyopic eyes. *Br. J. Ophthalmol.* 64:7–14.

Ciuffreda KJ, Hokoda SC, Hung GK, et al. (1983) Static aspects of accommodation in human amblyopia. *Am. J. Optom. Physiol. Opt.* 60:436–49.

Ciuffreda KJ, Hokoda SC, Hung GK, et al. (1984) Accommodative stimulus/response function in human amblyopia. *Doc. Ophthalmol.* 56:303–26.

Davidson DW, Eskridge JB. (1977) Reliability of visual acuity measures of amblyopic eyes. *Am. J. Optom. Physiol. Opt.* 54:756–66.

Flom MC. (1966) New concepts in visual acuity. *Optom. Weekly* 57:63–8.

Flom MC, Weymouth FW, Kahneman D. (1963) Visual resolution and contour interaction. *J. Opt. Soc. Am.* 53:1026–32.

Griffin JR. (1982) *Binocular Anomalies: Procedures for Vision Therapy.* Chicago: Professional Press.

Hokoda SC, Ciuffreda KJ. (1986) Different rates and amounts of vision function recovery during orthoptic therapy in an older strabismic amblyope. *Ophthalmic Physiol. Opt.* 6:213–20.

Lyle TK, Douthwaite C, Wilkinson J. (1960) *Reeducative Treatment of Suppression Amblyopia.* Edinburgh: Livingstone.

Phillips SR. (1974) Ocular Neurological Control Systems: Accommodation and the Near Response Triad. Ph.D. dissertation, University of California, Berkeley.

Schapero M. (1971) *Amblyopia.* Philadelphia: Chilton.

Selenow A, Ciuffreda KJ. (1983) Visual function recovery during orthoptic therapy in an exotropic amblyope with high unilateral myopia. *Am. J. Optom. Physiol. Opt.* 60:659–66.

Selenow A, Ciuffreda KJ. (1986) Visual function recovery during orthoptic therapy in an adult esotropic amblyope. *J. Am. Optom. Assoc.* 57:132–40.

Selenow A, Ciuffreda KJ, Mozlin R, Rumpf D. (1986) Prognostic value of laser interferometric visual acuity in amblyopia therapy. *Invest. Ophthalmol. Vis. Sci.* 27:273–77.

Thomas J. (1978) Normal and abnormal contrast sensitivity functions in central and peripheral retinas. *Invest. Ophthalmol. Vis. Sci.* 17:746–53.

von Noorden GK. (1965) Occlusion therapy in amblyopia with eccentric fixation. *Arch. Ophthalmol.* 73:776–81.

von Noorden GK. (1973) Experimental amblyopia in monkeys: Further behavioral observations and clinical correlations. *Invest. Ophthalmol.* 12:721–6.

Zurcher B, Lang J. (1980) Reading capacity in cases of "cured" strabismic amblyopia. *Trans. Ophthalmol. Soc. U.K.* 100:501–3.

Index